ELECTROCARDIOGRAPHY
FOR HEALTHCARE PROFESSIONALS

Fourth Edition

Kathryn A. Booth, RN-BSN, RMA (AMT), RPT, CPhT, MS
Total Care Programming, Inc.
Palm Coast, Florida

Thomas O'Brien, AS, CCT, CRAT, RMA
Remington College
Allied Health Programs Chair

Mc Graw Hill Education

ELECTROCARDIOGRAPHY FOR HEALTHCARE PROFESSIONALS, FOURTH EDITION

Published by McGraw-Hill Education, 2 Penn Plaza, New York, NY 10121.

This book is printed on acid-free paper.

7 8 9 0 LMN 21 20 19 18

ISBN 978-0-07-802067-4
MHID 0-07-802067-0

Senior Vice President, Products & Markets: *Kurt L. Strand*
Vice President, General Manager, Products & Markets: *Marty Lange*
Vice President, Content Design & Delivery: *Kimberly Meriwether David*
Managing Director: *Chad Grall*
Brand Manager: *William Mulford*
Director, Product Development: *Rose Koos*
Senior Product Developer: *Christine Scheid*
Executive Marketing Manager: *Roxan Kinsey*
Digital Product Analyst: *Katherine Ward*
Director, Content Design & Delivery: *Linda Avenarius*
Program Manager: *Angela R. FitzPatrick*
Content Project Managers: *April R. Southwood/Sherry Kane*
Senior Buyer: *Michael McCormick*
Design: *Srdjan Savanovic*
Content Licensing Specialists: *Lori Hancock*
Cover Image: *©Rivetti/Getty Images*
Compositor: *Laserwords Private Limited*
Printer: *LSC Communications*

Library of Congress Cataloging-in-Publication Data

Booth, Kathryn A., 1957- author.
Electrocardiography for healthcare professionals / Kathryn A. Booth, Thomas E. O'Brien. — Fourth edition.
p. ; cm.
Includes index.
ISBN 978-0-07-802067-4 (alk. paper) — ISBN 0-07-802067-0 (alk. paper)
I. O'Brien, Thomas E. (Thomas Edward), 1959- author. II. Title.
[DNLM: 1. Electrocardiography—methods—Problems and Exercises.
2. Arrhythmias, Cardiac—diagnosis—Problems and Exercises. WG 18.2]
RC683.5.E5
616.1'207547—dc23

2014019157

www.mhhe.com

Dedication

To the individuals using this book, you have chosen a worthwhile and rewarding career. Thank you; your skills and services are truly needed. To my youngest granddaughter, Harper Kathryn, so happy you are in my life.

Kathryn Booth

I want to thank my beautiful wife, Michele, and our wonderful children, Thomas, Robert, and Kathryn. Without their love and support, I would have nothing. They inspire me every day to make a difference in people's lives. I also want to express my sincere thanks to the faculty, staff, and students of Remington College for their encouragement and guidance. Today's students are the difference makers of tomorrow!

Thomas O'Brien

About the Author

Kathryn A. Booth, RN-BSN, RMA (AMT), RPT, CPhT, MS, is a registered nurse (RN) with CPR and ACLS training as well as a master's degree in education and certifications in phlebotomy, pharmacy tech, and medical assisting. She is an author, educator, and consultant for Total Care Programming, Inc. She has over 30 years of teaching, nursing, and healthcare work experience that spans five states. As an educator, Kathy has been awarded the teacher of the year in three states where she taught various health sciences. She serves on the American Medical Technologists registered Phlebotomy Technician Examinations, Qualifications, and Standards Committee. She stays current in the field by practicing her skills in various settings as well as by maintaining and obtaining certifications. In addition, Kathy volunteers at a free healthcare clinic and teaches online. She is a member of advisory boards at two educational institutions. Her larger goal is to develop up-to-date, dynamic healthcare educational materials to assist other educators as well as to promote the healthcare professions. In addition, Kathy enjoys presenting innovative new learning solutions for the changing healthcare and educational landscape to her fellow professionals nationwide.

Thomas E. O'Brien, AS, CCT, CRAT, RMA, is the Allied Health Program chairperson at Remington College, Fort Worth, Texas. Tom also works as an author of CME activities and editor with Practical Clinical Skills (www.practicalclinicalskills.com). He is also on the Board of Trustees and Exam Chair for the Certified Cardiographic Technician and Certified Rhythm Analysis Technician Registry Examinations working with Cardiovascular Credentialing International (CCI). His background includes over 24 years in the U.S. Air Force and U.S. Army Medical Corps. Tom's medical career as an Air Force Independent Duty Medical Technician (IDMT) has taken him all over the United States and the world. He has several years' experience working in the Emergency Services and Critical Care arena (Cardiothoracic Surgery and Cardiac Cath Lab). He was awarded Master Instructor status by the U.S. Air Force in 1994 upon completion of his teaching practicum. He now has over 15 years of teaching experience; subjects include Emergency Medicine, Cardiovascular Nursing, Fundamentals of Nursing, Dysrhythmias, and 12-Lead ECG Interpretation. His current position provides challenges to meet the ever-changing needs of the medical community and to provide first-rate education to a diverse adult education population.

Brief Contents

Contents

and infection control, operating the ECG machine, checking the tracing, reporting results, and equipment maintenance. Extra sections are included regarding pediatric ECG, cardiac monitoring, special patient circumstances, and emergencies. Procedure checklists are included to practice performing both an ECG and continuous monitoring.

- *Chapter 5 Rhythm Strip Interpretation and Sinus Rhythms* introduces the five-step criteria for classification approach to rhythm interpretation that will be utilized throughout Chapters 5 to 10. With updated, realistic rhythm strip figures, explanations, and Checkpoint Questions, the user learns to interpret the sinus rhythms, including criteria for classification, how the patient may be affected, basic patient care, and treatment.
- *Chapter 6 Atrial Dysrhythmias* provides an introduction to and interpretation of the atrial dysrhythmias, including criteria for classification, how the patient may be affected, basic patient care, and treatment.
- *Chapter 7 Junctional Dysrhythmias* provides an introduction to and interpretation of the junctional dysrhythmias, including criteria for classification, how the patient may be affected, basic patient care, and treatment.
- *Chapter 8 Heart Block Dysrhythmias* provides an introduction to and interpretation of the heart block dysrhythmias, including criteria for classification, how the patient may be affected, basic patient care, and treatment.
- *Chapter 9 Ventricular Dysrhythmias* provides an introduction to and interpretation of the ventricular dysrhythmias, including criteria for classification, how the patient may be affected, basic patient care, and treatment.
- *Chapter 10 Pacemaker Rhythms and Bundle Branch Block* provides an introduction to pacemaker rhythms, evaluation of pacemaker function, and complications related to the ECG tracing. An introduction to bundle branch block dysrhythmias, including criteria for classification, how the patient may be affected, basic patient care, and treatment, is also included.
- *Chapter 11 Exercise Electrocardiography* provides the information necessary to assist with the exercise electrocardiography procedure. The competency checklist provides the step-by-step procedure for practice and developing proficiency at the skill.
- *Chapter 12 Ambulatory Monitoring* includes the latest information about various types of ambulatory monitors and includes what you need to know to apply and remove a monitor. A procedure checklist is also provided for this skill.
- *Chapter 13 Clinical Presentation and Management of the Cardiac Patient* expands on the anatomy of the coronary arteries and relates them to typical and atypical cardiac symptoms. STEMI, non-STEMI, and heart failure are introduced. The chapter includes a section about sudden cardiac death as compared to myocardial infarction and finishes with assessment, immediate care, and continued treatment of the cardiac patient.
- *Chapter 14 Basic 12-Lead ECG Interpretation* provides an introduction to 12-lead ECG interpretation. It includes anatomic views of the coronary arteries and correlates the arteries with the leads and views obtained on a 12-lead ECG. It also identifies the morphologic changes in the tracing that occur as a result of ischemia, injury, and infarction. Axis deviation, bundle branch block, and left ventricular hypertrophy round out the chapter concepts. The last section helps users put all of these concepts together for 12-lead interpretation.

These chapters can be utilized in various careers and training programs. Following are some suggested examples:

- Telemetry technicians (Chapters 1–12, depending on requirements)
- EKG/ECG technicians (the entire book, depending on requirements)
- Medical assistants (the entire book, depending on where they work)
- Cardiovascular technicians working in any number of specialty clinics, such as cardiology or internal medicine (the entire book)
- Remote monitoring facilities personnel (transtelephonic medicine) (Chapters 1–10, 12–14)
- Emergency medical technicians (Chapters 2, 5–10, 14, possibly more depending on where they work)
- Paramedics (Chapters 2–14)
- Nursing, especially for cross-training or specialty training (Chapters 2–14)
- Patient care tech or nursing assistant (Chapters 2–4, 12, perhaps more depending on job requirements)
- Polysomnography technologist (Chapters 2–10)
- Echocardiography technologist (Chapters 2, 5–11)
- Cardiac cath lab technologist (Chapters 2–10, 14)

New to the Fourth Edition

- Over 25 new photos and revised figures for an improved, up-to-date, and realistic look that also provides additional student practice.
- Complete revision of Chapter 1 including new and expanded sections on safety and infection control and basic vital signs.
- Modified Bloom's specific learning outcomes providing one learning outcome per level 1 heading and corresponding questions to ensure student understanding and success.
- Added and updated content about the following essential topics: cardiac anatomy, lead descriptions, law and ethics, cardiac output, vagal tone, stroke volume, premature complexes, Wolff-Parkinson-White syndrome, Torsades de Pointes, pacemakers, exercise electrocardiography (including a new table for common stress test chemicals), and ambulatory monitoring.
- Modified and simplified descriptions of arrhythmias; changed the term *configuration* to *morphology* when appropriate for accuracy.

Features of the Text

- **Key Terms and Glossary:** Key terms are identified at the beginning of each chapter. These terms are in **bold, color** type within the chapter and are defined both in the chapter and in the glossary at the end of the book.
- **Checkpoint Questions:** At the end of each main heading in the chapter are short-answer Checkpoint Questions. Answer these questions to make sure you have learned the basic concepts presented.
- **Troubleshooting:** The Troubleshooting feature identifies problems and situations that may arise when you are caring for patients or performing a procedure. At the end of this feature, you are asked a question to answer in your own words.

- **Safety & Infection Control:** You are responsible for providing safe care and preventing the spread of infection. This feature presents tips and techniques to help you practice these important skills relative to electrocardiography.
- **Patient Education & Communication:** Patient interaction and education and intrateam communication are integral parts of healthcare. As part of your daily duties, you must communicate effectively, both orally and in writing, and you must provide patient education. Use this feature to learn ways to perform these tasks.
- **Law & Ethics:** When working in healthcare, you must be conscious of the regulations of HIPAA (Health Insurance Portability and Accountability Act) and understand your legal responsibilities and the implications of your actions. You must perform duties within established ethical practices. This feature helps you gain insight into how HIPAA, law, and ethics relate to the performance of your duties.
- **Real ECG Tracings:** Actual ECG tracings, or rhythm strips, have been provided for easy viewing and to make the task of learning the various dysrhythmias easier and more realistic. Use of these ECG rhythm strips for activities and exercises throughout the program improves comprehension and accommodates visual learners.
- **Chapter Summary:** Once you have completed each chapter, take time to read and review the summary table. It has been correlated to key concepts and learning outcomes within each chapter and includes handy page number references.
- **Chapter Review:** Complete the chapter review questions, which are presented in a variety of formats. These questions help you understand the content presented in each chapter. Chapters 4, 11, and 12 also include Procedure Checklists for you to use to practice and apply your knowledge.

Resources

Mc Graw Hill Education connect®

***A one-stop spot to present, deliver, and assess digital assets available from McGraw-Hill Education: McGraw-Hill Connect® for Booth/O'Brien:* Electrocardiography for Healthcare Professionals**

McGraw-Hill Connect® for Electrocardiography provides online presentation, assignment, and assessment solutions. It connects your students with the tools and resources they'll need to achieve success. With Connect you can deliver assignments, quizzes, and tests online. A robust set of questions and activities—including all of the end-of-chapter questions, additional algorithmic math exercises focused on the three calculation methods, and interactive exercises—are presented and aligned with the text's learning outcomes. As an instructor, you can edit existing questions and create entirely new problems. Connect enables you to track individual student performance—by question, by assignment, or in relation to the class overall—with detailed grade reports. You can integrate grade reports easily with Learning Management Systems (LMSs) such as Blackboard, Desire2Learn, or eCollege—and much more. **McGraw-Hill Connect® Electrocardiography** provides students with all the advantages of Connect Electrocardiography *plus* 24/7 online access to an eBook. This media-rich version of the textbook is available through the McGraw-Hill Connect platform and allows seamless integration of text, media, and assessments. To learn more, visit **http://connect.mheducation.com.**

The Best of Both Worlds

***A single sign-on with Connect and your Blackboard® course:* McGraw-Hill Education and Blackboard—for a premium user experience**

Blackboard, the web-based course management system, has partnered with McGraw-Hill to better allow students and faculty to use online materials and activities to complement face-to-face teaching. Blackboard features exciting social learning and teaching tools that foster active learning opportunities for students. You'll transform your closed-door classroom into communities where students remain connected to their educational experience 24 hours a day. This partnership allows you and your students access to McGraw-Hill Connect® and McGraw-Hill Create™ right from within your Blackboard course—all with a single sign-on. Not only do you get single sign-on with Connect and Create, but you also get deep integration of McGraw-Hill Education content and content engines right in Blackboard. Whether you are choosing a book for your course or building Connect assignments, all the tools you need are right where you want them—inside Blackboard. Gradebooks are now seamless. When a student completes an integrated Connect assignment, the grade for that assignment automatically (and instantly) feeds into your Blackboard grade center. McGraw-Hill and Blackboard can now offer you easy access to industry-leading technology and content, whether your campus hosts it or we do. Be sure to ask your local McGraw-Hill Education representative for details.

Using another Learning Management System but still want a single sign-on?

See how **MH Campus®** makes the grade by offering universal sign-on, automatic registration, gradebook synchronization, and open access to a multitude of learning resources—all in one place. MH Campus supports Active Directory, Angel, Blackboard, Canvas, Desire2Learn, eCollege, IMS, LDAP, Moodle, Moodlerooms, Sakai, Shibboleth, WebCT, BrainHoney, Campus Cruiser, and Jenzibar eRacer. Additionally, MH Campus can be easily connected with other authentication authorities and LMSs. Visit **http://mhcampus.mhhe.com/** to learn more.

At-a-glance analysis of your class's progress: Connect Insight

Connect Insight is the first and only analytical tool of its kind, which highlights a series of visual data displays—each framed by an intuitive question—to provide at-a-glance information regarding how your class is doing. As an instructor or administrator, you receive an instant, at-a-glance view of student performance on five key insights. It puts real-time analytics in your hands so you can take action early and keep struggling students from falling behind. It also empowers you with a more valuable, transparent, and productive connection between you and your students. Available on demand wherever and whenever it is needed, Connect Insight travels from office to classroom!

Create a textbook organized the way you teach: McGraw-Hill Create™

With **McGraw-Hill Create™**, you can easily rearrange chapters, combine material from other content sources, and quickly upload content you have written, such as your course syllabus or teaching notes. Find the content you need in Create by searching through thousands of leading McGraw-Hill Education textbooks. Arrange your book to fit your teaching style. Create even allows you to personalize your book's appearance by selecting the cover and adding your name, school, and course information. Order a Create book and you'll receive a complimentary print review copy in 3 to 5 business days or a complimentary electronic review copy (eComp) via e-mail in minutes. Go to **www.mcgrawhillcreate.com** today and register to experience how McGraw-Hill Create™ empowers you to teach *your* students *your* way.

Record and distribute your lectures for multiple viewing—Tegrity

McGraw-Hill Tegrity® records and distributes your class lecture with just a click of a button. Students can view it anytime and anywhere via computer, iPod, or mobile device. It indexes as it records your PowerPoint presentations and anything shown on your computer, so students can use keywords to find exactly what they want to study. Tegrity is available as an integrated feature of McGraw-Hill Connect Electrocardiography and as a stand-alone product.

McGraw-Hill LearnSmart® is one of the most effective and successful adaptive learning resources available on the market today and is now available for **Electrocardiography for Healthcare Professionals.** More than 2 million students have answered more than 1.3 billion questions in LearnSmart since 2009, making it the most widely used and intelligent adaptive study tool that's proven to strengthen memory recall, keep students in class, and boost grades. Studies show that students using LearnSmart are 13% more likely to pass their classes and are 35% less likely to drop out. This revolutionary learning resource is available only from McGraw-Hill Education. See the power of LearnSmart for yourself by trying it today at **http://learnsmartadvantage.com/trial.**

New from McGraw-Hill Education, **LearnSmart Advantage™** is a series of adaptive learning products fueled by McGraw-Hill LearnSmart®, the most widely used and intelligent adaptive learning resource proven to improve learning since 2009. Developed to deliver demonstrable results in boosting grades, increasing course retention, and strengthening memory recall, the LearnSmart Advantage series spans the entire learning process from course preparation through final exams. LearnSmart Advantage also provides the first and only adaptive reading experience in SmartBook™. Distinguishing what students know from what they don't, and honing in on concepts they are most likely to forget, each product in the series helps students study smarter and retain more knowledge. A smarter learning experience for students coupled with valuable reporting tools for instructors, and available in hundreds of course areas, LearnSmart Advantage is advancing learning like no other products in higher education today. **Go to www.LearnSmartAdvantage.com** for more information.

SmartBook® is the first and only adaptive reading experience available today. SmartBook personalizes content for each student in a continuously adaptive reading experience. Reading is no longer a passive and linear experience, but an engaging and dynamic one in which students are more likely to master and retain important concepts, coming to class better prepared. Valuable reports provide instructors with insight on how students are progressing through textbook content, and are useful for shaping in-class time or assessment. As a result of the adaptive reading experience found in SmartBook, students are more likely to retain knowledge, stay in class, and get better grades. This revolutionary technology is available only from McGraw-Hill Education and for hundreds of courses—including **Electrocardiography for Healthcare Professionals**—as part of the LearnSmart Advantage series.

Performing the actual ECG procedure is not difficult; however, it must be performed competently. The tracing of the electrical current of the heart must be accurate because it is used to make decisions about a patient's care. An inaccurate tracing could result in a wrong decision about the patient's medication or treatment. These decisions could result in a negative outcome for the patient.

Checkpoint Questions (LO 1.1)

1. What is the leading cause of death in the United States?

____

____

2. Who is credited with determining that the human heart produces electrical currents that can be recorded?

____

____

1.2 Uses of an ECG

healthcare providers Physicians and other medically trained personnel who are licensed by individual states to provide healthcare to patients. The scope of practice for each type of healthcare provider is determined by the state license.

Healthcare providers study the ECG tracing to determine many things about the patient's heart. They look for changes from the normal ECG tracing or from a previous ECG tracing. The American Heart Association (AHA) recommends that individuals over the age of 40 have an ECG done annually as part of a complete physical. This baseline tracing assists the physician in diagnosing abnormalities of the heart. A sample of a normal tracing is shown in Figure 1-2. Normal and abnormal ECG tracings are discussed in the chapters *The Cardiovascular System* and *Rhythm Strip Interpretation and Sinus Rhythms.*

Electrocardiography can be performed in a number of healthcare settings. The type of ECG tracing produced depends on the setting and the type of ECG machine used.

Figure 1-2 A normal ECG tracing is a horizontal line with upward and downward spikes or deflections that indicate electrical activity within the heart.

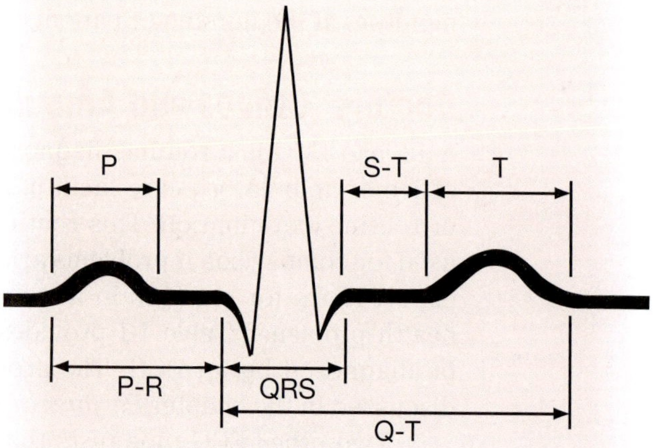

Code Blue A common name for an alert that notifies healthcare providers that a patient is unresponsive and needs assistance immediately.

stat Immediately.

In the Hospital (Acute Care)

A 12-lead ECG is one of the most commonly used ECGs in the hospital setting. A 12-lead ECG provides a tracing of the electrical activity in the patient's heart at the exact time the ECG tracing is done. In the hospital, a 12-lead ECG is done as a routine procedure or during an emergency frequently called a **Code Blue.** An emergency ECG may be required **stat,** or immediately. These are done when a patient experiences chest pain or has a change in cardiac rhythm. Routine ECGs are also frequently done before surgery.

Troubleshooting

Remain Calm

It is essential that you remain calm when recording a stat ECG. Remaining calm is necessary to avoid stress to the patient and to reduce confusion during the emergency.

What would be an appropriate way to tell a patient you are doing a stat ECG?

____

____

Another use of the ECG tracing in the hospital is during continuous monitoring. The purpose of continuous monitoring is to observe the pattern of the electrical activity of the patient's heart over time. During continuous monitoring, electrodes are attached to the patient's chest and the tracing is viewed on a monitor. Patients on continuous monitoring are usually in an intensive care unit (ICU), coronary care unit or cardiac care unit (CCU), surgical intensive care unit (SICU), or emergency department (ED). Continuous monitoring is also done routinely during surgery.

Another type of continuous monitoring done in a hospital is known as *telemetry monitoring.* Telemetry monitors are small boxes with electrodes and lead wires attached to the chest. The monitor is usually housed in a case and is attached to the patient so he or she can move about. The ECG tracing is transmitted to a central location for evaluation. When several patients are on a telemetry unit, the tracings of all the patients are recorded on multiple monitors at the nursing or patient care station.

Doctors' Offices and Ambulatory Care Clinics

A 12-lead ECG is a routine diagnostic test performed in almost any doctor's office or ambulatory care facility. It may be performed as part of a general or routine examination. This routine ECG provides a baseline tracing to be used for comparison if problems arise with a patient. The physician or trained expert looks for changes in a tracing that may indicate different types of health problems. Table 1-1 provides a complete list of conditions that may be diagnosed by an ECG. The procedure for performing a 12-lead ECG is discussed in the chapter *Performing an ECG.*

Two other ECG-type tests that may be performed in an office include treadmill stress testing and the ambulatory monitor, or Holter monitor,

TABLE 1-1 Conditions Evaluated by the ECG

- Disorders in heart rate or rhythm and the conduction system.
- Presence of electrolyte imbalance.
- Condition of the heart prior to defibrillation.
- Damage assessment during and after a myocardial infarction (heart attack).
- Symptoms related to cardiovascular disorders, including weakness, chest pain, or shortness of breath.
- Diagnosis of certain drug toxicities.
- Diagnosis of metabolic disorders such as hyper- or hypokalemia, hyper- or hypocalcemia, hyper- or hypothyroidism, acidosis, and alkalosis.
- Heart condition prior to surgery for individuals at risk for undiagnosed or asymptomatic heart disease.
- Damage assessment following blunt or penetrating chest trauma or changes after trauma or injury to the brain or spinal cord.
- Assessment of the effects of cardiotoxic or antiarrhythmic therapy.
- Suspicion of congenital heart disease.
- Evaluation of pacemaker function.

testing (Figure 1-3 and Figure 1-4). The treadmill stress test, also known as *exercise electrocardiography,* is done to determine whether the heart gets adequate blood flow during stress or exercise. The stress test is discussed in more detail in the chapter *Exercise Electrocardiography.*

A Holter monitor, or ambulatory monitor, is a small box that is strapped to a patient's waist, neck, or shoulder to monitor the heart for 24 to 48 hours or even up to 30 days as the patient performs normal daily activities. After the monitoring period, the ECG tracing is then analyzed and interpreted by the physician. The ambulatory monitor is discussed in detail in the chapter *Ambulatory Monitoring.*

Figure 1-3 This patient is performing a treadmill stress test, also known as exercise electrocardiography. During the exercise, the patient's heart and blood pressure are monitored carefully.

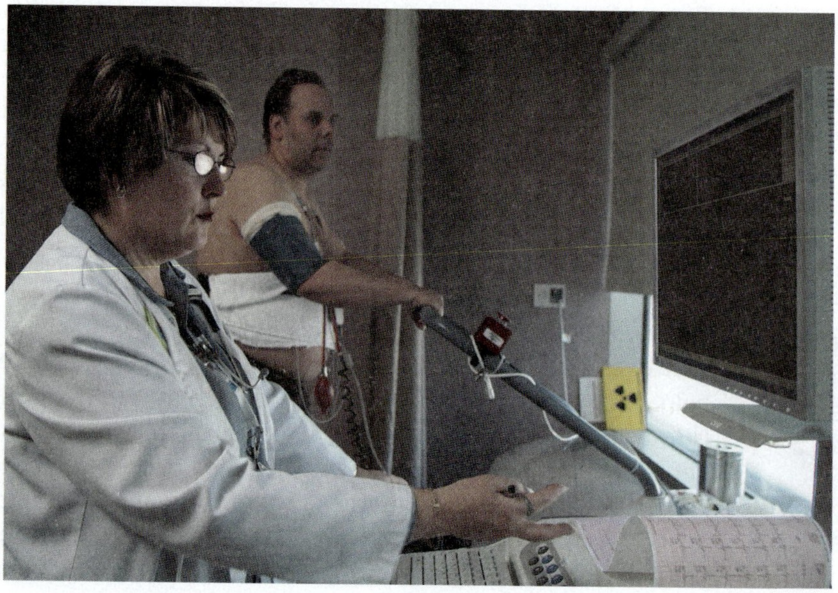

Figure 1-4 The Holter, or ambulatory, monitor allows the patient to participate in routine daily activities while the electrical activity of the heart is being recorded.

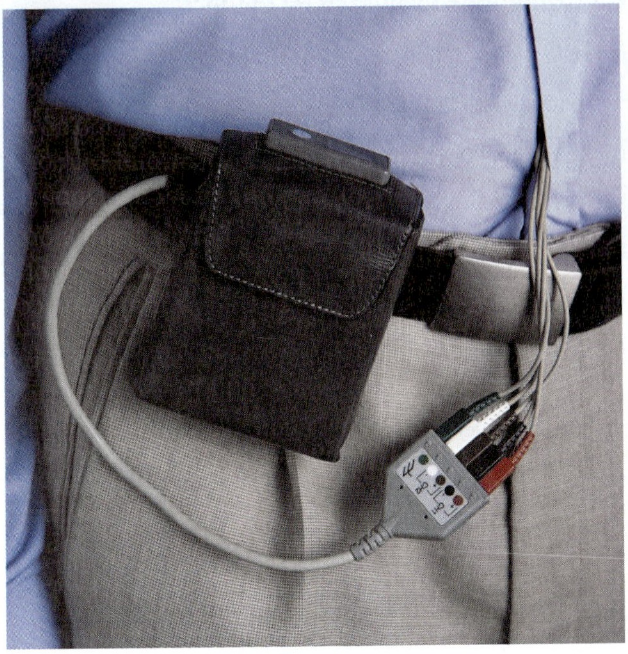

Outside of a Healthcare Facility

Outside of a healthcare facility, the ECG is used during cardiac emergencies such as a myocardial infarction. Emergency medical technicians and paramedics are equipped with portable ECG machines that can produce an ECG tracing at the site of the emergency. Whether the patient is at home, in a car, or in a crowded football stadium, emergency personnel can trace and monitor the electrical activity of the heart. Figure 1-5 shows one example of a portable ECG machine. In an emergency setting, the tracing can be evaluated for an abnormal ECG pattern. It is either transmitted back to the physician for evaluation or assessed by the emergency medical personnel at the scene. An abnormal pattern may require immediate treatment.

Defibrillators

defibrillator A machine that produces and sends an electrical shock to the heart in an attempt to correct the electrical pattern of the heart.

Treatment for abnormal rhythms includes use of a defibrillator and/or administration of cardiac medications. A **defibrillator** produces an electrical shock to the heart that is intended to correct the heart's electrical pattern. A defibrillator is commonly used in emergencies such as a Code Blue in the hospital or other care facilities or at the site of the emergency by appropriate personnel. If the heart is not beating effectively, the heart must be defibrillated quickly. The survival rate of the victim decreases by 7% to 10% for every minute a normal heartbeat is not restored.

Automatic External Defibrillators

automatic external defibrillator (AED) A lightweight, portable device that recognizes an abnormal rhythm and determines whether it is considered a "shockable rhythm."

dysrhythmia Abnormal heartbeat.

Automatic external defibrillators (AEDs) have enabled lay rescuers to help patients with sudden cardiac arrest and serious **dysrhythmias** (Figure 1-6). AEDs are available in public and private places where large numbers of people gather or live. They may also be kept by people who are at high risk for heart attacks. An AED is a lightweight, portable device that recognizes an abnormal rhythm and determines if the rhythm is considered a "shockable rhythm." The equipment is placed only on patients who are

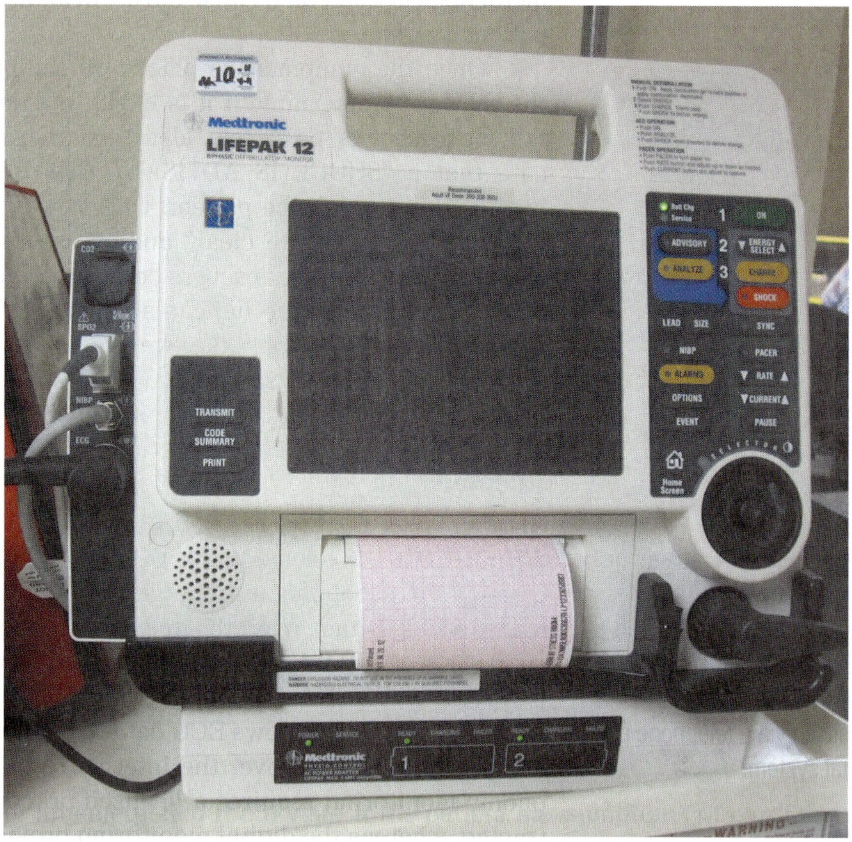

Figure 1-5 A portable ECG monitor is transported to the scene during a cardiac emergency and is attached to the patient. The ECG tracing is recorded and viewed by the emergency personnel. In addition, the tracing can be transmitted to the hospital, where a physician can evaluate and determine the necessary drugs and treatment for the patient based upon the heart rhythm viewed and the report from the emergency personnel.

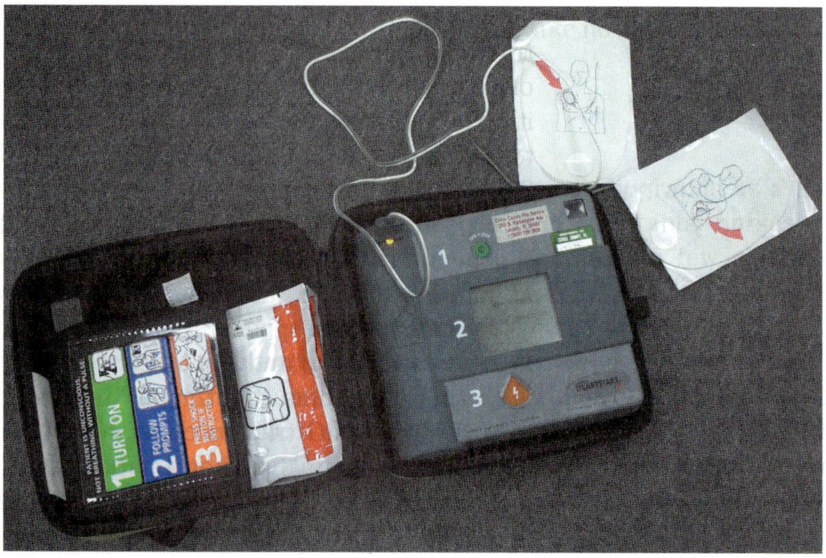

Figure 1-6 Automatic external defibrillators (AEDs) can deliver an electrical impulse that may correct an abnormal heart rhythm and increase the survival rate of myocardial infarction victims. AEDs can be found in public places and require minimal training to operate.

cardiopulmonary resuscitation (CPR) The provision of ventilations (breaths) and chest compressions (blood circulation) for a person who shows no signs of breathing or having a heartbeat.

unresponsive to stimulation (who cannot be aroused) and have no evidence of breathing or a pulse. AEDs shock only abnormal rhythms that do not produce a heartbeat. Learning about normal and abnormal rhythms is part of rhythm strip interpretation which is discussed in later chapters. When the machine recognizes other rhythms that cause the patient to be unresponsive, the AED recommends beginning **cardiopulmonary resuscitation (CPR).** Individuals using an AED should consider safety for themselves and the patient. A healthcare-provider-level CPR course is best for learning this technique. The patient should be checked for nitroglycerin patches, pacemakers, and

Figure 1-8 Multiple patients can be monitored on a single monitor screen. The patients being monitored may be in a hospital or at home depending upon the type of monitoring device they are using.

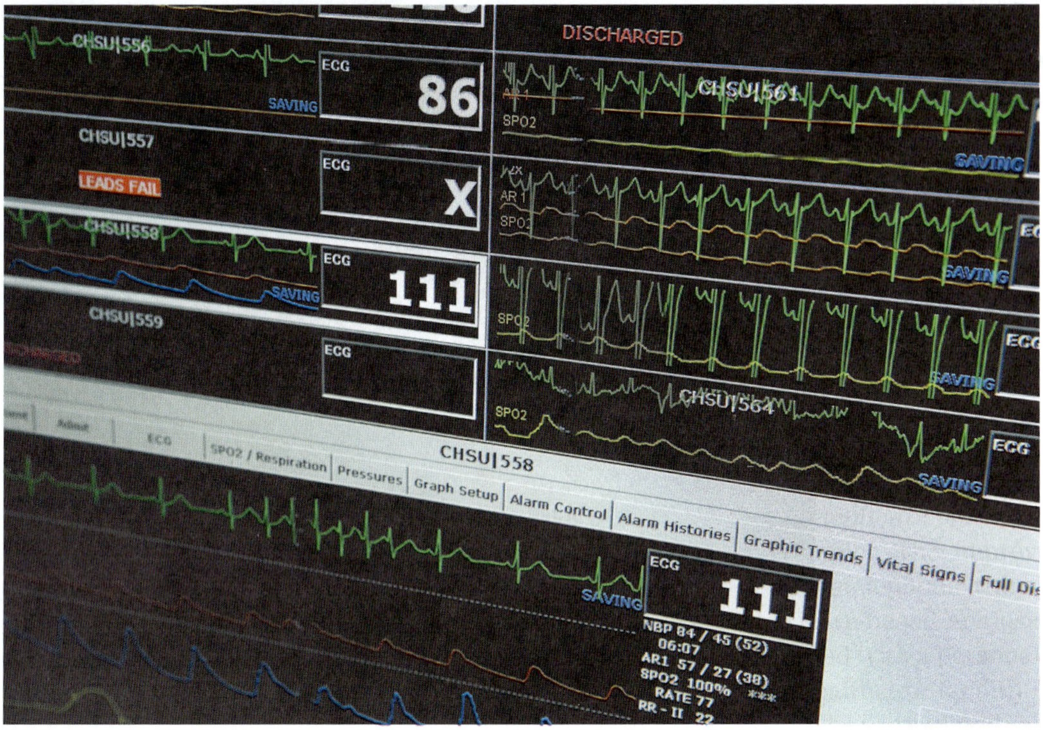

rhythm occurs, alert the healthcare professional who can treat the abnormality. ECG monitor technicians must be able to evaluate the ECG tracing. They must understand the various heart rhythms and recognize abnormal ones. They may also be asked to perform other duties, such as maintaining patient records and recording ECGs.

cardiovascular technologist An individual who has advanced skills and can assist physicians with invasive cardiovascular diagnostic tests, such as angioplasty or heart surgery.

If you enjoy the field of electrocardiology and want to advance your skills or education, you may choose to be a **cardiovascular technologist.** Technologists require more extensive training than technicians. They may assist physicians with invasive cardiovascular diagnostic tests such as angioplasty, heart surgery, or implantation of electronic, artificial pacemakers. Another specialization for cardiovascular technologists is performing ultrasounds on the blood vessels. Ultrasound equipment transmits sound waves and then collects the echoes to form an image on a screen. As part of their duties, cardiovascular technologists may also perform ECGs.

Checkpoint Questions (LO 1.2)

1. An automatic external defibrillator (AED) is used to treat what conditions?

____

____

2. Briefly describe the role of an ECG technician.

____

____

1.3 Preparing for an ECG

Preparing for an ECG involves more than just making sure the equipment is in order. You must be aware of legal and ethical issues, and you must also communicate appropriately with the patient to make sure the patient understands the procedure.

Legal and Ethical Issues

law A rule of conduct that is enforced by a controlling authority such as the government.

ethics Standards of behavior and concepts of right and wrong; based on moral values formed through the influence of family, culture, and society.

Laws are rules of conduct that are enforced by a controlling authority such as the government. An unlawful act can result in loss of your job, a fine, or other penalty such as time in jail. **Ethics** are standards of behavior and concepts of right and wrong. They are based on moral values that are formed through the influence of the family, culture, and society. Unethical acts may result in poor job evaluations or even job loss. When comparing law and ethics, you should understand that illegal acts are always unethical, but unethical acts are not always illegal.

Protecting Patient Information: HIPAA

In 1996, the Health Insurance Portability and Accountability Act (HIPAA) was established in response to patient information that was being transferred electronically for medical transactions. This act established a national standard for electronic healthcare transactions and also for providers, health plans, and employers. Its purpose was to ensure that the widespread use of electronic data was limited and secured. The patient can specify who can see information and what information is protected. A patient's information cannot be shared among healthcare professionals unless it is necessary for the patient's treatment.

Law & Ethics

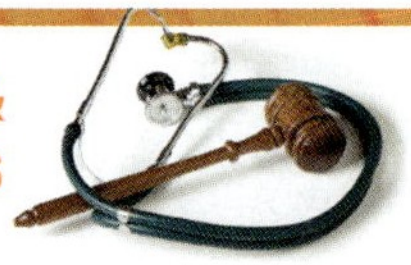

Keep Information Private

The patient's chart or a computer screen with patient data should not be left out or open in an area where other patients or visitors may be able to view it. This is a breach of confidentiality and HIPAA.

Practicing Ethics

Many professions have a *code of ethics*. These are standards of behavior or conduct as defined by the professional group. As a healthcare professional, you must follow the standards of behavior or code of ethics set forth by your profession and place of employment. The following are some basic ethics you should practice.

Confidentiality is an essential part of patient care. You may collect information about a patient for use during his or her care and treatment; however, this information should not be made public. Confidentiality is a basic right of every patient. You should not speak about your patient or allow information about your patient to be heard or seen by anyone other than those caring for him or her. A breach in confidentiality is both unethical and illegal.

Treat all patients with respect and dignity. You should respect the privacy of patients at all times. Avoid exposing your patient's body when performing any procedure by closing the door, pulling the curtain, and/or draping the patient. In some cases, it may be necessary for a male healthcare professional to have a third person present when performing an ECG on a female. Check the policies at the facility where you are employed. Practicing ethics also includes acting professionally and cooperating with co-workers, supervisors, and other healthcare professionals. Maintain your professionalism by continuing your education and training to provide the highest level of care for your patients.

Professional Liability

medical professional liability Healthcare professionals are legally responsible for their performance.

Medical professional liability means that a healthcare professional is legally responsible for his or her performance. Healthcare professionals can be held accountable for performing unlawful acts, performing legal acts improperly, or simply failing to perform an act when they should. For example, if you find a patient's wallet after he or she leaves and you decide to keep it, this is an illegal act. While you are assisting with a treadmill stress test, if you report the blood pressure results incorrectly, resulting in the patient having a severe heart attack, this is performing a legal act improperly. If you decide to take a break when you are supposed to be monitoring a patient's heart rhythm and during the time you are gone the patient experiences an abnormal heart rhythm resulting in death from lack of prompt treatment, you have failed to perform your duties as required.

Slander and Libel

You will be speaking and writing about patients as part of your job as an electrocardiographer; you should never speak defamatory words about patients even when they upset you. Making derogatory remarks about a patient—or anyone else—that jeopardizes his or her reputation or means of livelihood is called **slander.** Slander is an illegal and unethical act that could cause you to lose your job. If you write defamatory words, this is known as **libel,** which is also illegal and unethical.

slander Making derogatory remarks or speaking defamatory words about someone; both illegal and unethical.

libel Writing defamatory words about someone; both illegal and unethical.

Documentation

Medical care and treatment must be documented as part of the medical record. The medical record can be used in court as evidence in a medical professional liability case. To protect yourself legally and to provide continuity of patient care, be sure to include complete information in the medical record. Table 1-2 contains a complete list of the information that needs to be documented in the medical record.

Consent

Before you can perform an ECG on any patient, the patient must agree, or consent, to having the procedure done. Consent is often implied between the patient and healthcare professional, such as a physician in an office. For example, when a patient comes to the physician's office, he or she is agreeing to be treated by the physician. This is implied consent. When a patient agrees to the ECG procedure, this is also implied consent.

TABLE 1-2 Required Entries for Medical Records

- Patient identification, including full name, Social Security number, birth date, full address and telephone number, marital status, and place of employment, if applicable.
- Patient's medical history.
- Dates and times of all appointments, admissions, discharges, and diagnostic tests (such as an ECG).
- Diagnostic test results.
- Information regarding symptoms and reasons for appointment, diagnostic tests, and admissions.
- Physician examinations and records of results, including patient instructions.
- Medications and prescriptions given, including refills.
- Documentation of informed consent when required.
- Name of legal guardian or representative, if patient is unable to give informed consent.

Troubleshooting

Obtaining Consent

When a patient who cannot read is required to sign a consent form, you will need to explain the procedure to both the patient and a family member or the patient's legal guardian or representative. The patient then signs the consent form unless he or she has been determined to be incompetent. If this is not possible, or if the patient cannot write, explain the procedure to the patient with a witness present. Ask the patient to place an *X* on the form in the witness's presence, and then have the witness sign.

Who should sign the consent form if a patient cannot read or write?

____

____

Certain diagnostic procedures, including a treadmill stress test, require *informed consent.* The patient must understand the procedure and its associated risks, alternative procedures and their risks, and the potential risks to the patient if he or she refuses treatment. Informed consent requires the patient to sign a consent form.

Patient Education and Communication

Communicating with your patients is key to recording an ECG successfully. You must develop a positive relationship and atmosphere to reduce apprehension and anxiety during an ECG. You can reduce the patient's fears and make the ECG a positive experience by practicing effective communication techniques. Maintain a friendly, confident manner while interacting with your patient.

Helping the patient understand the procedure and follow instructions is essential. When explaining the procedure, use simple terms and speak slowly and distinctly. Encourage the patient to ask questions and repeat the instructions. This process will help ensure patient understanding. Your patient will be more cooperative if he or she trusts that you are competent to perform your job.

Patient Education & Communication

Improving Communication

When speaking to a patient who is hard of hearing, look directly at the patient and speak slowly and distinctly. The patient may be able to read your lips. If the patient speaks another language, you may want to ask an interpreter or family member to assist you with communication, thus reducing apprehension and anxiety.

Troubleshooting

Critical Thinking and Problem Solving

Being able to troubleshoot situations that arise during the ECG procedure is essential. Troubleshooting requires critical thinking. Critical thinking is the process of thinking through the situation or problem and making a decision to solve it. The problem-solving process includes the following steps:

1. Identify and define the problem.
2. Identify possible solutions.
3. Select the best solution.
4. Implement the selected solution.
5. Evaluate the results.
6. If, in step 5, you determine that the problem has not been solved, repeat steps 2 through 5 until an acceptable solution is reached.

While performing an ECG, you may need to troubleshoot actual or potential complications using the steps of the problem-solving process. These problems may arise from the patient's condition, patient communication, equipment failure, or other complications. For example, suppose that you are about to perform an ECG, and the patient refuses to let you attach the lead wires. As part of troubleshooting, you ask the patient why she is refusing. The patient states, "I do not want that electricity going through me!" In a calm manner, you explain that the machine does not produce or generate electricity, and it is not harmful. After your explanation, the patient agrees to have the ECG. You have performed successful troubleshooting.

The previous example concerns a problem with communication. However, you may also need to troubleshoot problems that occur with the equipment or tracing produced. Throughout this text, the Troubleshooting boxes will provide a variety of problems or situations you may encounter and then ask for your solution. Use your critical thinking and problem-solving skills to answer each question. In each chapter, review the "What Should You Do?" questions to check your ability to think critically and troubleshoot.

Checkpoint Question (LO 1.3)

1. Explain how you would employ the steps of the problem-solving process if a patient refuses to have an ECG.

____

____

____

1.4 Safety and Infection Control

To perform an ECG, you need to be able to transport and operate the ECG machine. You must have the ability to lift and move the patient, if necessary. These actions require using proper body mechanics and getting assistance when needed. **Body mechanics** is using movements that maintain proper posture and avoid muscle and bone injuries (Table 1-3). In addition, you must understand the basic principles of safety and infection control.

body mechanics Using movements that maintain proper posture and avoid muscle and bone injuries.

Safety

When performing healthcare procedures you must always maintain the patient's safety, as well as your own safety. Follow general safety guidelines. These specific precautions are discussed in more detail in the chapter *Performing an ECG.*

Infection Control

Preventing the spread of infection is an essential part of providing healthcare and performing an ECG. This is for your safety as well as the safety of your patients. The Centers for Disease Control and Prevention (CDC) has implemented two levels of precautions to prevent infections—standard precautions and isolation precautions.

standard precautions Procedures, such as performing hand hygiene and wearing gloves, that are used with all patients and are designed to prevent the spread of infection.

Standard precautions include a combination of performing hand hygiene and wearing gloves when there is a possibility of exposure to blood and body fluids, nonintact skin, or mucous membranes (Figure 1-9). Standard precautions apply to blood, all body fluids, secretions, and excretions (except sweat), regardless of whether they contain visible blood. Standard precautions reduce the risk of transmission of microorganisms from both

TABLE 1-3 Proper Body Mechanics

Movement	Your Action
Maintain a wide base of support.	Keep your feet shoulder-width apart at all times.
Avoid twisting.	Face the direction in which you intend to move.
Protect your back.	Bend at your hips and knees, and keep your back straight at all times.
Use stronger muscles for lifting.	Lift with your legs, not your back. Use both arms.
Maintain body alignment.	Keep your chin up and shoulders back, and avoid unnecessary reaching. Keep heavy weights as close to your body as possible.

Figure 1-9 A. Handwashing, especially between patients, is essential to prevent the spread of infection. B. The use of an alcohol-base rub on hands without visible soilage is an accepted technique for preventing infection.

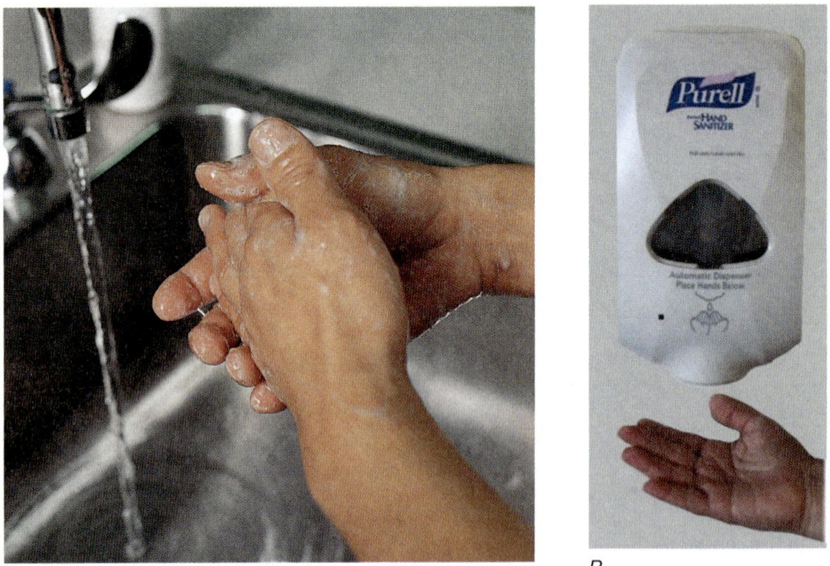

personal protective equipment (PPE) Devices such as gloves, gowns, face masks or shields, and eye protection designed to protect a healthcare worker from sources of infection.

recognized and unrecognized sources of infection. In addition to performing hand hygiene and wearing gloves, practices may include using **personal protective equipment (PPE)** such as a gown, mask, and eye protection (Figure 1-10).

In addition, the CDC advises healthcare workers not to wear artificial nails because they are more likely to harbor gram-negative pathogens than natural nails, both before and after handwashing. Natural nails should be no more than 1/4-inch long.

Safety & Infection Control

Hand Hygiene

Performing proper hand hygiene is the single most important thing you can do to prevent the spread of infection. Wash your hands or use an alcohol-based rub (if no visible soilage is present) between patients and procedures and before and after you use gloves. *Note:* Certain types of infections, such as *Clostridium difficile,* require handwashing because the use of alcohol-based hand rubs is not sufficient to kill all the infectious organisms. Always use the method of hand hygiene that is most appropriate for the patient's condition.

isolation precautions The second level of steps taken to prevent the spread of infection; used when a specific infection is known or suspected. Examples include separating the infected person from others and using personal protective equipment.

The second level includes **isolation precautions,** which are based on how the infectious agent is transmitted. Isolation precautions include the following:

- Airborne precautions—require special air handling, ventilation, and additional respiratory protection (HEPA or N95 respirators).
- Droplet precautions—require mucous membrane protection (goggles and masks).

Figure 1-10 Wearing appropriate personal protective equipment (PPE) reduces the risk of transmission of infection. PPE includes items such as gloves, mask, gown, and eye protection.

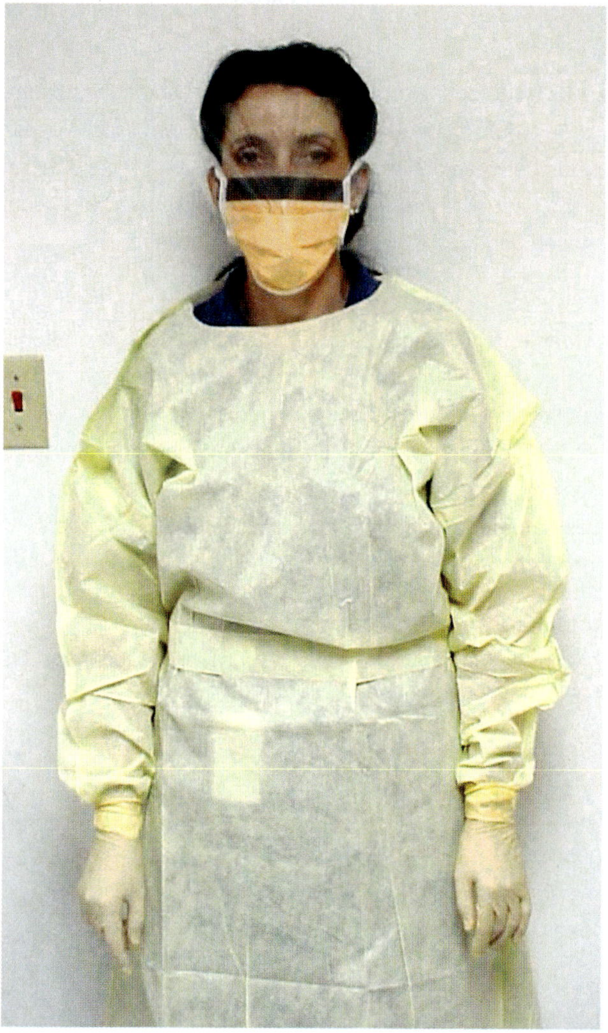

- Contact precautions—require gloves and gowns for direct skin-to-skin contact or for contact with contaminated linen, equipment, and so on.

Standard precautions are practiced in all employment situations in which exposure to blood or body fluids is likely. Isolation precautions are used less often and only with patients who have specific infections. When isolation precautions are in place for a patient during an ECG, you will be required to follow the specific guidelines for the type of precautions implemented. Table 1-4 provides a list of standard precautions that should be practiced when recording an ECG. See the appendix *Standard and Isolation Precautions* for additional information about these precautions.

Checkpoint Question (LO 1.4)

1. What measures would you use to prevent the spread of infection to you and your patients?

____

____

____

TABLE 1-4 Standard Precautions Related to Electrocardiography

Hand Hygiene
- Wash your hands after touching blood, body fluids, secretions, excretions, and contaminated items.
- Wash your hands before putting on gloves and after removing gloves.
- Wash your hands between patient contacts.
- Wash your hands between tasks and procedures on the same person.
- Use alcohol-based hand rub if you have no visible soilage.

Gloves
- Wear gloves when touching blood, body fluids, secretions, excretions, and contaminated items.
- Wear gloves when touching mucous membranes and nonintact skin.
- Change gloves between procedures and patients.
- Change gloves after contacting materials that are highly contaminated.
- Remove gloves promptly after use.
- Remove gloves before touching uncontaminated surfaces or items.
- Wash your hands immediately after glove removal.

Masks, Eye Protection, and Face Shields
- Wear mask, eye protection, and face shield during procedures and tasks that are likely to cause splashes or sprays of blood, body fluids, secretions, and excretions.

Gowns
- Wear a gown to protect the skin and clothing.
- Wear a gown during procedures and activities that are likely to cause splashes or sprays of blood, body fluids, secretions, or excretions.
- Remove a soiled gown promptly.
- Wash your hands immediately after gown removal.

Equipment
- Handle used equipment carefully. It may be soiled with blood, body fluids, secretions, and excretions.
- Prevent skin and mucous membrane exposure and clothing contamination.
- Clean, disinfect, or sterilize reusable equipment before it is used on another person.
- Discard single-use equipment promptly.

Environmental Control
- Follow facility procedures for the routine care, cleaning, and disinfection of surfaces. This includes environmental surfaces, nonmovable equipment, and other frequently touched surfaces.

Occupational Health and Bloodborne Pathogens
- Use resuscitation devices for mouth-to-barrier resuscitation.

1.5 Vital Signs

vital signs Temperature, pulse, respiration, blood pressure, and pain assessment.

A patient's **vital signs**—pulse, respiration, blood pressure, temperature, and pain assessment—are among the most important assessments for determining a patient's current health status. Changes in the vital signs can indicate an abnormality, or they can be a normal response to exertion, heat, stress, or other environmental factors. This section focuses on adult pulse, respirations, and blood pressure because these vital signs may be checked or monitored by ECG professionals. Table 1-5 shows the normal ranges for vital signs in adults.

TABLE 1-5 Normal Vital Signs in Adults

Vital Sign	Adult Normal Range
Pulse (beats per minute)	60–100
Respirations (per minute)	12–20
Blood pressure (mmHg)	
Systolic	Less than 120
Diastolic	Less than 80

Pulse and Respiration

Pulse and respiration are related because the circulatory and respiratory systems work together. Pulse is measured as the number of times the heart beats in 1 minute. Respiration is the number of times a patient breathes in 1 minute. One breath, or respiration, equals one inhalation and one exhalation. Usually, if either the pulse or respiration rate is high or low, the other is also.

Pulse

cardiac output The amount of blood the heart pumps per minute.

A pulse rate gives information about the patient's cardiovascular system. It is an indirect measurement of the patient's **cardiac output,** or the amount of blood the heart is able to pump in 1 minute. If the pulse is weak, irregular, or abnormally fast or slow, the patient may show signs of low cardiac output.

Measure the pulse of adults at the radial artery, where it can be felt in the groove on the thumb side of the inner wrist (Figure 1-11). Press lightly on this pulse point with the pads of your fingers. Do not use your thumb because your thumb has a pulse, which you may feel instead of the patient's pulse. Count the number of beats you feel in 1 minute and note the rhythm and volume. The rhythm can be regular or irregular. The volume can be weak, strong, or bounding. A bounding pulse feels like it is leaping out and then quickly disappearing with each pulse beat.

In some instances you will not be able to feel a pulse at the wrist, especially if the patient is very weak or has unstable vital signs. In these cases, you can check for a pulse at the carotid artery. This artery is located on the

Figure 1-11 Place your fingers in the groove on the thumb side of the inner wrist to check a patient's pulse.

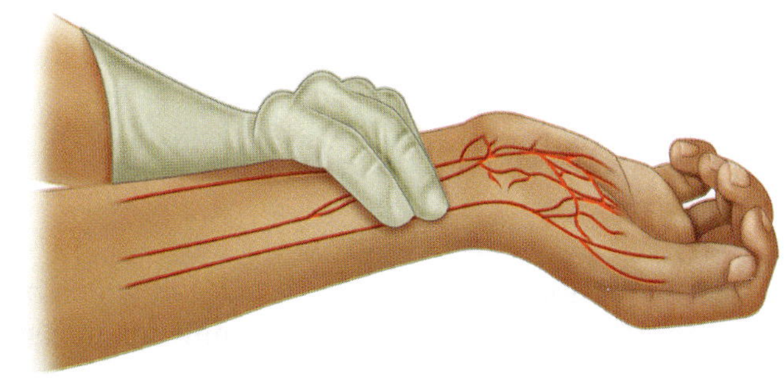

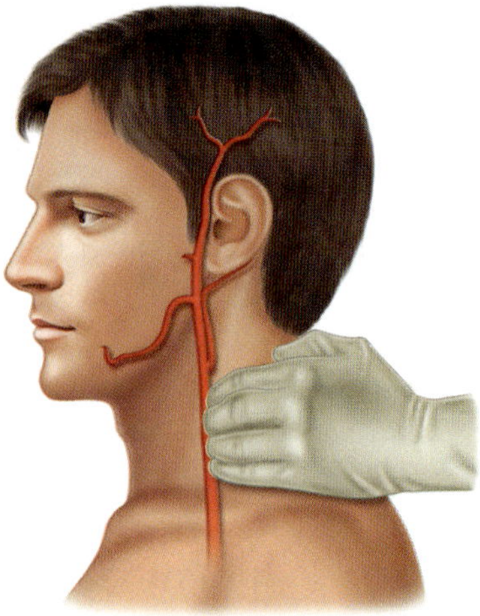

Figure 1-12 To check the carotid pulse, place your fingers on the side of the neck next to the airway.

side of the neck next to the airway (Figure 1-12). This is the same pulse location that is used for adults during basic life support.

Respiration

A patient's respiration rate indicates how well the patient's body is providing oxygen to tissues. The best way to check respiration is by watching, listening, or feeling the movement at the patient's chest, stomach, back, or shoulders. If you cannot see the chest movement, then place your hand over the patient's chest, shoulder, or abdomen and listen and feel for the movement of air. Respirations also may be counted with a stethoscope. Place the stethoscope on one side of the spine in the middle of the back to count respirations.

You need to count respirations subtly because once the patient is aware that respiration is being measured, he may unintentionally alter his breathing. If you are using a stethoscope, tell the patient that you want to listen to his lungs. If you are not using a stethoscope, count the respirations while you have your hand on the pulse site.

Respirations are counted for 1 full minute to determine the rate, rhythm, and effort (quality). Counting for less than a minute may cause you to miss certain breathing abnormalities. The rhythm should be regular. The quality or effort should be normal, shallow, or deep. Irregularities such as *hyperventilation* (excessive rate and depth of breathing), *dyspnea* (difficult or painful breathing), *tachypnea* (rapid breathing), or *hyperpnea* (abnormally rapid, deep, or labored breathing) are indications of possible disease and should be noted.

Rales and rhonchi are types of noisy breathing that can indicate an abnormality. Rales—crackling sounds—may indicate fluid in the lungs and can be heard in patients with pneumonia, congestive heart failure, and other conditions. Rhonchi are wheezing or snorelike sounds that occur when the airways are narrowed or obstructed.

Blood Pressure

Blood pressure is the force at which blood is pumped against the walls of the arteries. The standard unit for measuring blood pressure is millimeters of mercury (mmHg). The pressure measured when the left ventricle of the heart

systolic blood pressure The blood pressure measured when the left ventricle of the heart contracts.

diastolic blood pressure The blood pressure measured when the heart relaxes; the minimum amount of pressure exerted against the vessel walls at all times.

hypertension High blood pressure.

hypotension A lower-than-normal blood pressure that can cause reduction of blood flow to vital organs.

contracts is known as the **systolic blood pressure.** The pressure measured when the heart relaxes is known as the **diastolic blood pressure.** The diastolic pressure indicates the minimum amount of pressure exerted against the vessel walls at all times.

Factors Affecting Blood Pressure

Many factors can affect blood pressure. Internal factors such as cardiac output, blood volume (amount of blood in the body), vasoconstriction (constriction of the veins), and blood viscosity (thickness) regulate the blood pressure within the body.

If a patient's blood pressure reading is consistently elevated after two or more visits to the physician, the patient may be diagnosed with **hypertension,** or high blood pressure. Hypertension may be categorized as essential or secondary. *Essential hypertension* has no identifiable cause. According to the Joint National Committee on Prevention, Detection, Evaluation, and Treatment of High Blood Pressure, part of the National Heart, Lung, and Blood Institute in the National Institutes of Health, 95% of all hypertension is essential. *Secondary hypertension* occurs as a result of some other condition, such as kidney or heart disease.

Hypotension, or low blood pressure, is not generally a chronic health problem. Slightly low blood pressure may be normal for some patients and does not usually require treatment. Severe hypotension may be present with shock, heart failure, severe burns, and excessive bleeding.

Measuring Blood Pressure

Blood pressure is measured using a *sphygmomanometer,* or blood pressure cuff. To measure blood pressure, wrap the blood pressure cuff around the patient's upper arm, 1 to 2 inches above the pulse point of the brachial artery (Figure 1-13). This pulse point is located in the bend of the elbow, called the *antecubital space.* Never apply the blood pressure cuff over clothing.

When measuring blood pressure, you should first determine the palpatory pressure that represents the target peak inflation. Inflate the cuff as you palpate the radial pulse. Palpation provides an approximation of the systolic blood pressure to ensure an adequate level of inflation when the actual measurement is made. It also helps prevent overinflation, which is uncomfortable for the patient. Inflate the cuff until you can no longer feel the radial pulse

Figure 1-13 *A.* Place the blood pressure cuff about 2 inches above the bend in the patient's elbow. *B.* Palpate the blood pressure at the antecubital space.

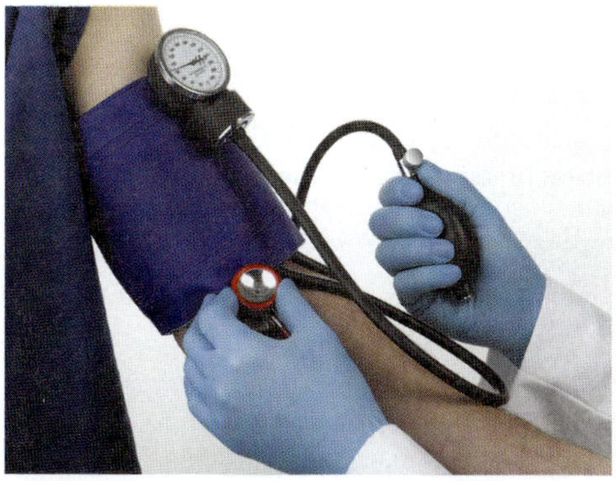

A.

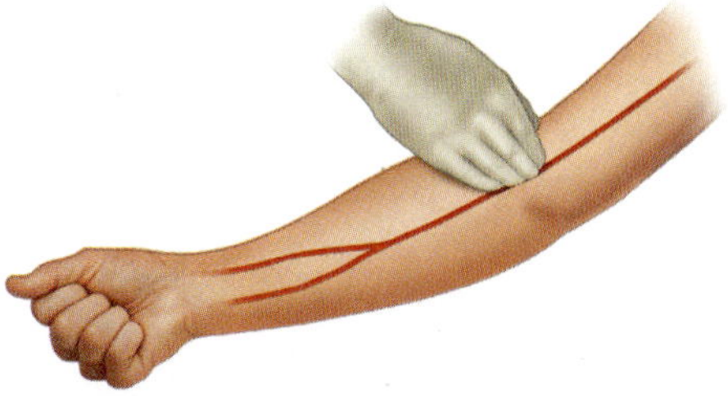

B.

auscultated blood pressure Blood pressure determined while listening with a stethoscope.

and note the pressure at that point. Release the air from the cuff and allow the arm to rest for 30 to 60 seconds, or remove the cuff entirely and replace it after 30 to 60 seconds. To determine the **auscultated blood pressure,** inflate the cuff to 30 mmHg above the palpatory result, generally in the range of 180 to 200 mmHg. Then, while you slowly release the air in the cuff (2 to 4 mmHg/second), listen with the stethoscope placed over the brachial pulse point. You will hear vascular sounds that will change. These sounds are called *Korotkoff sounds.* Record the first sound you hear as the systolic number. Record the final sound you hear as the diastolic number.

Checkpoint Questions (LO 1.5)

1. Which three vital signs are of particular importance to ECG technicians?

   ____

2. What is the difference between a palpated blood pressure and an auscultated blood pressure?

   ____

   ____

Chapter Summary

Learning Outcomes	Summary	Pages
1.1 Describe the history and the importance of the ECG.	An ECG is a tracing of the heart's electrical activity made using an electrocardiograph. Willem Einthoven is credited with developing the first electrocardiograph. Today the machine is used to diagnose cardiovascular disease, which is the number one cause of death in America.	2–3
1.2 Identify the uses of an ECG and opportunities for an electrocardiographer.	The ECG is used routinely in hospitals before surgery, during emergencies, and as part of continuous monitoring. In an outpatient setting, an ECG is part of an exam or is used during stress tests or Holter monitoring. Outside of the healthcare facility, the ECG is used to evaluate patients during emergencies. Career opportunities in electrocardiography include ECG technician, ECG monitor technician, and cardiovascular technologist.	3–10

(Continued)

Learning Outcomes	Summary	Pages
1.3 Troubleshoot legal, ethical, patient education, and communication issues related to the ECG.	Legal and ethical issues include protecting patient information in accordance with HIPAA, preventing situations that lead to professional liability, avoiding slander and libel, documenting all procedures thoroughly, and obtaining the patient's consent before performing any procedure. Communicating with and educating the patient are an important part of preparing for an ECG. Troubleshooting may involve solving problems with the patient, the equipment, or the tracing produced.	11–15
1.4 Perform safety and infection control measures required for the ECG.	Working safely includes using proper body mechanics and getting assistance when needed to move heavy objects. Follow all safety and infection control guidelines at your facility, including standard precautions and isolation precautions as necessary. Performing proper hand hygiene is the single most important thing you can do to prevent the spread of infection.	15–18
1.5 Compare basic vital sign measurements related to the ECG.	The vital signs include pulse, respiration, blood pressure, temperature, and pain assessment. ECG technicians are commonly asked to check or monitor the pulse, respiration, and blood pressure of adults. Normal vital signs for most adults are a pulse of 60–100 beats per minute, 12–18 respirations per minute, and a blood pressure of less than 120 mmHg (systolic) over 80 mmHg (diastolic).	18–22

Chapter Review

Matching

Match the term on the left with its definition on the right.

_______ **1.** cardiovascular disease (LO 1.1)

_______ **2.** electrocardiogram (LO 1.1)

_______ **3.** coronary artery disease (LO 1.1)

_______ **4.** standard precautions (LO 1.4)

_______ **5.** electrocardiograph (LO 1.1)

_______ **6.** defibrillator (LO 1.2)

_______ **7.** AED (LO 1.2)

_______ **8.** isolation precautions (LO 1.4)

a. an instrument used to record the electrical activity of the heart

b. a tracing of the signal produced by the heart's electrical activity and used for diagnostic evaluation of the heart

c. The second level of protection against the transmission of disease; based on how the infectious agent is transmitted

d. narrowing of the heart's blood vessels that causes a reduction of blood flow to the heart

e. used to analyze the heart rhythm and produce a shock if necessary

f. disease related to the heart and blood vessels (veins and arteries)

g. a machine that delivers an electrical shock to the heart that is intended to correct the abnormal electrical pattern of the heart

h. guidelines that apply to blood, body fluids, secretions, and excretions (except sweat); followed when there is a possibility of exposure to blood or body fluids

True/False

Read each statement and determine if it is true or false. Circle the T or F. For false (F) statements, correct them on the line provided.

T F 9. An ECG machine produces and records the electrical activity of the heart. (LO 1.1)

____

____

T F 10. Standard precautions are guidelines written for healthcare providers to help prevent the spread of infection. (LO 1.4)

____

____

T F 11. Libel is the act of making derogatory remarks about someone. (LO 1.3)

____

____

T F **12.** A transtelephonic monitor transmits an ECG over the Internet. (LO 1.2)

____

____

Multiple Choice

Circle the correct answer.

13. The normal range for an adult's pulse is (LO 1.5)
- **a.** 40–80 beats per minute.
- **b.** 50–60 beats per minute.
- **c.** 60–100 beats per minute.
- **d.** 90–120 beats per minute.

14. Which physician received a Nobel Prize for inventing the electrocardiograph? (LO 1.1)
- **a.** Augustus D. Waller
- **b.** Sir Thomas Lewis
- **c.** Willem Einthoven
- **d.** Joseph Lister

15. The main responsibility of an ECG monitor technician is to (LO 1.2)
- **a.** view and evaluate ECG tracings on an oscilloscope and alert healthcare professionals when abnormalities appear.
- **b.** attach the ECG electrodes to patients who will be monitored remotely.
- **c.** assist physicians with angioplasty, heart surgery, and implantation of artificial pacemakers.
- **d.** perform ultrasounds on patients' blood vessels.

16. Which of the following is *not* a reason for performing an ECG? (LO 1.2)
- **a.** To evaluate heart conditions
- **b.** To check for problems with the flow of electricity through the heart
- **c.** To see how well the heart is contracting and pumping
- **d.** To evaluate the rate and rhythm of breathing

17. A defibrillator can be used (LO 1.2)
- **a.** to treat an abnormal heart rhythm.
- **b.** without training.
- **c.** to produce an electrical rhythm.
- **d.** to record the patient's breathing pattern.

18. Transtelephonic monitoring allows for information to be (LO 1.2)
- **a.** reviewed immediately by the patient.
- **b.** transmitted over a telephone.
- **c.** submitted for billing purposes only.
- **d.** recorded by a computerized device.

19. A continuous ECG monitor is used most commonly in a(n) (LO 1.2)
- **a.** physician's office.
- **b.** hospital.
- **c.** assisted-living center.
- **d.** clinic.

2 The Cardiovascular System

Learning Outcomes

2.1 Explain how circulation occurs in relation to the ECG.

2.2 Recall the structures of the heart including valves, chambers, and vessels.

2.3 Differentiate among pulmonary, systemic, and coronary circulation.

2.4 Explain the cardiac cycle including the difference between systole and diastole.

2.5 Describe the parts and function of the heart and conduction system and how they relate to the ECG.

2.6 Describe the heart activity that produces each part of the ECG waveform.

Key Terms

action potential
aorta
aortic semilunar valve
atrioventricular (AV) node
atrium (pl. atria)
automaticity
Bachmann's bundle
bundle branches
bundle of His (AV bundle)
cardiac cycle
chordae tendineae
complexes
conductivity
contractility
coronary circulation
deoxygenated blood
depolarization
diastole
excitability
interval
interventricular septum
ischemia
isoelectric
left atrium
left ventricle
mitral (bicuspid) valve
myocardial
oxygenated blood
papillary muscles
parasympathetic
pericardium
polarization
pulmonary artery
pulmonary circulation
pulmonary semilunar valve
pulmonary veins
Purkinje fibers
Purkinje network
repolarization
right atrium

right ventricle
segment
semilunar valve
sinoatrial (SA) node
sympathetic
systemic circulation
systole
tricuspid valve
vena cava (pl. venae cavae)

2.1 Circulation and the ECG

The function of the heart is to pump blood to and from all the tissues of the body. Blood supplies the tissues with nutrients and oxygen and removes carbon dioxide and waste products. The process of transporting blood to and from the body tissues is known as *circulation.* The heart's powerful muscular pump performs the task of circulation. Circulation of the blood depends on the heart and its ability to contract or beat. Each electrical activity of the heart is recorded on the ECG. Knowledge of the heart, its functions, and what produces the ECG tracing will provide you with a clear understanding of the tasks you will be performing as an ECG healthcare professional.

Checkpoint Questions (LO 2.1)

1. What is circulation?

____

____

2. What is recorded on the ECG strip?

____

____

2.2 Anatomy of the Heart

The heart lies near the center of the chest, under the sternum, and between the lungs. Two-thirds of it lies to the left of the sternum. The heart varies in size and weight depending on a person's weight, physical condition, and gender. The average heart is approximately the size of your fist and weighs about 10.6 ounces or 300 grams (Figure 2-1).

The heart is a powerful muscular pump that beats an average of 72 times per minute, 100,000 times per day, and 22.5 billion times in the average lifetime. Each ventricle pumps about 70 milliliters (mL) of blood per beat, for a total output of roughly 5 liters (L) per minute. Each day the heart pumps approximately 7,250 liters or 1,800 gallons of blood. This is enough to fill an average-size bathtub about 36 times.

pericardium A two-layered sac of tissue enclosing the heart.

The heart consists of three layers: the endocardium, myocardium, and epicardium (or visceral pericardium) (Table 2-1 and Figure 2-2). The entire heart is enclosed in a sac of tissue called the **pericardium.** This sac consists of two layers: the tough, outer layer is called the *parietal layer,* and the inner layer is called the *visceral layer.* The visceral pericardium adheres closely to the heart. It is also referred to as the *epicardium,* the outermost layer of the heart. The purpose of the pericardium is to protect the heart from infection

Figure 2-1 The heart is tipped to the right side of the body with about two-thirds of it located on the left side of the chest.

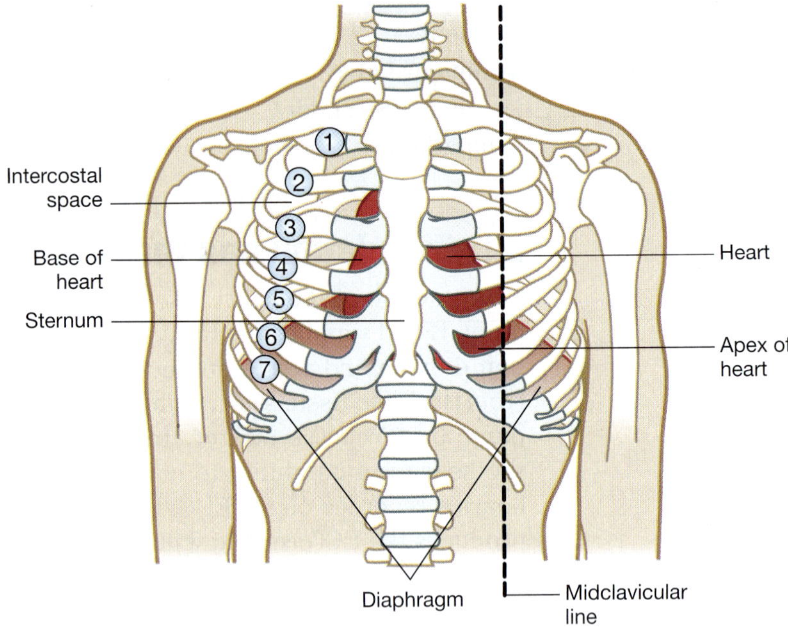

right atrium The right upper chamber of the heart, which receives blood from the body.

left atrium The left upper chamber of the heart, which receives blood from the lungs.

right ventricle The right lower chamber of the heart, which pumps deoxygenated blood to the lungs.

left ventricle The left lower chamber of the heart, which pumps oxygenated blood through the body. It is the biggest and strongest chamber, known as the workhorse of the heart.

interventricular septum A partition or wall (septum) that divides the right and left ventricles.

atrium (pl. atria) Top two chambers of the heart.

and trauma. The space between the two layers is called the *pericardial space.* It contains about 10 to 20 mL (about ½ ounce) of fluid, which cushions the heart against blows and decreases friction between the layers created by the pumping heart.

Chambers and Valves

The heart is divided into four chambers. The top chambers are the **right atrium** and **left atrium.** The bottom chambers are the **right ventricle** and **left ventricle.**

Between the right and left ventricles is a partition known as the **interventricular septum.** The myocardium varies in thickness between chambers. It is thin in the **atria** (sing. atrium), thick in the right ventricle, and thickest in the left ventricle. The thicker the myocardium of a chamber is, the

TABLE 2-1 Heart Layers

Layer	Location and Function
Endocardium	Inner layer of the heart that lines the chambers and valves. The Purkinje fibers are located just below this layer.
Myocardium	Middle, thickest muscular layer, responsible for heart contraction.
Epicardium (also called the visceral pericardium)	Outside, thin layer of the heart that contains the coronary arteries; it is also known as the inner layer of the pericardium.
Pericardium (made up of the visceral pericardium and the parietal pericardium)	A double-layer sac that encloses the heart. The inner layer, or visceral pericardium, is also called the epicardium; the outer layer is the parietal pericardium.

Figure 2-2 Three distinct layers can be identified on the heart. A sac called the *pericardium* protects it.

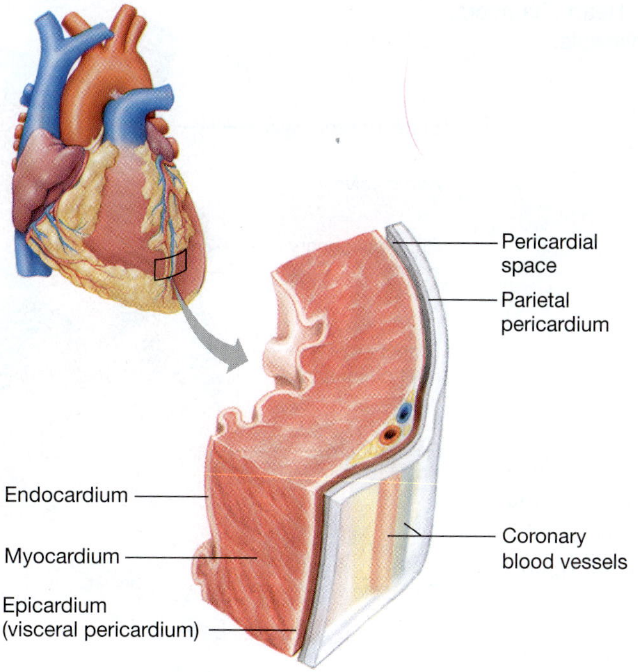

tricuspid valve Valve located between the right atrium and right ventricle; it prevents backflow of blood into the right atrium.

mitral (bicuspid) valve Valve with two cusps or leaflets located between the left atrium and left ventricle; it prevents backflow of blood into the left atrium.

chordae tendineae Structures that connect the atrioventricular valves to the papillary muscles and prevent them from opening in the wrong direction.

papillary muscles Muscles in the ventricles that anchor the chordae tendineae and atrioventricular valves.

pulmonary artery Large artery that transports deoxygenated blood from the right ventricle to the lungs. This is the only artery in the body that carries deoxygenated blood.

aorta The largest artery of the body, which transports oxygenated blood from the left ventricle of the heart to the entire body.

semilunar valve A valve with half-moon-shaped cusps that open and close, allowing blood to travel only one way; located in the pulmonary artery and the aorta.

stronger the muscular contraction of that chamber. The left ventricle is sometimes known as the "workhorse of the heart" because of its thick myocardium and powerful muscular contraction.

Between the right atrium and right ventricle is the **tricuspid valve.** Between the left atrium and left ventricle is the **mitral (bicuspid) valve.** These two valves are known as *atrioventricular (AV) valves* because they divide the atria from the ventricles. **Chordae tendineae** connect the atrioventricular (tricuspid and mitral) valves to the papillary muscles (sometimes referred to as "heartstrings"). The chordae tendineae prevent the valves from opening in the wrong direction. The **papillary muscles** are structures within the ventricles that are attached to the chordae tendineae and serve as the anchor for both the chordae tendineae and the AV valves.

The **pulmonary artery** and the **aorta** each has a **semilunar valve.** They are called *semilunar* because the valve flaps look like a half (*semi*) moon (*lunar*). These valves are called the **aortic semilunar valve** and the **pulmonary semilunar valve** (Table 2-2 and Figure 2-3). The semilunar valves separate the ventricles from the arteries leading to the lungs or body. These one-way valves in the heart keep the blood flow headed in the right

TABLE 2-2 **Heart Valves and Their Locations**

Name	Valve Type	Location
Aortic	Semilunar	Between left ventricle and aorta
Pulmonary	Semilunar	Between right ventricle and pulmonary artery
Tricuspid	Atrioventricular	Separates right atrium and right ventricle
Mitral (bicuspid)	Atrioventricular	Separates left atrium and left ventricle

Figure 2-3 Heart chambers, valves, and vessels.

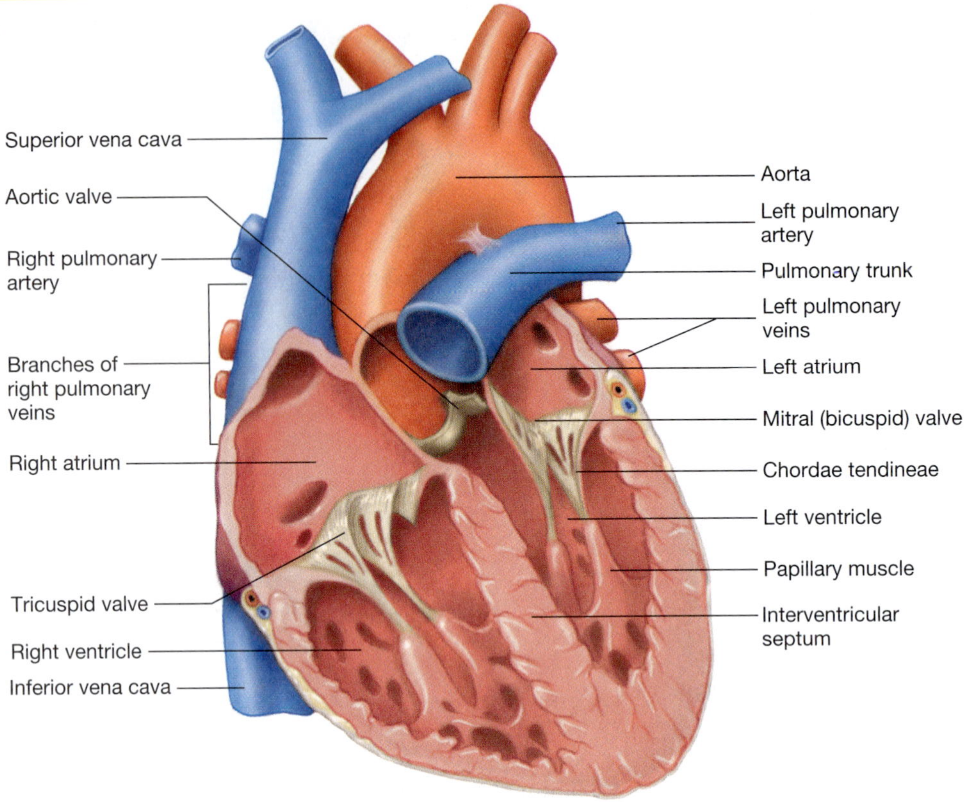

aortic semilunar valve Valve located in the aorta that prevents the backflow of blood into the left ventricle.

pulmonary semilunar valve Valve found in the pulmonary artery that prevents backflow of blood into the right ventricle.

vena cava Largest vein in the body, which provides a pathway for deoxygenated blood to return to the heart; its upper portion, the superior vena cava, transports blood from the head, arms, and upper body; and its lower portion, the inferior vena cava, transports blood from the lower body and legs.

direction. The flaps or "cusps" open to allow the blood to flow, then close to prevent the backflow of blood (Figure 2-4).

The Major Vessels to and from the Heart

Blood vessels are the veins and arteries that transport blood all over the body. The major blood vessels that transport blood to and from the heart are the venae cavae, pulmonary artery, pulmonary veins, and aorta.

Blood travels from the body tissue through the veins toward the heart. The blood is returned through the largest vein of the body, the **vena cava**

Figure 2-4 Valves viewed from a cross section of the heart.

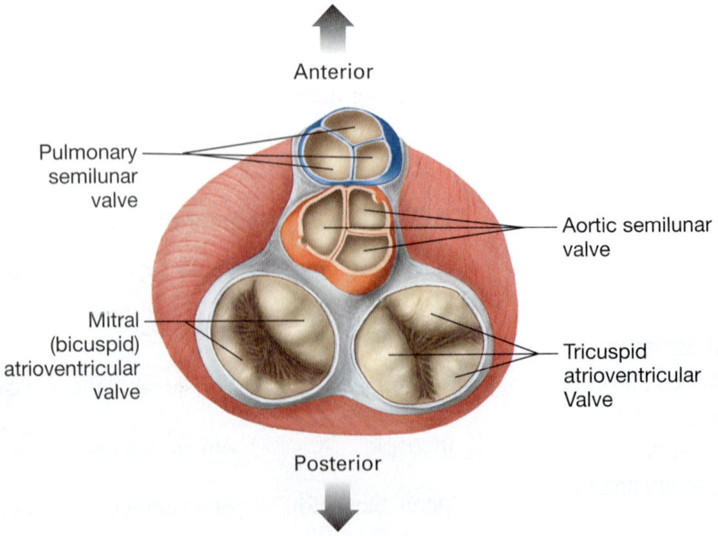

deoxygenated blood Blood that has little or minimal oxygen (oxygen-poor blood).

pulmonary veins Transport oxygenated blood back into the left atrium of the heart. These are the only veins that carry oxygenated blood.

oxygenated blood Blood having oxygen (oxygen-rich blood).

(pl. venae cavae), to the right atrium. The superior vena cava transports blood from the head, arms, and upper body. The inferior vena cava transports blood from the lower body and legs (Figure 2-5).

When the heart contracts, the right ventricle pumps **deoxygenated blood** (blood that has little or minimal oxygen) to the lungs via the pulmonary artery. In the lungs, the exchange of carbon dioxide and oxygen occurs to enrich the blood with oxygen. The **pulmonary veins** transport **oxygenated blood** (blood containing oxygen) back to the heart into the left atrium. Transporting blood to the entire body is the function of the aorta. When the left ventricle contracts, the blood is pumped into the aorta. The first vessels to branch off the aorta are the coronary arteries. Coronary arteries are part of the coronary circulation, which supplies blood to the muscular heart pump (Figure 2-5).

Figure 2-5 Pathways for blood through the heart.

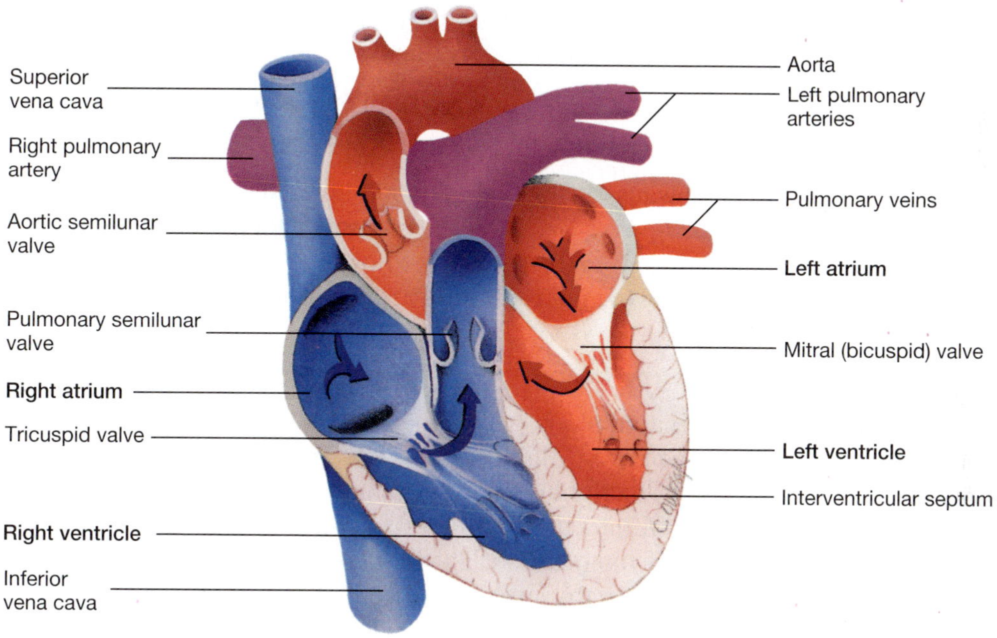

A. Major blood vessels to and from the heart.

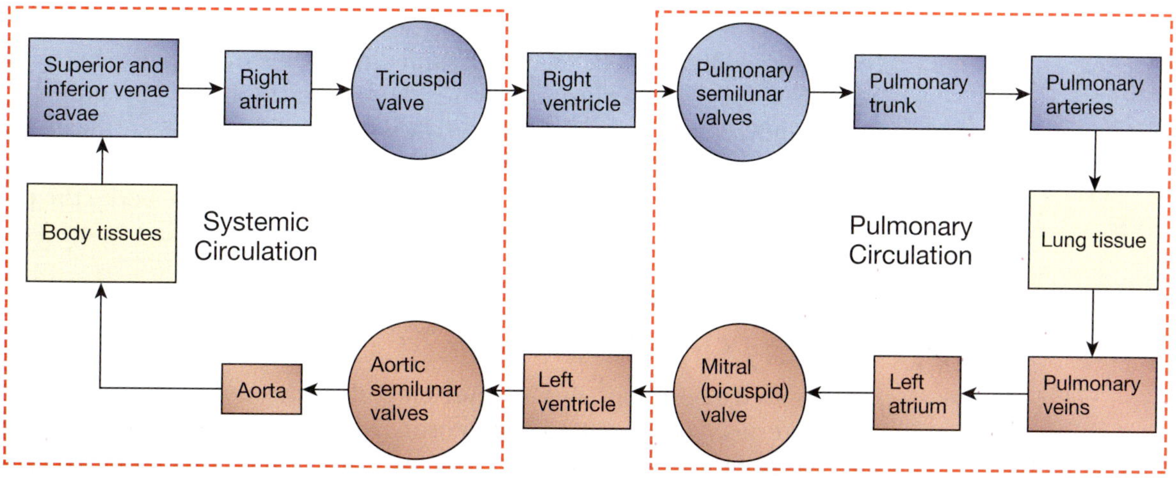

B. Blue = deoxygenated blood; red = oxygenated blood.

Checkpoint Questions (LO 2.2)

1. What is the name of the middle layer of the heart (the muscular layer)?

____

____

2. Which valve is located between the left atrium and left ventricle?

____

____

2.3 Principles of Circulation

The heart is actually a two-sided pump. The left side of the heart is a high-pressure pump that pumps oxygenated blood to the body tissue. The right side of the heart is a low-pressure pump that pumps deoxygenated blood to the lungs. Think of the heart like this:

left side ⟶ high oxygen concentration
right side ⟶ low oxygen concentration

The pathways for pumping blood to and from the lungs are known as **pulmonary circulation.** The pathways for pumping blood throughout the body and back to the heart are known as **systemic circulation.** The circulation of blood to and from the heart muscle is known as **coronary circulation.**

pulmonary circulation The transportation of blood to and from the lungs; blood is oxygenated in the lungs during pulmonary circulation.

systemic circulation The pathways for pumping blood throughout the body and back to the heart.

coronary circulation The circulation of blood to and from the heart muscle.

Pulmonary Circulation: The Heart and Lung Connection

Deoxygenated blood enters the right atrium through the superior and inferior venae cavae. Blood travels through the tricuspid valve into the right ventricle. The right ventricle pumps the blood through the pulmonary semilunar valve into the pulmonary artery, then into the lungs. In the lungs, the blood is oxygenated. The blood returns to the heart through the pulmonary veins into the left atrium. The left atrium is the last step of pulmonary circulation.

Systemic Circulation: The Heart and Body Connection

Oxygenated blood enters the left atrium and travels through the mitral valve into the left ventricle. The left ventricle pumps the blood through the aortic semilunar valve into the aorta. The aorta provides the pathway for the blood to circulate through the body. In the body, the oxygen in the blood is exchanged with carbon dioxide. After traveling through the body, the deoxygenated blood returns to the heart through the superior and inferior venae cavae (Figure 2-6).

Coronary Circulation: The Heart's Blood Supply

Oxygenated blood from the left ventricle travels through the aorta to the coronary arteries. There are two main coronary arteries, the left coronary artery and the right coronary artery. These arteries branch to supply oxygenated

Figure 2-6 Pulmonary and systemic circulation.

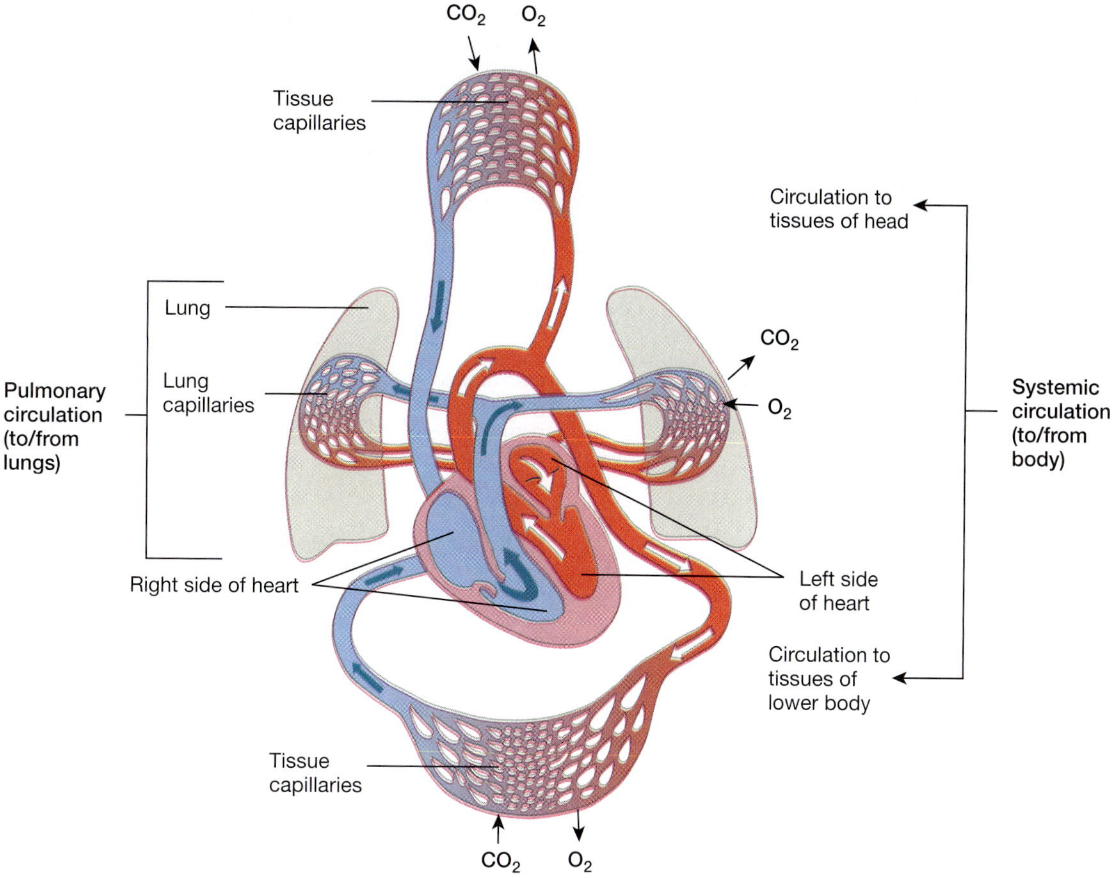

blood to the entire heart. The left coronary artery has more branches than the right because the left side of the heart is more muscular and requires more blood supply. The deoxygenated blood travels through the coronary veins and is collected in the coronary sinus, which empties the blood directly into the right atrium (Figure 2-7).

The Heart as a Pump

The heart is an amazing pump that distributes blood throughout the body. The average heart beats 72 times a minute. Each ventricle pumps about 70 mL of blood during contraction. The volume of blood ejected with each contraction is referred to as *stroke volume*. This amount can vary depending on things such as a person's gender, size, level of physical fitness, disease state, or genetics. The volume of blood pumped each minute is referred to as *cardiac output*. The average cardiac output is approximately 5 L per minute. When the volume of blood decreases, the heart rate increases; similarly, if the contractile force of the heart decreases, the stroke volume is decreased. In such cases, patients show signs of decreased or low cardiac output, including pallor, confusion, low blood pressure, nausea, and dizziness. A patient's cardiac output is estimated by multiplying heart rate by stroke volume ($HR \times SV = CO$).

Figure 2-7 Coronary circulation.

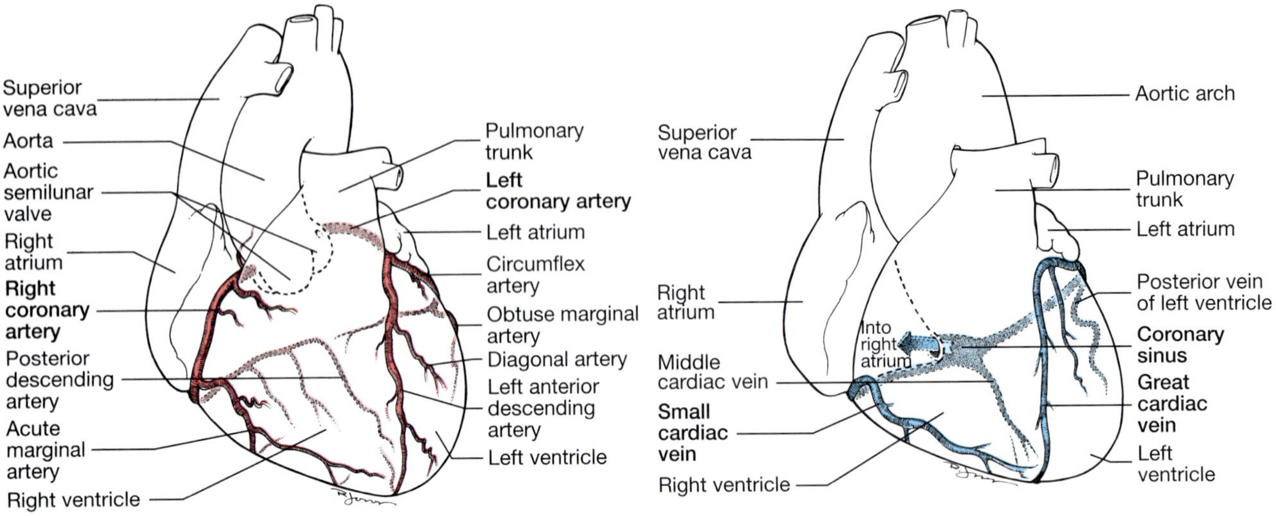

A. Branches of the coronary arteries supply blood to the heart tissue.

B. Branches of the cardiac veins drain blood from the heart tissue.

Checkpoint Questions (LO 2.3)

1. What are the first vessels to branch off the aorta called?

____

____

2. Describe the three types of circulation.

____

____

____

3. What is cardiac output?

____

____

cardiac cycle The contraction and relaxation of the heart.

diastole The phase of the cardiac cycle when the heart is expanding and refilling; also known as the relaxation phase.

systole The contraction phase of the cardiac cycle, during which the heart is pumping blood out to the pulmonary (lungs) and systemic (body) circulation.

2.4 The Cardiac Cycle

Each beat of the heart has two phases that correspond to the contraction and the relaxation periods of the heart. The contraction and relaxation of the heart together make up the **cardiac cycle.** When the heart contracts, it is squeezing blood out to the pulmonary (lungs) and systemic (body) circulation. As the heart relaxes, it is expanding and refilling. The relaxation phase of the heart is known as **diastole.** The contraction phase is known as **systole.**

Diastole: Relaxation of the Heart

During diastole the heart chambers are relaxing and filling. Blood from the vena cava fills the right atrium, pushing open the tricuspid valve. This allows blood to flow into the right ventricle. At the same time, blood is returning from the lungs via the pulmonary veins to the left atrium. This blood fills the left atrium and forces the mitral valve open to allow blood to flow into the left ventricle.

Systole: Contraction of the Heart

During the systolic phase, the heart muscle contracts, creating pressure to open the pulmonary and aortic valves. Blood from the right ventricle is pushed into the lungs to exchange oxygen and carbon dioxide. Blood from the left ventricle is pushed through the aorta to be distributed throughout the body to provide oxygen for tissues and remove carbon dioxide (Figure 2-8).

In adults, the average heart beats approximately 60 to 100 times per minute. In general, women have a faster heartbeat than men. Children's heart rates are usually faster than an adult's heart rate and depend on the age and size of the child.

If you listen to the heart with a stethoscope, you will hear two sounds: "lubb" and "dupp." These sounds are made by the closing of the heart valves, which is caused by the contraction and relaxation of the heart. The "lubb" you hear is the sound made during the systolic phase by the contraction of the ventricles and the closing of the mitral and tricuspid valves. The "dupp" sound is made during the diastolic phase. It is shorter and occurs during the beginning of ventricular relaxation. This sound is from the closure of the pulmonary and aortic valves. Each complete "lubb-dupp" you hear is actually one beat of the heart.

Checkpoint Questions (LO 2.4)

1. What is the cardiac cycle?

____

____

2. How are diastole and systole different from one another?

____

____

Figure 2-8 Diastole and systole.

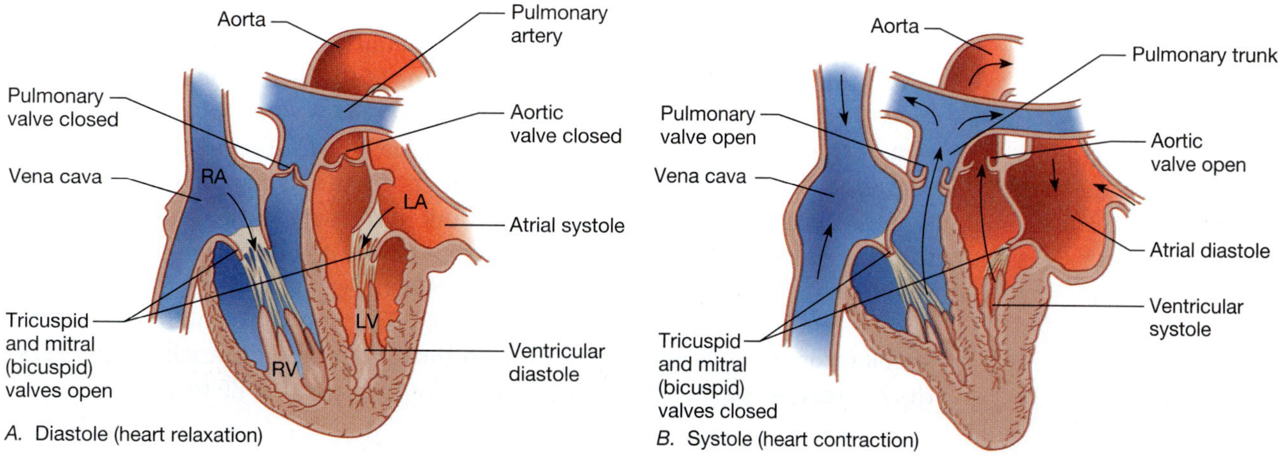

2.5 Conduction System of the Heart

The pumping cycle is controlled by electrical impulses: electrical impulses stimulate contraction of the heart muscle, and the absence of electrical impulses allows the heart muscle to relax. These electrical impulses are initiated by specialized pacemaker cells in the heart. The electrical impulses are transferred through the heart by the electrical conduction system. The working cells of the heart respond by shortening, causing cardiac contraction and blood flow. The conduction system is necessary for the heart to pump continuously and rhythmically.

Unique Qualities of the Heart

The conduction system is a network of conducting tissue that creates the heartbeat and establishes a pattern for the electrical activity of the heart. The conducting tissue of the heart has several unique qualities that control the beat of the heart and produce the electrical wave. They include automaticity, conductivity, contractility, and excitability.

automaticity The ability of the heart to initiate an electrical impulse without being stimulated by another or independent source.

myocardial Pertaining to the heart (*cardi*) muscle (*myo*).

conductivity The ability of the heart cells to receive and transmit an electrical impulse.

contractility The ability of the heart muscle cells to shorten in response to an electrical stimulus.

excitability The ability of the heart muscle cells to respond to an impulse or stimulus; also called irritability.

Automaticity is the ability of the heart to initiate an electrical impulse without being stimulated by a source outside the heart. Automaticity is a form of the word *automatic*, which is exactly how the heart beats—automatically. The heart tissue has its own innate ability to initiate an electrical impulse.

The heartbeat relies on the ability of the **myocardial** cells to conduct electrical impulses. **Conductivity** is the ability of the heart cells to receive and transmit an electrical impulse. The electrical impulse is initiated by automaticity and then travels through the rest of the heart due to the conductivity of the heart cells.

When the heart muscle cells are stimulated by an electrical impulse, they contract. This ability of the heart muscle cells to shorten in response to an electrical stimulus is known as **contractility.** The contraction of the heart muscle cells produces the heartbeat or pumping of the heart.

Excitability (also referred to as irritability) is the ability of the heart muscle cells to respond to an impulse or stimulus. Without the quality of excitability, the heart would not react to the electrical impulses that are initiated within the heart.

As you can see, the heart's unique qualities are essential to the rhythmic contraction of the heart muscle and the circulation of blood through the body. Without these qualities, the heart would not beat.

Regulation of the Heart

sympathetic The part of the ANS that causes an increase in the heart rate.

In addition to automaticity, the heartbeat is controlled by the *autonomic nervous system (ANS)*. Like the unique qualities of the heart, the ANS is involuntary. This means you have no conscious control over its functions. The **sympathetic** branch of the ANS increases the heart rate and contractility by secreting norepinephrine. This happens automatically when you are under stress or become frightened. You can think of the automaticity of the heart as the cruise control in your car. In a normal heart, it automaticity sets the rate of the heart to 60 to 100 beats a minute. When the sympathetic branch of the ANS is stimulated, it speeds up the heart. When you take your foot off the accelerator (remove the stimulation to the sympathetic branch of the ANS), the heart rate coasts down to the cruise control speed of 60 to 100.

parasympathetic The part of the ANS that helps slow the heart rate.

The **parasympathetic** branch of the ANS exerts a depressant effect on the heart by secreting acetylcholine. The vagus nerve is the major nerve of the parasympathetic system and exerts an effect on many of the body organs. It is widespread throughout the body. Stimulation of the vagus nerve slows the heart, acting like a brake to the heart rate. When a patient is experiencing an abnormally fast heart rate, stimulation of the vagus nerve is used to bring the heart back to its normal cruise control rate.

Other factors can affect the heart. For example, exercise, stress, or a fever can increase the heart rate. The cardiac control center, located in the brain, sends impulses to decrease the heart rate when the blood pressure rises. When the blood pressure falls, it sends impulses to increase the heart rate. The levels of the electrolytes potassium and calcium play a role in the control of the heart. When there is a low concentration of potassium ions in the blood, the heart rate decreases; but a high concentration causes an abnormal heart rate or rhythm. A low concentration of calcium ions in the blood depresses heart actions, but a high concentration of calcium causes heart contractions that are longer than normal heart contractions.

Pathways for Conduction

sinoatrial (SA) node An area of specialized cells in the upper right atrium that initiates the heartbeat.

Bachmann's bundle The structure that relays the electrical impulse from the SA node to the left atrium in a normal heart.

atrioventricular (AV) node Delays the electrical impulse to allow the atria to complete their contraction.

bundle of His (AV bundle) Located next to the AV node; provides the transfer of the electrical impulse from the atria to the ventricles.

bundle branches Left and right branches of the bundle of His that conduct impulses down either side of the interventricular septum to the left and right ventricles.

The heart's conduction system consists of the sinoatrial (SA) node, atrioventricular (AV) node, bundle of His (AV bundle), bundle branches, and the Purkinje fibers in the ventricles. The SA and AV nodes are small, round structures that consist of many specialized cardiac cells. Normal conduction in the heart begins with the **sinoatrial (SA) node,** which is located in the upper portion of the right atrium. It is the pacemaker of the heart and initiates the heartbeat. The electrical impulse travels through the internodal pathways and stimulates the right atrium and is simultaneously relayed to the left atrium through **Bachmann's bundle.** The automaticity of the cells in the atria causes them to contract. In a normal heart, the SA node fires at about 60 to 100 times per minute.

On the floor of the right atrium is another mass of specialized cardiac cells known as the **atrioventricular (AV) node.** Impulses travel to the AV node because of the unique quality of conductivity through a specialized pathway through the atria. The AV node itself causes a delay (slowdown) in the electrical impulse. This process is important for three reasons. First, it provides time for additional blood to travel from the atria to the ventricles before they contract. This additional blood is known as the *atrial kick.* The atrial kick increases the cardiac output. Second, the delay in the electrical impulse reduces the number of electrical impulses transmitted to the ventricles. This is important when the atria are firing too fast. It prevents an excessive rate of electrical impulses from reaching the ventricles. A third benefit to the delay in contraction of the atria is that it allows the ventricles to contract from the bottom up to avoid conflicting contractions between atria and ventricles. The delay aids in coordinated contraction of the heart. The AV node can also act as the pacemaker if the SA node is not working. It will fire at a rate of 40 to 60 times per minute. This is known as the *inherent rate* of the AV node.

The **bundle of His (AV bundle),** located next to the AV node, transfers the electrical impulse from the atria to the ventricles. When the impulse reaches the ventricles, it divides into the **bundle branches,** located along the left and right sides of the interventricular septum. The left and right bundle

Purkinje fibers The fibers within the heart that distribute electrical impulses from cell to cell throughout the ventricles.

Purkinje network Spreads the electrical impulse throughout the ventricles by means of the Purkinje fibers.

branches are like a fork in the road, and the electrical impulse splits and travels down both sides to stimulate the left and right ventricles to contract. Impulses traveling down the left bundle branch also stimulate the interventricular septum to contract in a left-to-right pattern.

Purkinje fibers form a network, the **Purkinje network,** that spreads the electrical impulse throughout the ventricles. These fibers provide an electrical pathway for each of the cardiac cells. The electrical impulses accelerate and activate the right and left ventricles at the same time to cause the ventricles to contract. The electrical impulse produces an electrical wave, resulting in contraction of the ventricles (Table 2-3 and Figure 2-9).

TABLE 2-3 Parts of the Conduction System

Part	Function
Sinoatrial (SA) node (pacemaker)	Electrical impulses occur at a rate of 60 to 100 beats per minute
Atrioventricular (AV) node	Delays the electrical impulse to allow for the atria to complete their contraction and ventricles to fill before the next contraction; also serves as a secondary pacemaker if the SA node fails
Bundle of His (AV bundle)	Conducts electrical impulses from the atria to the ventricles
Bundle branches	Conduct impulses down both sides of the interventricular septum
Purkinje fibers (network)	Distribute the electrical impulses through the right and left ventricles

Figure 2-9 Conduction pathways.

1. The heartbeat originates in the sinoatrial (SA) node; it travels across the wall of the atrium through the internodal pathways to the atrioventricular (AV) node and Bachmann's bundle to the left atrium.
2. The impulse passes through the AV node into the AV bundle (bundle of His) to the interventricular septum.
3. The impulse is divided between the right and left bundle branches and travels to the apex of the heart through the interventricular septum via the bundle branches.
4. The Purkinje fibers carry the impulse through the right and left ventricles, causing them to contract.

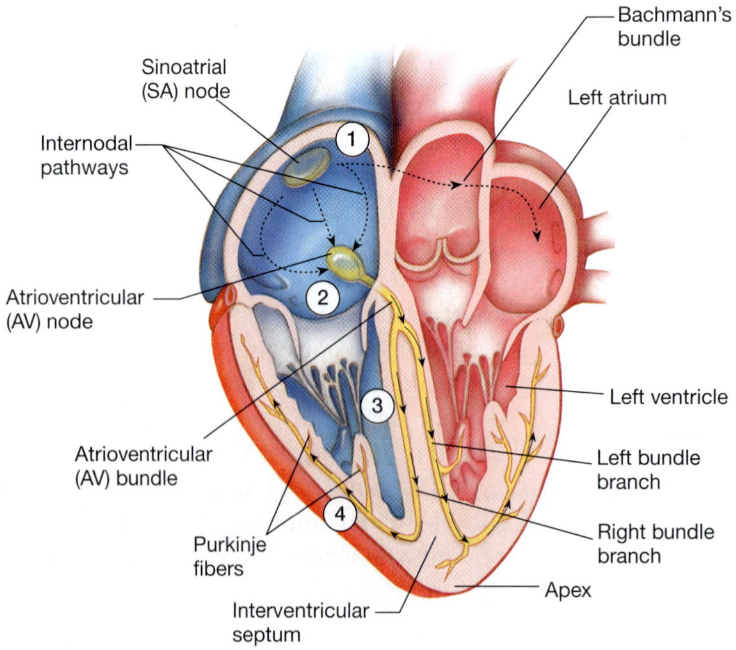

Checkpoint Questions (LO 2.5)

1. List the parts of the conduction system in the order the electrical impulse travels.

____

____

2. What term refers to the ability of the heart muscle cells to respond to a stimulus?

____

____

3. Where does the electrical impulse get delayed to allow all the blood to leave the atria before the ventricles contract?

____

____

2.6 Electrical Stimulation and the ECG Waveform

polarization The state of cellular rest in which the inside is negatively charged and the outside is positively charged.

depolarization The electrical activation of the cells of the heart that initiates contraction of the heart muscle.

action potential The change in the electrical potential of the heart muscle when it is stimulated.

repolarization The return of heart muscle cells to their resting electrical state, causing the heart muscle to relax.

Polarization is the state during which the heart cells are at their peak resting energy. During this portion of the cycle, the cells (in their resting state) are electrically polarized. This means the inside of the cardiac cell is negatively charged in relation to the outside of the cell. This is much like the opposite ends of a battery. One is negative and one is positive. This state of cellular rest, polarization, is the ready phase of the heart.

Depolarization, on the other hand, is a state of cellular stimulation that precedes contraction. It is the electrical activation of the cells of the heart when the electrical charge is reversed across the cell membrane so the interior becomes positively charged. This rapid change in polarization is known as **action potential.** The action potential is brought on by a rapid change in the cell membrane permeability to certain ions (they lose their internal negativity) in response to the electrical impulse from the SA node. Depolarization moves from cell to cell through the electrical pathways under normal circumstances. Depolarization is the most important electrical event in the heart—it causes the myocardial cells to shorten and contract and under normal circumstances pump blood to the body.

Repolarization is a state of cellular recovery that follows each contraction. The cardiac cells return to their resting phase of internal negativity. After depolarization, the cardiac cells return to this state in order to prepare for another depolarization. During repolarization, the heart relaxes and allows the chambers of the heart to refill.

The cycle of polarization, depolarization, and repolarization is often compared to a camera with an automatic flash. When the little light on the back of the camera is lit, this is just the same as polarity or peak resting energy. When you press the button to take a picture, energy is released, causing the light to flash. This is the same as depolarization and the wave of energy that spreads throughout the myocardium, causing contraction and the pumping action of the heart. After the picture has been taken, you may have noticed a quiet sound as the energy is building in the capacitor in the camera as it prepares for the next picture. This event is the same as repolarization or the resting, reenergizing phase of action potential.

isoelectric The period when the electrical tracing of the ECG is at zero or a straight line, and no positive or negative deflections are seen.

The ECG waveform is recorded from the electrical activity produced during depolarization and repolarization of the heart. The waveform on the electrocardiogram is a series of up-and-down deflections off a straight line known as an **isoelectric** line. The isoelectric line represents the period when no electrical activity is occurring in the heart and is known as a *baseline.* Deflections, which appear as waves on the ECG tracing, indicate electrical activity in the heart. The deflections that go up are positive; the deflections that go down are negative. The discussion of the direction of the deflections in this chapter is based on lead II of the ECG.

When Willem Einthoven first discovered the waveform, he labeled the waves of the electrocardiogram P, Q, R, S, and T. Legend holds that he chose the letters from the center of the alphabet because he did not know what the waves meant or whether other waves preceding the P wave or following the T wave would be discovered. The U wave was added after Einthoven's discovery. Each of these waves indicates specific activity in the heart.

interval The period of time between two activities within the heart.

segment A portion or part of the electrical tracing produced by the heart.

complexes Atrial or ventricular contractions as they appear on the ECG; complete ECG waveforms.

In addition to the waves, the ECG waveform contains **intervals, segments,** and **complexes.** Each of these elements indicates specific activity within the heart. The elements include the QRS complex, the ST segment, the PR interval, and the QT interval (Table 2-4).

What Each Part of the Waveform Represents

The first deflection is positive and is known as the P wave. The P wave is generated when the atria depolarize. The P wave is small (compared to the other waves of the ECG), rounded, and is the first wave of the normal complex.

During the delay of conduction that occurs at the atrioventricular node, a short baseline segment is seen on the waveform. There is no electrical activity occurring (depolarization or repolarization); thus, no wave or deflection is seen. It is during this time that atrial kick occurs.

TABLE 2-4 ECG Components

Component	Appearance	Heart Activity
P wave	Upward small curve	Atrial depolarization with resulting atrial contraction
QRS complex	Q, R, and S waves	Ventricular depolarization and resulting ventricular contraction (larger than the P wave); atrial repolarization occurs (not seen)
T wave	Small upward-sloping curve	Ventricular repolarization
U wave	Small upward curve	Repolarization of the bundle of His and Purkinje fibers (not always seen); may be seen in instances of electrolyte imbalance
PR interval	P wave and baseline prior to QRS complex	Beginning of atrial depolarization to the beginning of ventricular depolarization
QT interval	QRS complex, ST segment, and T wave	Period of time from the start of ventricular depolarization to the end of ventricular repolarization
ST segment	End of QRS complex to the beginning of T wave	Time between ventricular depolarization and the beginning of ventricular repolarization

The next three waves occur together as the QRS complex representing ventricular depolarizations. The Q wave represents the conduction of the impulse down the interventricular septum. It is a negative deflection before the R wave. It is not unusual or abnormal for a QRS complex not to have a Q wave. A normal Q wave is less than one-fourth of the height of the R wave. The R wave is the first positive wave of the QRS complex. It represents the conduction of electrical impulse to the left ventricle. It is usually the easiest wave to locate on the ECG tracing. The S wave is the first negative deflection after the R wave. It represents the conduction of the electrical impulse through both ventricles. The Q, R, and S waves together form the QRS complex. The QRS complex represents ventricular depolarization. It reflects the time it takes for the impulses to depolarize the interventricular septum down through the ventricular myocardium, causing the ventricles to contract (Figure 2-10).

ischemia Occurs when there is a sudden loss or reduction in blood supply (oxygen) to a region of the heart tissue. This occurs due to the presence of atherosclerotic plaque, blood clot, emboli, or even vascular spasm (Prinzmetal's angina).

The ST segment is measured from the end of the S wave to the beginning of the T wave. This segment should normally be on the isoelectric line. It indicates the end of ventricular depolarization and the beginning of ventricular repolarization. The reason this segment is studied in a 12-lead ECG recording is to determine whether there is any ischemia or myocardial (heart) damage. **Ischemia,** which occurs when there is a sudden loss or reduction in blood supply (oxygen) to a region of heart tissue, can result in a change in the ST segment. The ST segment becomes elevated or depressed, depending on the extent of the ischemia and the amount of damage to the cardiac cells. A change in the ST segment typically indicates some form of injury to the heart

Figure 2-10 Electrical activity in the heart.

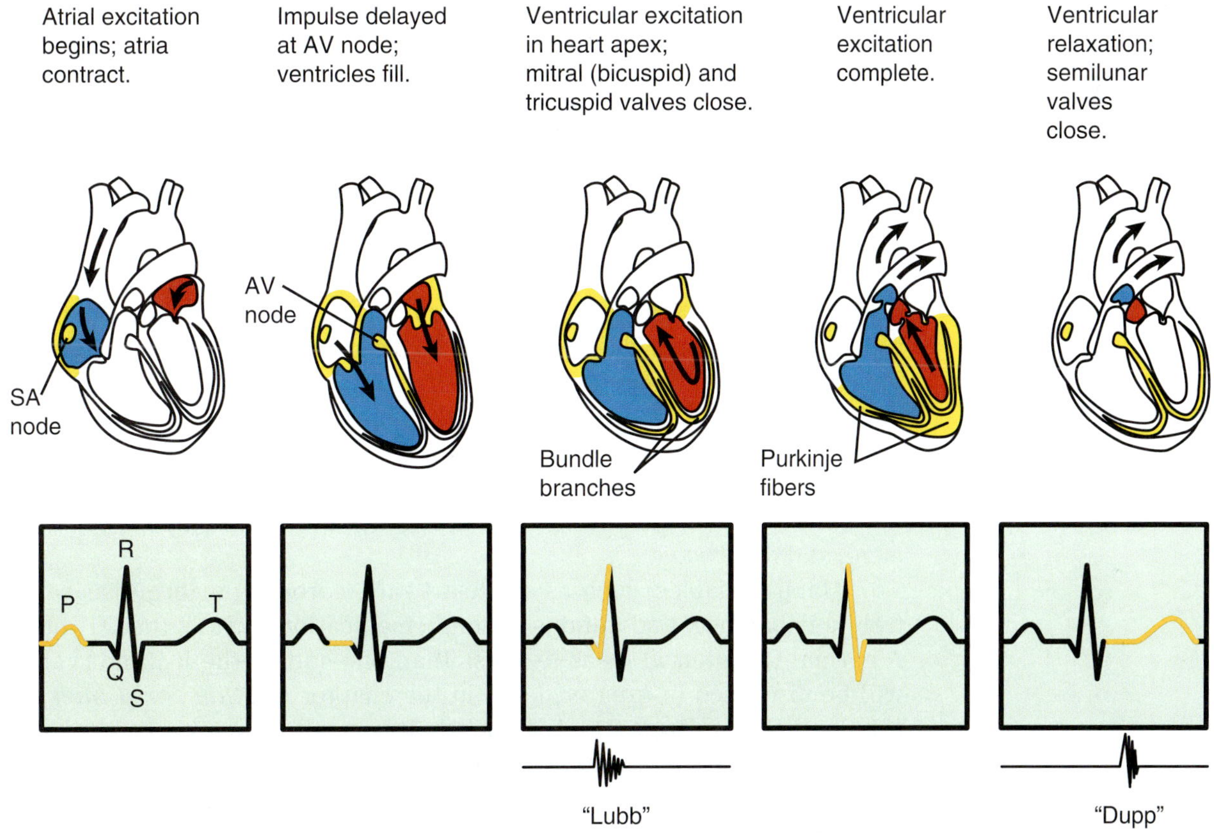

Figure 2-11 The ECG waveform and heart activity.

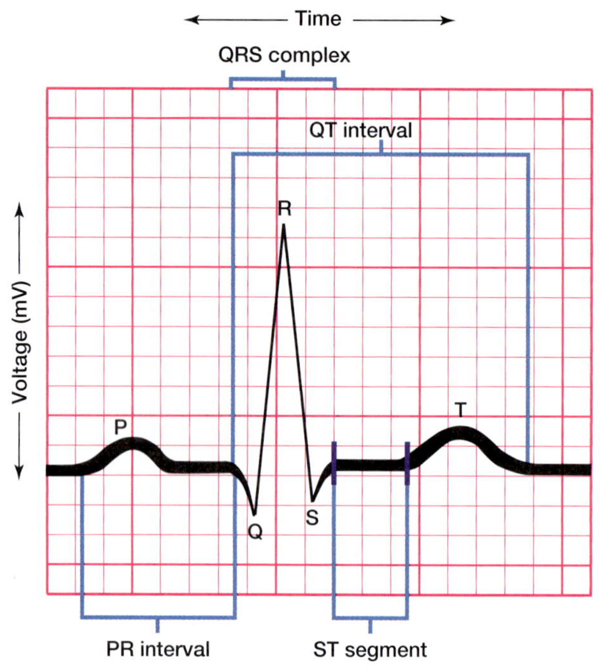

muscle. These changes are studied when interpreting an ECG. More information about interpreting an ECG is included in the chapter *Rhythm Strip Interpretation and Sinus Rhythms.*

The T wave represents ventricular repolarization. As repolarization occurs, the ventricular muscles relax. Normal T waves are in the same direction as the P wave. A normal QRS complex goes in both directions. A normal T wave on a 12-lead ECG tends to peak toward the end instead of the middle. Unlike the symmetrical mountain shape of the P wave, the T wave looks like a mountain with one sloping side.

The U wave follows the T wave. The U wave represents repolarization of the bundle of His and Purkinje fibers. It will be in the same direction as the T wave in most cases; it is more prominent when the heart rate is slow. The U wave does not always show up on the ECG; however, its presence can indicate an electrolyte imbalance.

The PR interval is measured from the beginning of the P wave to the beginning of the QRS complex. The normal length of time for the PR interval is 0.12 to 0.20 second. The PR interval on a normal ECG should be consistent. This time interval represents the time from initiation of the electrical impulse until the ventricles are stimulated by the impulse to start the contraction.

The QT interval is the time required for ventricular depolarization and repolarization to take place. It begins at the beginning of the QRS complex and ends at the end of the T wave. It includes the QRS complex, the ST segment, and the T wave.

Many variables, such as the heart rate, coronary artery disease, electrolyte imbalance, and antidysrhythmic medications, affect the QT interval. A normal QT interval measures less than one-half of the R-R interval. This will be discussed in greater detail in the chapter *Rhythm Strip Interpretation and Sinus Rhythms.* A longer-than-normal QT interval may indicate that the patient is at an increased risk for certain ventricular dysrhythmias and sudden cardiac death. When the heart rate exceeds 100 beats per minute (bpm), the QT interval is of little clinical significance due to the intervals closing as a result of the increased heart rate.

The R-R interval is the time from the start of a QRS complex in a rhythm to the start of the next adjacent QRS complex. R waves are readily seen on the ECG and are used to calculate the heart rate in a regular rhythm. We discuss this in the chapter *The Electrocardiograph.*

The junction of the QRS interval and the ST interval is the J point. This represents the end of the QRS complex and ventricular depolarization. The J point is important when measuring the length of the QRS complex and interpreting the ECG tracing. A normal QRS complex occurs within 0.06 to 0.1 second (Figure 2-11).

Checkpoint Questions (LO 2.6)

1. Which electrical event normally results in contraction of the heart?

____

____

2. Which wave represents the atrial depolarization? Ventricle repolarization?

____

____

3. What is ischemia?

____

____

Chapter Summary

Learning Outcomes	Summary	Pages
2.1 Explain how circulation occurs in relation to the ECG.	The heart action creates circulation; circulation provides nutrients and oxygen to the tissues and removes waste and carbon dioxide; the ECG waveform is a measurement of the heart's electrical activity.	29
2.2 Recall the structures of the heart including valves, chambers, and vessels.	The heart consists of four chambers (two atria and two ventricles) and four major valves (mitral [bicuspid], tricuspid, and two semilunar valves). The major vessels to and from the heart include the venae cavae, pulmonary artery and veins, and aorta.	29–34

Learning Outcomes	Summary	Pages
2.3 Differentiate among pulmonary, systemic, and coronary circulation.	Pulmonary circulation is the circulation from the right ventricle through the blood vessels of the lungs to the left atrium. Systemic circulation is the circulation from the left ventricle through the blood vessels of the body to the right atrium. Coronary circulation supplies blood within the heart through the coronary arteries and coronary sinus.	34–36
2.4 Explain the cardiac cycle, including the difference between systole and diastole.	The contraction and relaxation period of the heart together make up the cardiac cycle. Diastole is the relaxation phase of the cardiac cycle when blood fills the heart. Systole is the contraction phase of the cardiac cycle when blood leaves the heart.	36–37
2.5 Describe the parts and function of the heart and conduction system and how they relate to the ECG.	The conduction system of the heart includes the SA node, Bachmann's bundle, internodal pathways, AV node, AV bundle, bundle branches, and Purkinje fibers, which together create and maintain the electrical activity of the heart. The conducting tissue of the conduction system has qualities that control the beat of the heart, including automaticity, conductivity, contractility, and excitability. The conduction system of the heart creates the electrical activity and thus creates the ECG waveform.	38–41
2.6 Describe the heart activity that produces each part of the ECG waveform.	The ECG waveform includes the P wave, QRS complex, T wave, U wave (not always seen), PR interval, QT interval, and ST segment. The parts of the ECG waveform are created by the electrical activity of the heart, including atrial and ventricular depolarization and repolarization.	41–45

Chapter Review

Matching I

Match the valves, vessels, and chambers of the heart on the left with their definitions on the right. (LO 2.2)

_______ **1.** left ventricle
_______ **2.** tricuspid valve
_______ **3.** left atrium
_______ **4.** aorta
_______ **5.** pulmonary trunk
_______ **6.** right atrium
_______ **7.** right ventricle
_______ **8.** semilunar valve
_______ **9.** pulmonary vein
_______ **10.** mitral (bicuspid) valve

a. artery that transports blood to the entire body
b. type of valve located in the aorta and the pulmonary artery
c. atrioventricular valve between the left atrium and left ventricle
d. heart chamber that pumps blood to the body, known as the workhorse of the heart
e. heart chamber that receives blood from the lungs
f. chamber of the heart that receives blood from the body
g. chamber of the heart that pumps blood to the lungs
h. blood vessel that transports blood from the lungs to the left atrium
i. valve located between the right atrium and right ventricle
j. blood vessel that provides a pathway for deoxygenated blood to return to the lungs

Matching II

Match the conduction system parts and unique qualities of the heart on the left with their definitions on the right. (LO 2.5)

_______ **11.** excitability
_______ **12.** automaticity
_______ **13.** bundle branches
_______ **14.** SA node
_______ **15.** contractility
_______ **16.** depolarization
_______ **17.** AV node
_______ **18.** Purkinje fibers
_______ **19.** repolarization
_______ **20.** conductivity

a. delays the electrical conduction through the heart
b. ability of the heart to initiate an electrical impulse
c. branches off the bundle of His that conduct impulses to the left and right ventricles
d. ability of the heart cells to receive and transmit an electrical impulse
e. an electrical current that initiates the contraction of the heart muscle
f. ability of the heart muscle cells to shorten in response to an electrical stimulus
g. ability of the heart muscle cells to respond to an impulse or stimulus
h. heart muscle cells return to their resting electrical state and the heart muscle relaxes
i. initiates the heartbeat
j. distribute electrical impulses from cell to cell throughout the ventricles

Multiple Choice

Circle the correct answer.

21. The PR interval is usually (LO 2.6)
- **a.** 0.06 to 0.10 second.
- **b.** 0.12 to 0.20 second.
- **c.** greater than 0.20 second.
- **d.** less than 0.06 second.

22. What part of the ECG tracing represents the repolarization of the Purkinje fibers? (LO 2.6)
- **a.** T wave
- **b.** PR interval
- **c.** U wave
- **d.** P wave

23. What part of the ECG tracing represents the time from the start of the atrial activity to the start of ventricular activity? (LO 2.6)
- **a.** QRS complex
- **b.** J point
- **c.** QT interval
- **d.** PR interval

24. What part of the ECG tracing is measured from the end of the S wave to the beginning of the T wave and is normally on the isoelectric line? (LO 2.6)
- **a.** ST segment
- **b.** QT segment
- **c.** U wave
- **d.** QRS complex

25. What wave on the ECG tracing is not always seen and sometimes, when seen, can indicate an electrolyte imbalance? (LO 2.6)
- **a.** U wave
- **b.** P wave
- **c.** Q wave
- **d.** R wave

26. The heart's ability to create its own electrical impulse is known as (LO 2.5)
- **a.** conductivity.
- **b.** contractility.
- **c.** automaticity.
- **d.** excitability.

27. When stimulated, the sympathetic system of the body causes the heart rate to (LO 2.5)
- **a.** increase.
- **b.** decrease.
- **c.** remain the same.
- **d.** increase, then decrease.

28. Which vessel of the body contains the highest concentration of oxygen? (LO 2.2)

a. Aorta
b. Pulmonary artery
c. Superior vena cava
d. Inferior vena cava

29. The heart is contained inside a sac also known as the (LO 2.2)

a. endocardium.
b. pericardial sac.
c. myocardium sac.
d. fluid sac.

30. Which of the following would most likely decrease the heart rate? (LO 2.5)

a. Stress, exercise, and fever
b. High concentration of potassium in the blood
c. Decreased blood pressure
d. Increased blood pressure

Matching III

Match the circulation and cardiac cycle terms on the left to their definitions on the right.

_______ **31.** deoxygenated blood (LO 2.2)

_______ **32.** cardiac cycle (LO 2.4)

_______ **33.** systole (LO 2.4)

_______ **34.** coronary circulation (LO 2.3)

_______ **35.** systemic circulation (LO 2.3)

_______ **36.** oxygenated blood (LO 2.2)

_______ **37.** diastole (LO 2.4)

_______ **38.** pulmonary circulation (LO 2.3)

a. period from the beginning of one beat of the heart to the beginning of the next
b. circulation of blood through the heart and heart muscle
c. blood that has little or no oxygen
d. phase of the cardiac cycle when the heart is expanding and refilling; also known as the relaxation phase
e. blood having oxygen
f. circulation between the heart and the entire body, excluding the lungs
g. transportation of blood between the heart and lungs
h. contraction phase of the cardiac cycle, when the heart is pumping blood out to the body

Label the Parts

39. a.–r. Label the vessels, valves, chambers, and muscles of the heart by writing the letters on the lines provided. (LO 2.2)

a. Right atrium
b. Aorta
c. Right ventricle
d. Right pulmonary veins
e. Left atrium
f. Left ventricle
g. Superior vena cava
h. Pulmonary trunk
i. Aortic valve
j. Tricuspid valve
k. Right pulmonary artery
l. Mitral (bicuspid) valve
m. Inferior vena cava
n. Left pulmonary veins
o. Left pulmonary artery
p. Interventricular septum
q. Chordae tendineae
r. Papillary muscle

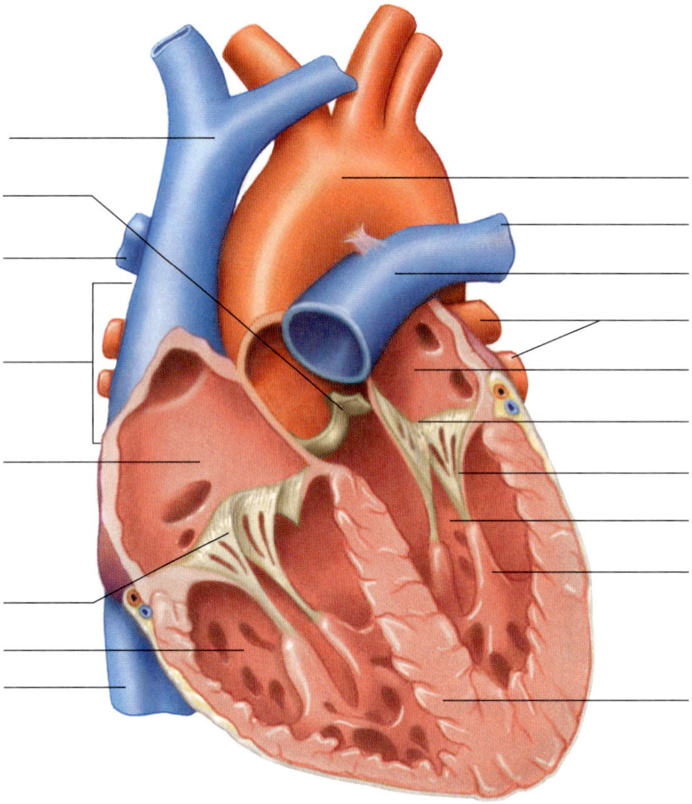

40. a.–m. Label the following diagram representing the flow of blood through the heart by writing the letters in the appropriate circles or boxes. (LO 2.3)

a. Superior and inferior venae cavae
b. Right atrium
c. Aorta
d. Right ventricle
e. Pulmonary semilunar valves
f. Left atrium
g. Mitral (bicuspid) valve
h. Pulmonary trunk
i. Pulmonary veins
j. Tricuspid valve
k. Left ventricle
l. Aortic semilunar valve
m. Pulmonary arteries

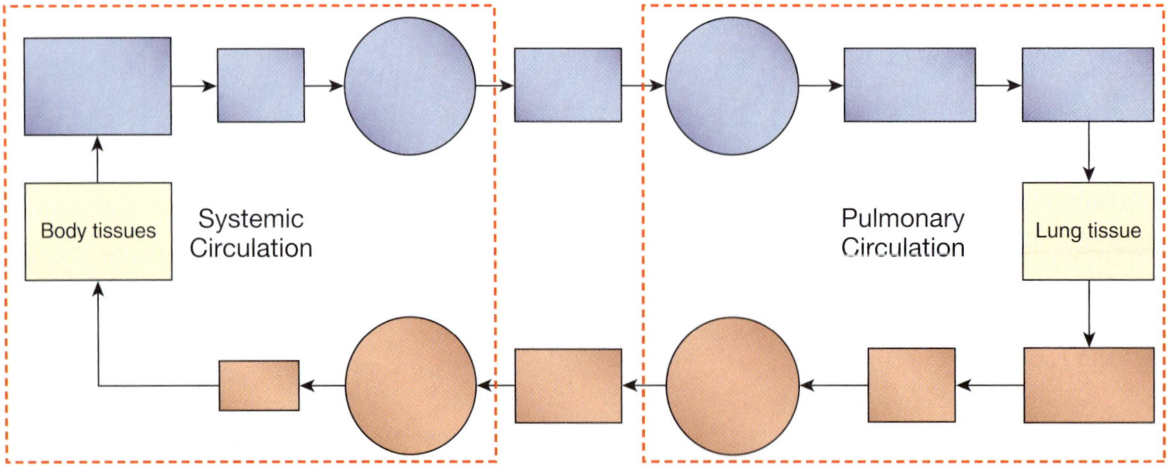

41. a.–j. Label the parts of the conduction system by writing the letters on the lines provided. (LO 2.5)

- **a.** Interventricular septum
- **b.** Left bundle branch
- **c.** Purkinje fibers
- **d.** AV node
- **e.** SA node
- **f.** AV bundle
- **g.** Right bundle branch
- **h.** Apex
- **i.** Bachmann's bundle
- **j.** Internodal pathways

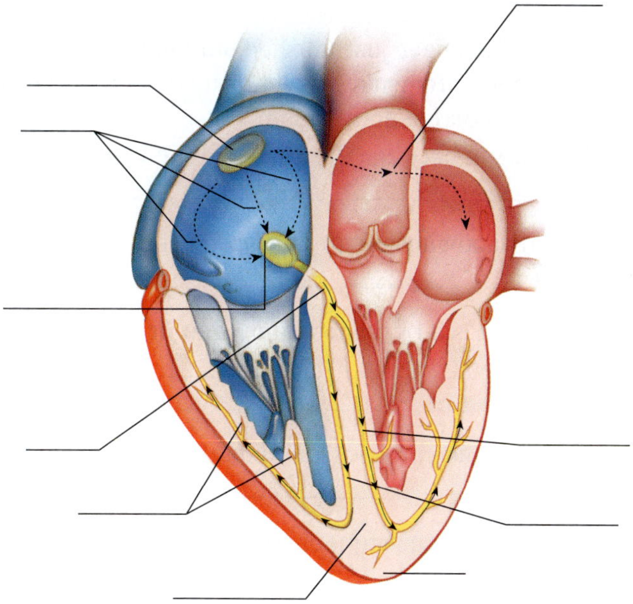

42. a.–i. Label the waves, complexes, intervals, and segments of the ECG waveform by writing the letters in the appropriate boxes. (LO 2.6)

- **a.** S wave
- **b.** R wave
- **c.** P wave
- **d.** T wave
- **e.** Q wave
- **f.** QT interval
- **g.** ST segment
- **h.** QRS complex
- **i.** PR interval

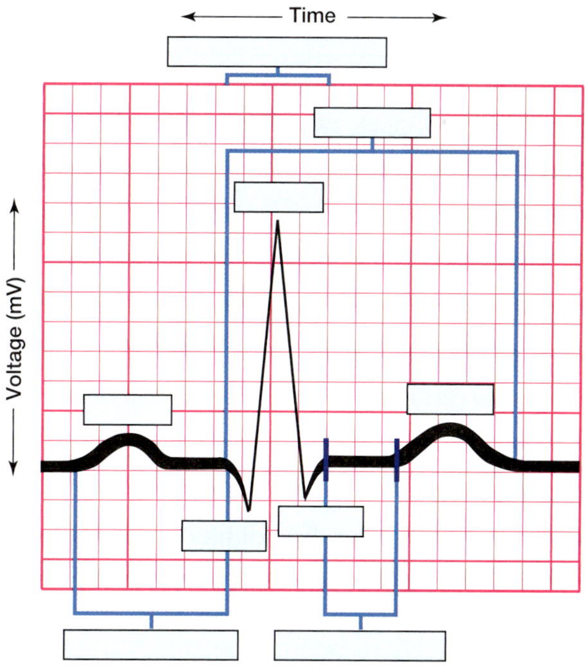

Right or Wrong?

43. You and a friend have just finished studying this chapter. Your friend makes the following statements. Are his or her statements correct or incorrect? If the statement is incorrect, write down what you would say to correct your friend.

a. "The valves between the atria and the ventricles are semilunar." (LO 2.2)

b. "The atria always pump the blood." (LO 2.2)

c. "The heart is a two-sided pump that produces pulmonary circulation and systemic circulation." (LO 2.4)

d. "The coronary arteries carry deoxygenated blood." (LO 2.2)

e. "The pulmonary artery carries oxygenated blood." (LO 2.2)

f. "The waves on the ECG waveform are positive when they go up from the baseline and negative when they go down from the baseline." (LO 2.6)

g. "If you are a man, you will have a faster heartbeat." (LO 2.5)

h. "The top chambers of the heart are the ventricles, and the bottom chambers of the heart are the atria." (LO 2.2)

i. "The right ventricle is sometimes known as the workhorse of the heart." (LO 2.2)

j. "The waves of the ECG waveform are P, Q, R, S, T, and sometimes a U." (LO 2.6)

Voyage Through the Heart

44. For each of the following statements, identify the vessel or structure you are in. Write only in the space provided. (LO 2.3)

a. Imagine that you are a drop of blood traveling through the heart. Returning from the brain, you are about ready to enter the heart. What vessel are you in?

b. After you enter the right atrium, you must go through a door to enter the right ventricle. What is the name of this door?

c. You have made it to the lungs successfully and are traveling back to the heart. What vessels are you in?

d. When you get to the heart, where will you be?____

e. You have finally made it to the last chamber of the heart. The left ventricle pumps you into the entire body. After entering the aorta, what are the very first vessels you will travel into?

Critical Thinking Application *What Should You Do?*

Read the following situations, and use your critical thinking skills to determine how you would handle each. Write your answer in detail in the space provided.

45. Sometimes when atrial cells other than the SA node trigger atrial contractions, atrial flutter or atrial fibrillation may occur. When these heart rhythms occur, the ventricles do not beat at the same rate as the atria. What part of the conduction system prevents the ventricles from beating as fast as the atria, and how does it occur? (LO 2.5)

46. You are working in the emergency department recording an ECG when the electricity goes out. There is a short period of darkness followed by a very loud noise. When you regain power, both your heart and the patient's are beating extremely fast. What part of the cardiovascular system is responsible for this increased heart rate? Should you continue recording the ECG now or later, and why? (LO 2.5)

connect® Now that you have completed the material in the chapter text, go to Connect and complete any chapter activities you have not yet done.

3 The Electrocardiograph

Learning Outcomes

3.1 Explain the three types of leads and how each is recorded.
3.2 Identify the functions of common ECG machines.
3.3 Explain how each ECG machine control is used.
3.4 Recognize common electrodes.
3.5 Describe the ECG graph paper.
3.6 Calculate heart rates using an ECG tracing.

Key Terms

artifact
augmented lead
bipolar lead
bradycardia
Einthoven triangle
electrodes
gain
hertz (Hz)
input
lead
limb lead
millimeter (mm)
millivolt (mV)
multichannel recorder
output display
precordial lead
serial ECG comparison
signal processing
speed control
tachycardia
unipolar lead

3.1 Producing the ECG Waveform

In this chapter, we discuss the electrocardiograph and the equipment needed to perform an ECG and record the ECG waveform. You will discover how the 12-lead system works and how to read the measurements on the ECG graph paper. Learning the equipment and lead system thoroughly and correctly will prepare you to record your first ECG.

The electrical impulse that is produced by the heart's conduction system is measured with the ECG machine. The ECG machine interprets the impulse and produces the ECG waveform. The waveform indicates how the heart is functioning electrically.

A single heart rhythm tracing views the heart from one angle. Because the heart is three-dimensional, it is necessary to view the electrical impulse from different sides to obtain a complete assessment of its electrical activity. A 12-lead ECG provides a complete picture, not of the heart's structure, but of its electrical activity. It records the heart's electrical activity from 12 different

TABLE 3-1 Lead Identification

Identifying Letters	Lead Wire Placement	Designated Color
RA	Right arm	White
LA	Left arm	Black
RL	Right leg	Green
LL	Left leg	Red
V1–V6	Chest leads	Brown*

*V1 to V6 lead colors may vary.

angles, as you might look at a sculpture from several different points of view. The 12 views provide information about how the electrical impulses travel through various parts of the heart.

A 12-lead ECG is actually recorded using only 10 lead wires, which, when attached to the chest and the limbs, provide the 12 different views for the 12-lead tracing. Six of these leads attach to the chest electrodes, and the other four attach to the electrodes on the arms and legs or shoulders and lower abdomen. **Electrodes** are small sensors placed on the skin to detect the electrical activity from the heart, and **leads** are covered wires that conduct the electrical impulse from the electrodes to the ECG machine. The lead wires are identified by color and are labeled with letters to match the correct position on the patient's body (Table 3-1 and Figure 3-1). The term *lead* also refers to the view on the ECG tracing as well as the physical location where the electrode is placed on the patient. For example, lead V2 refers to the labeled cable, the second intercostal space at the right sternal margin, and the V2 tracing on the printed ECG. Context is the clue to dealing with terms like these that have different meanings.

electrodes Small sensors placed on the skin to detect the electrical activity from the heart.

leads Covered wires that conduct the electrical impulse from the electrodes to the ECG machine.

The 10 lead wires produce 12 different circuits consisting of one or more wires from the electrodes to the electrocardiograph. The 12 circuits produce 12 different tracings or views of the heart. The combination of electrodes identifies each of the 12 leads. The 12 leads include three different lead types: three standard limb leads, three augmented leads, and six chest leads.

Troubleshooting

Check the Lead Wires

Each of the lead wires is coded by color and letter. If you place the lead wires incorrectly, the ECG will not record at all or it will record the waveforms improperly. Always check and double-check the lead wires before you begin the tracing. An ECG recording produced with the lead wires attached incorrectly is not acceptable and will have to be repeated.

If you attempt to record an ECG and no tracing appears, what should you do?

____

____

Figure 3-1 When attaching the lead wires, check carefully for the correct color- and letter-coded wire.

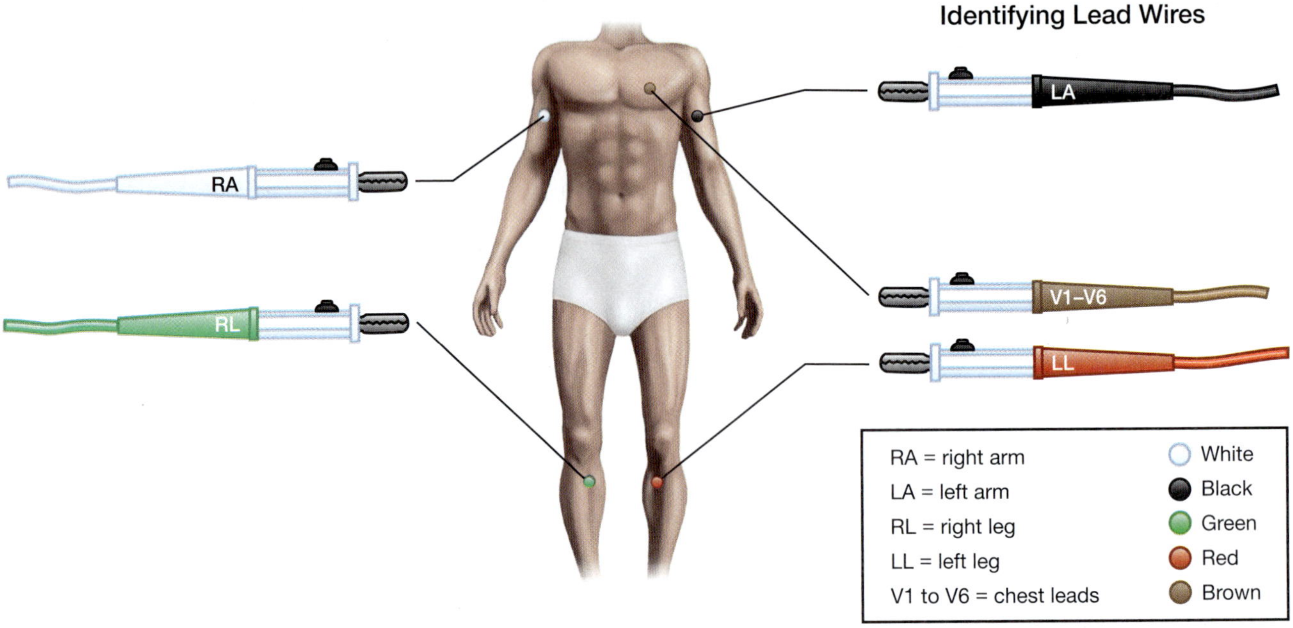

Einthoven triangle A triangle formed by three of the limb electrodes—the left arm, the right arm, and the left leg; it is used as a reference for the first six leads of the 12-lead ECG.

To understand the circuits for the first six leads (three standard and three augmented), we can use the Einthoven triangle. Einthoven is the scientist credited with developing the first ECG machine. The **Einthoven triangle** is formed by three of the limb electrodes: those on the right arm, the left arm, and the left leg. The right leg is used only as a ground or reference electrode (Figure 3-2).

The electrical current created by the heart is measured between the positive and negative electrodes placed on the body. If no current is flowing, the waveform is flat, or isoelectric. If the current moves toward the positive electrode, the ECG waveform will be positive (above the isoelectric baseline). If the current moves away from the positive electrode/toward the negative electrode, the ECG waveform will be negative (downward, below the isoelectric baseline).

Figure 3-2 *A.* The Einthoven triangle helps us understand the reference points for the 12-lead ECG. *B.* The black arrows indicate the direct and reverse views of each lead in this illustration.

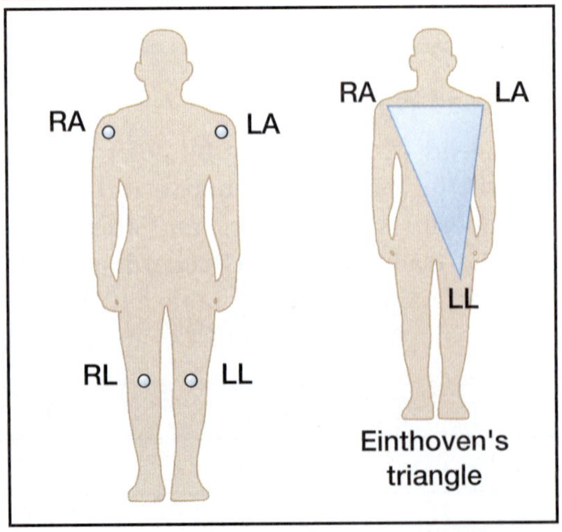

A.

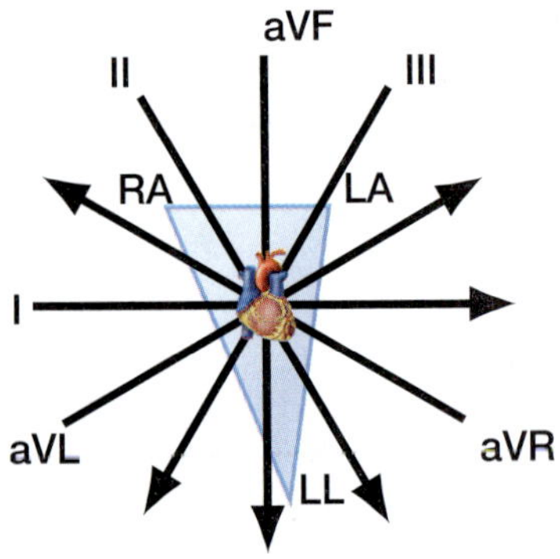

B.

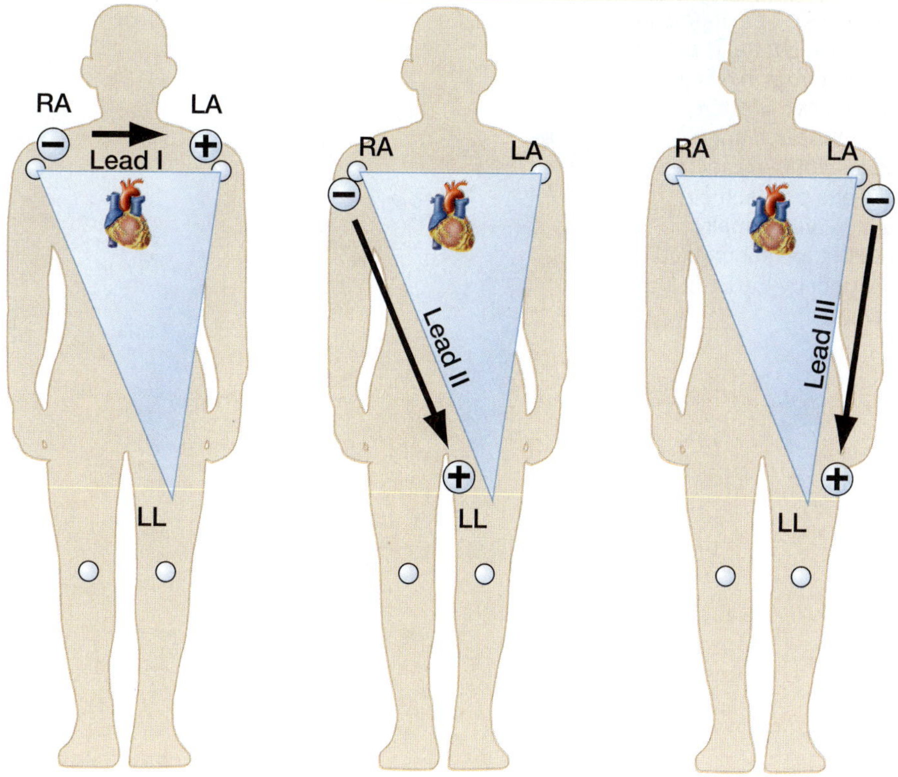

Figure 3-3 Leads I, II, and III are standard limb leads and are recorded from these reference points on the Einthoven triangle, producing a positive deflection.

Standard Limb Leads

limb lead Lead that attaches to the arms or legs.

bipolar lead A type of ECG lead that measures the flow of electrical current in both directions.

The first three leads are known as standard **limb leads.** They are also known as **bipolar leads** because they measure the flow of electrical current in both directions at the same time. These first three leads are called lead I, lead II, and lead III. In the Einthoven triangle, leads I, II, and III are positioned at the same distance from the heart's electrical activity. Lead I records the tracing from the right arm (−) to the left arm (+); lead II records the tracing from the right arm (−) to the left leg (+); and lead III records the electrical activity from the left arm (−) to the left leg (+) (Figure 3-3). All three leads produce positive deflections.

Augmented Leads

augmented lead Normally small ECG lead tracings that are increased in size by the ECG machine in order to be interpreted.

unipolar lead A type of ECG lead that measures the flow of electrical current in one direction only.

The next three leads are known as **augmented leads.** The voltage is very low in the augmented leads because of the angle of measurement; therefore, the ECG waveform will be very small. The ECG machine must increase (augment) the size of the waveforms for these leads to be readable on the ECG tracing. They are also known as **unipolar leads** because they measure toward one electrode on the body. They are called aVR, aVL, and aVF. The R, L, and F refer to the direction the lead is measuring: R is right arm, L is left arm, and F is foot (left leg/foot) (Figure 3-4). Lead aVR records electrical activity from the heart to the right arm. Lead aVL records electrical activity from the heart to the left arm. Lead aVF records electrical activity from the heart to the left leg.

Lead aVR is usually a negative deflection. If it does not produce a negative deflection, you might have the electrodes or lead wires placed incorrectly. To ensure accuracy of electrode and lead wire placement, check the aVR tracing produced when recording the 12-lead ECG; if it is not a negative deflection, verify the placement of the electrodes and lead wires to correct it.

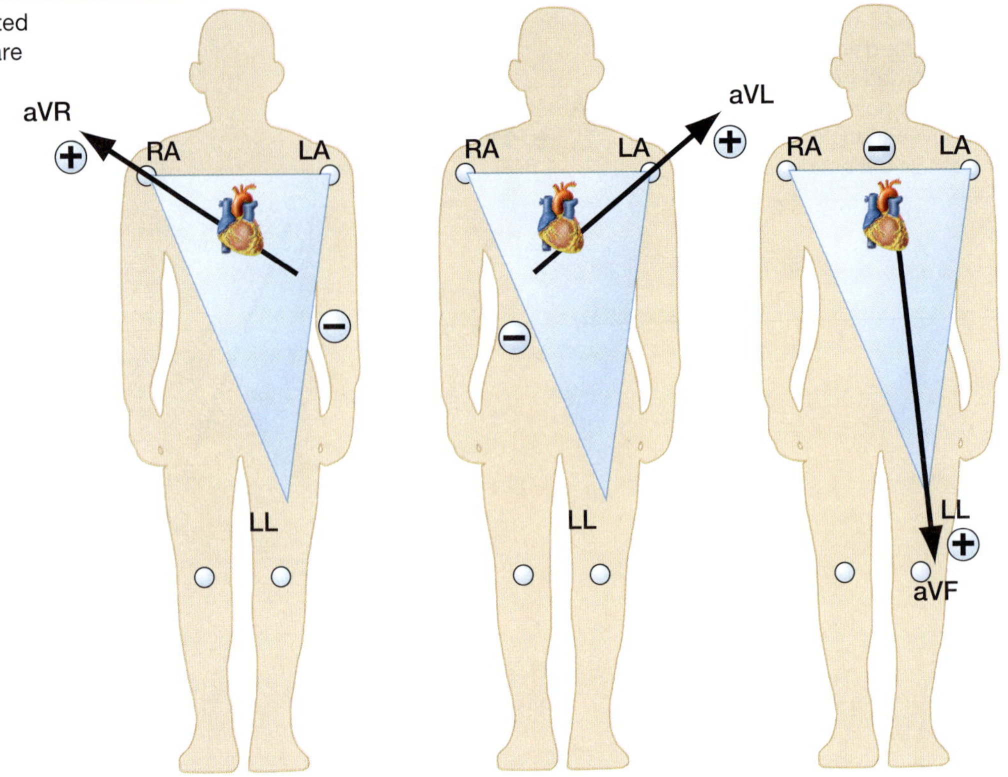

Figure 3-4 The augmented leads aVR, aVL, and aVF are recorded from midway between two points on the Einthoven triangle. Because of the lead reference points, their tracings are normally small but are augmented (enlarged) by the ECG machine.

Figure 3-5 Front and cross-sectional views of chest lead placement.

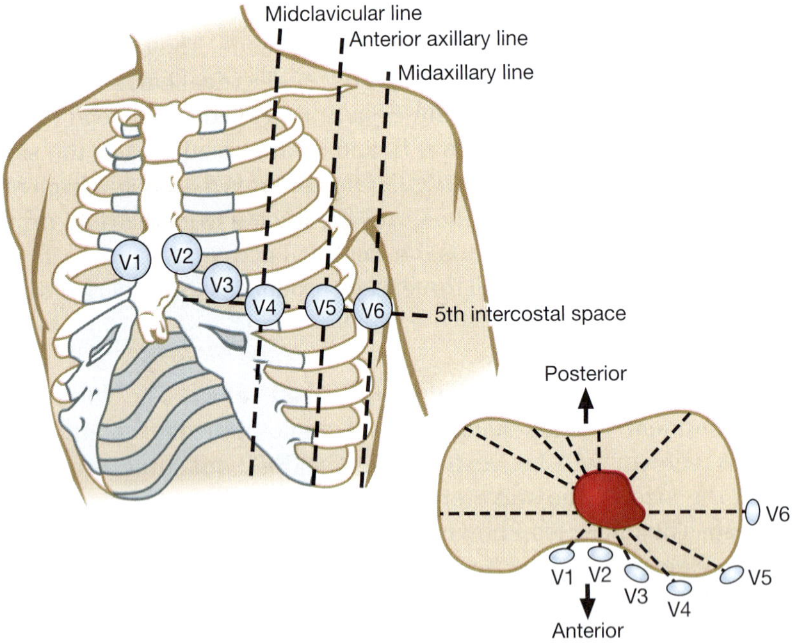

V1—Fourth intercostal space, right sternal border
V2—Fourth intercostal space, left sternal border
V3—Halfway between V2 and V4
V4—Fifth intercostal space at the midclavicular line
V5—On the same horizontal level with V4, at the anterior axillary line
V6—On the same horizontal level with V4 and V5, at the midaxillary line

Chest Leads

precordial lead A type of lead placed on the chest in front of the heart; known as a V lead.

The last six leads are the chest leads. Also known as **precordial leads,** these leads are located in front of (*pre*) the heart (*cor*). The chest leads are unipolar because they are measured in one direction only. They are placed on specific sites on the chest. Each of the chest leads begins with the letter V and is numbered from V1 to V6. These leads record activity between six points on the chest and within the heart. You can view the placements in Figure 3-5. The procedure for placing electrodes is discussed in the chapter *Performing an ECG.*

The 12-lead ECG tracings can be interpreted separately or in conjunction with each other. When an ECG is being recorded, each of the 12 leads must be identified on the tracing. Older machines required that the ECG tracing strip be coded with identifying marks manually. Most machines in use today identify each lead tracing automatically. Each lead tracing looks slightly different and presents a different picture of the heart. This allows the physician to determine damage or problems in specific areas of the heart (Figure 3-6).

Checkpoint Questions (LO 3.1)

1. What test is done to view the heart at 12 different angles?

___

___

2. How many lead wires are used to obtain a 12-lead ECG tracing?

___

___

3. Name the three augmented leads.

___

___

3.2 ECG Machines

Machines used today to measure an ECG weigh less than 10 pounds; some are as small as a credit card. All ECG machines vary slightly, but most have the same basic parts. The typical ECG machine sits on a small cart that can be pushed to the person requiring the ECG. You should become familiar with the type of machine you will be using by reading the manufacturer's instructions.

The **multichannel recorder** is a three-channel ECG machine that monitors all 12 leads but records three leads at once and switches leads automatically, recording each of the four sets of three leads (Figure 3-7). It produces a full page showing all 12 lead tracings. The actual recording time for this machine is approximately 10 seconds. Some multichannel ECG machines can record up to six lead tracings at one time. In most cases, electronic copies of 12-lead tracings and interpretations are stored and transmitted electronically via telecommunications.

multichannel recorder An ECG machine that monitors all 12 leads but records three leads at a time and switches automatically, recording each of the four sets of three leads.

input Data entered into an ECG machine, usually through electrodes on the skin surface.

signal processing The process within the ECG machine that amplifies the electrical impulse and converts it to a mechanical action that appears as a waveform on the output display.

Functions

The electrocardiograph has three basic functions: input, signal processing, and output display. Sensors in the ECG machine serve as receiving devices for the electrical activity of the heart. Electrodes placed on the patient's skin direct the impulses to the ECG instrument, providing the **input** for the ECG machine.

Signal processing occurs inside the ECG machine. It amplifies the electrical impulse and converts it into a form that can be shown on the display.

Figure 3-6 A 12-lead ECG produced on a multichannel ECG machine. Each lead is identified on the printout. Note that each lead tracing (I, II, III, aVR, aVL, aVF, and V1 to V6) looks different.

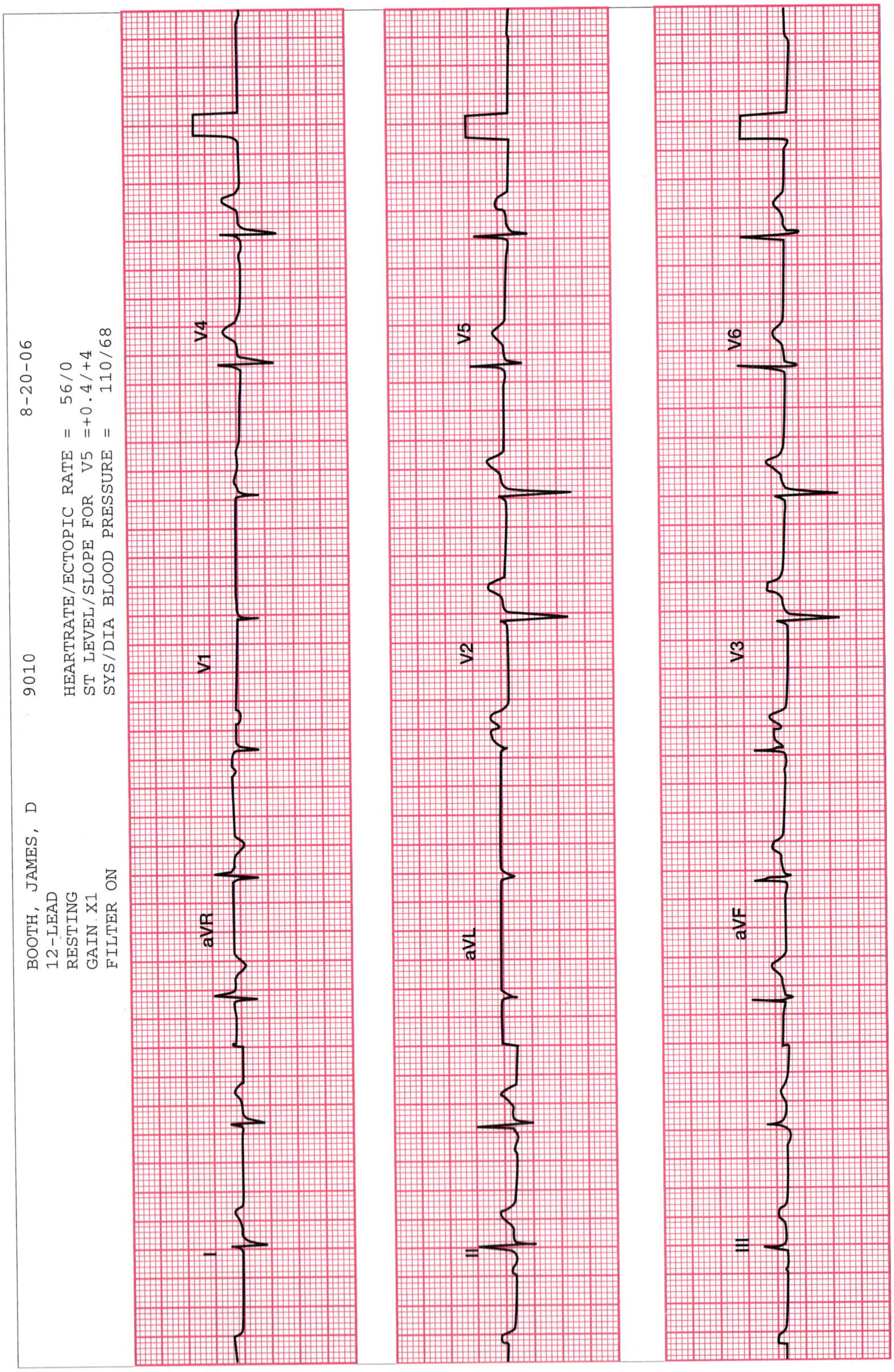

Figure 3-7 A multichannel ECG machine records three, four, or six leads at a time on a large sheet of ECG graph paper.

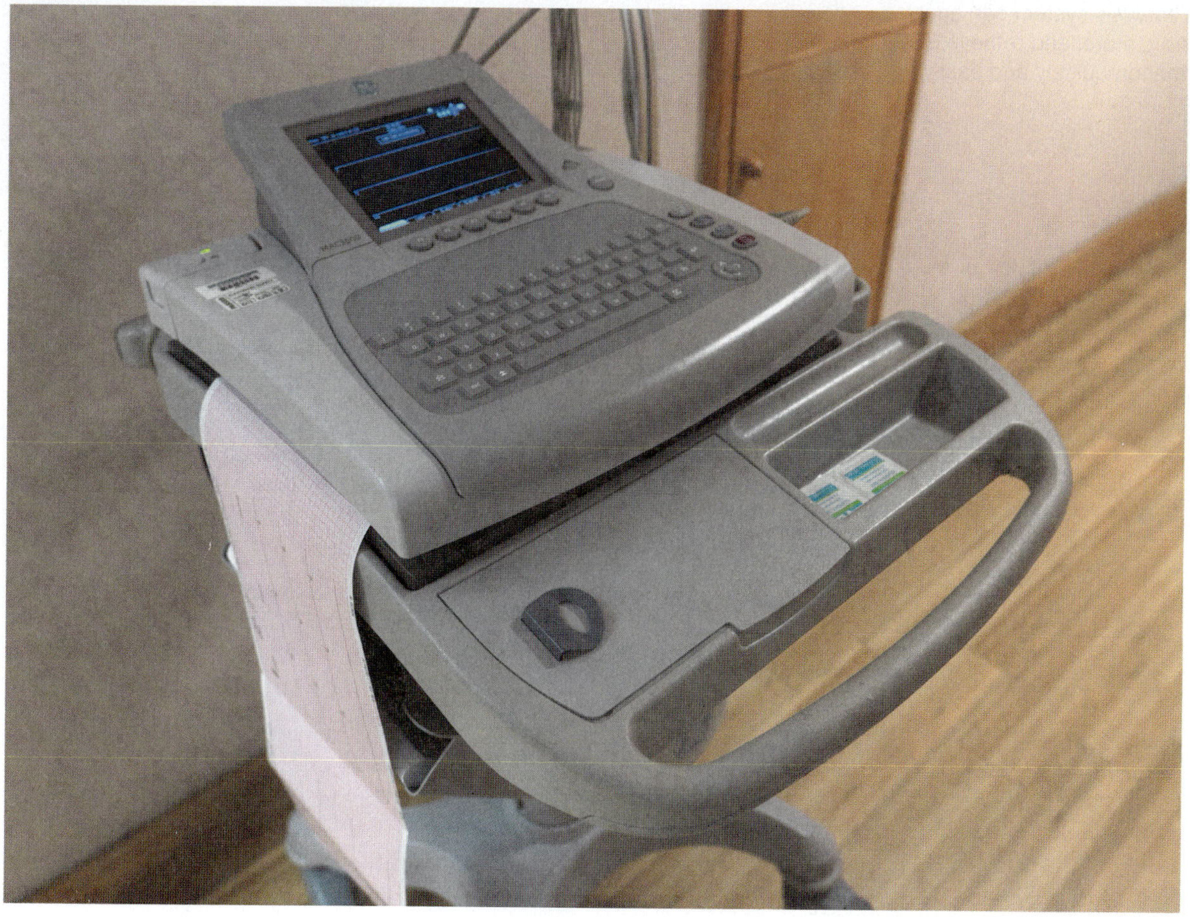

A complex collection of transistors, resistors, and circuitry amplifies and prepares the signal for transfer to the output display.

output display The part of the ECG machine that displays the tracing for the electrical activity of the heart, usually in electronic or a printed form on a 12-lead ECG machine.

The **output display** is the result of the ECG tracing. The output is typically on a computer or other electronic screen. The output can also appear on an LED screen, which is frequently found on a cardiac monitor or a defibrillator.

ECG machines perform other functions as well, including computerized measurement and analysis, storage, and communication. Computerized measurement and analysis provide a machine interpretation of the ECG tracing. This interpretation is not meant to replace the physician's interpretation. However, the computer interpretation can distinguish between a normal and abnormal recording quickly and may provide a second opinion. All computerized interpretations should be manually confirmed by a physician.

Some ECG machines store ECG results, which then can be recalled and printed later. ECG machines are also equipped to transmit results over the telephone, fax, or Internet.

Advancing Technologies

Technology has advanced all around us. Advances have impacted the fields of cardiology and electrocardiology. ECG machines have undergone many advances over the past 30 years. They have gone from single-channel to 3-lead machines, to our current 12-lead machines and wireless technology (Figure 3-8). The 12-lead ECG machines 30 years ago seem primitive compared to modern equipment.

Figure 3-8 The MAC 5500 resting ECG analysis system can analyze, transmit, store, and retrieve ECG information quickly and easily.

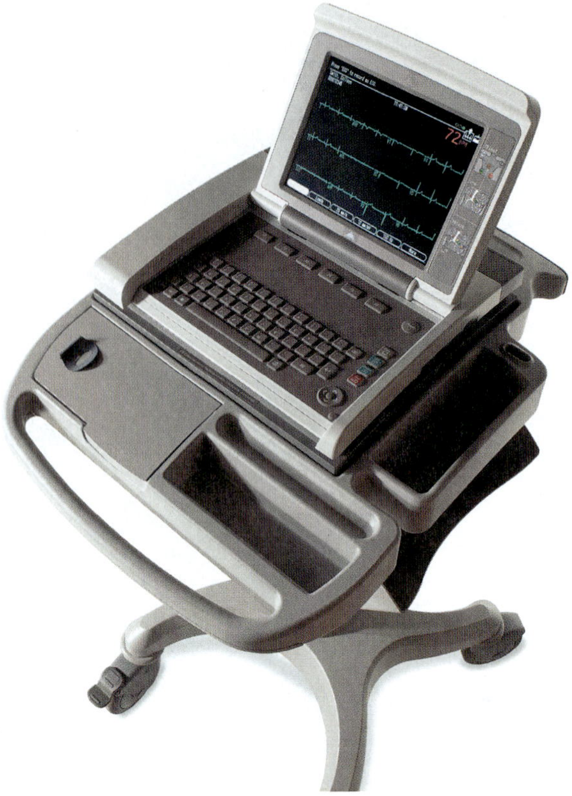

One of the more recent advances in medicine is the area of digital technology. Many ECG machines are now able to not only acquire and store the tracings but also transmit a digital image of the 12-lead for storage in a central location. This is particularly beneficial when patients are seen in hospitals other than the one where the 12-lead ECG was obtained. Access to this vital information is much more readily available than at any time in the past.

One such digital storage system is the MUSE Cardiology Information System developed by GE Healthcare (Figure 3-9). This system is able to integrate, manage, and streamline the flow of cardiac information, such as resting 12-lead ECG, exercise stress ECG, and Holter devices. This system provides faster data delivery, distribution of information, and analysis. The MUSE digital storage system allows the provider easy access to patient information. Devices like this make the healthcare system more efficient due to their ability to communicate between the hospital information system, electronic health records, and the ECG devices themselves.

serial ECG comparison Multiple and frequent ECG tracings recorded at intervals based on the patient's condition and compared to monitor changes.

This system allows you to retrieve the current ECG and older ECGs for **serial ECG comparison.** The retrieved 12-lead on the computer screen looks just like the printed record (Figure 3-9). The screen has a simple toolbar to make accessing common features quick and clear. These features help with viewing and printing the ECG. The ability to view serial ECGs is important for detecting subtle changes that may indicate myocardial abnormalities (such as ischemia, injury, or infarction).

Systems such as the MUSE support the progressive paperless electronic health record initiative. Computer advances in medicine improve efficiency, billing accuracy, and time from test to diagnosis, and they reduce personnel demands. Ultimately, the use of MUSE and electronic health records improves

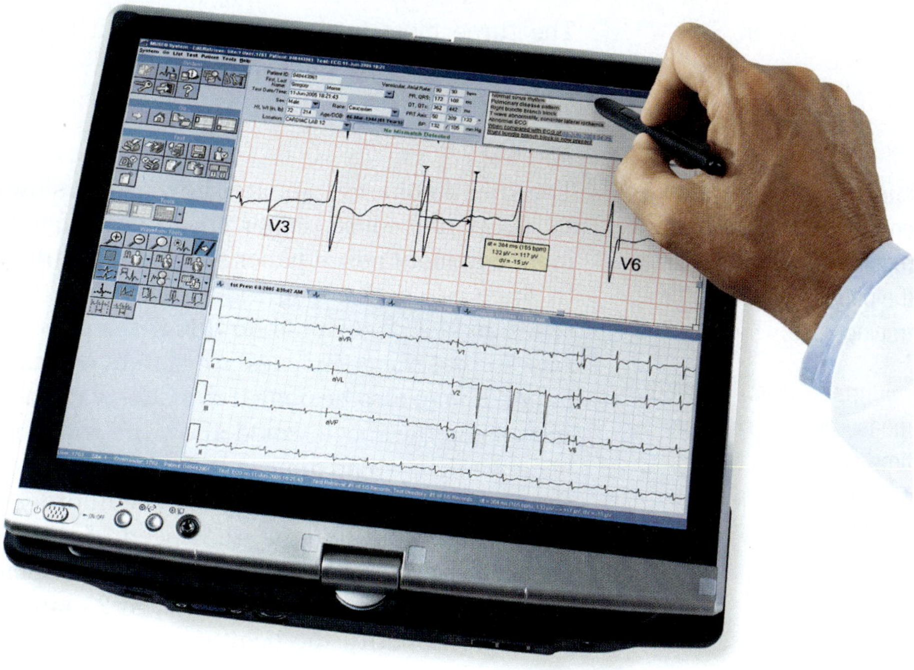

Figure 3-9 The electronically stored ECG retrieved by the MUSE Cardiology Information System by GE Healthcare looks just like the printed record.

the speed and quality of medical care, where quick access to critical cardiac information is essential to patient care. Every second can count in reducing the long-term damage that can result from heart trauma. As technology advances, it is essential to stay current with any equipment you will be using.

Law & Ethics

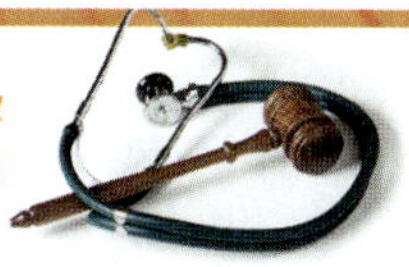

Protecting ECG Records

Two primary purposes of HIPAA are to improve the efficiency and effectiveness of healthcare delivery and protect and enhance the rights of patients by controlling the inappropriate use or disclosure of patient information. Transmitting, retrieving, and storing the ECG tracing provide for quick access and improved delivery of care to patients. The electronic ECG recording is part of the patient record and just like the rest of the electronic health record must be password protected and handled confidentially.

Checkpoint Questions (LO 3.2)

1. A multichannel ECG monitors all 12 leads but usually records how many leads at one time?

____

____

2. What are the three basic functions of an ECG?

____

____

3.3 ECG Controls

The three most important controls on the electrocardiograph include the speed, gain, and artifact filter.

Speed

speed control A control on the ECG machine that regulates how fast or slow the paper runs during the tracing.

millimeter (mm) A unit of measurement to indicate time on the ECG tracing. Time is measured on the horizontal axis.

The **speed control** regulates how fast or slow the paper or data runs during the ECG procedure. Paper speed is measured in **millimeters (mm).** The most commonly used paper speed is 25 millimeters per second (25 mm/sec). In some cases, you may want to increase the speed to 50 mm/sec, which is twice as fast. You would do this if the patient has an unusually rapid heart rate so that the complexes are spread over a greater distance on the graph paper. It may also be done if the ECG waveform parts are too close together. Increasing the speed would allow the waveform to be analyzed more easily because they would appear wider. Some ECG machines allow you to reduce the speed to 5 mm/sec or 10 mm/sec in order to analyze the ECG recording more carefully. Changing the speed of the recorder is usually done at the request or preference of the physician. Remember, if you change the speed to anything other than the standard 25 mm/sec, you must note this on the tracing and notify the healthcare provider who will interpret the tracing, if possible.

Troubleshooting

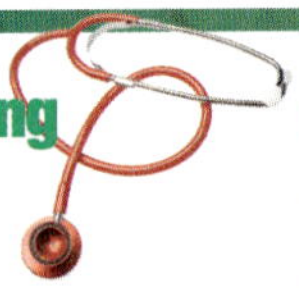

Changing the ECG Tracing Speed

When the patient's heart rate is very fast, it is difficult to read the ECG tracing because the waveform parts are close together. Set the speed control at 50 mm/sec to widen the complexes so the ECG can be interpreted more easily. *Circle or note the speed setting and, when possible, verbally tell the healthcare provider who will be interpreting the results about the change in speed.* This notification is essential to avoid misinterpretation of the ECG; for example, a normal ECG set to double speed can sometimes look like an abnormal rhythm known as a heart block.

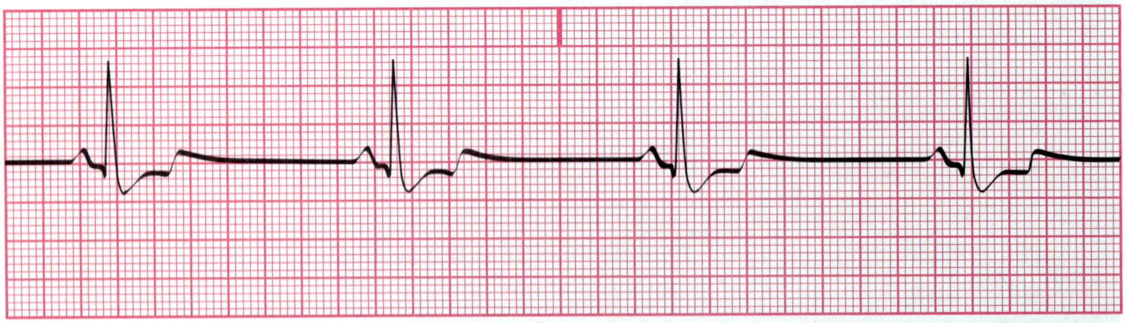

This ECG tracing was produced at a speed of 50 mm/sec. What should you do?

____

____

gain A control on the ECG machine that increases or decreases the size of the deflections on the ECG tracing.

millivolt (mV) A unit of measurement to indicate voltage on the ECG tracing. Voltage is measured on the vertical axis.

Gain

The **gain** control regulates the output or height of the ECG waveform. Voltage on an ECG tracing is measured in **millivolts (mV).** The normal setting is 10 mm/mV (millivolts are the units of measurement used to indicate voltage on the ECG tracing). By setting the gain to 20 mm/mV, you can double the size; by setting the gain to 5 mm/mV, you reduce the size by half. Some machines will let you change the gain, depending on which lead you are tracing. Because the tracing size can vary between leads, setting the gain will allow the ECG waveform to be readable for any lead tracing. If you change the gain setting during any lead tracing, you must record this change on the ECG report. Digital machines standardize the wave output height automatically. Calibration marks are seen at either the beginning or the end of a 12-lead ECG tracing (Figure 3-10). These open-ended rectangular shapes are used as a reference to compare with the cardiac complexes to determine the amount of electricity (voltage) being generated in the atria and ventricles of the heart during each cardiac complex. This is similar to an old-fashioned map on which a certain measurement, such as 1 inch, is equal to a certain number of miles.

Figure 3-10 The calibration mark on the ECG tracing must be verified to ensure accuracy. The first rectangular waveform on the ECG tracing is indicating the standardization of the machine for the recorded ECG.

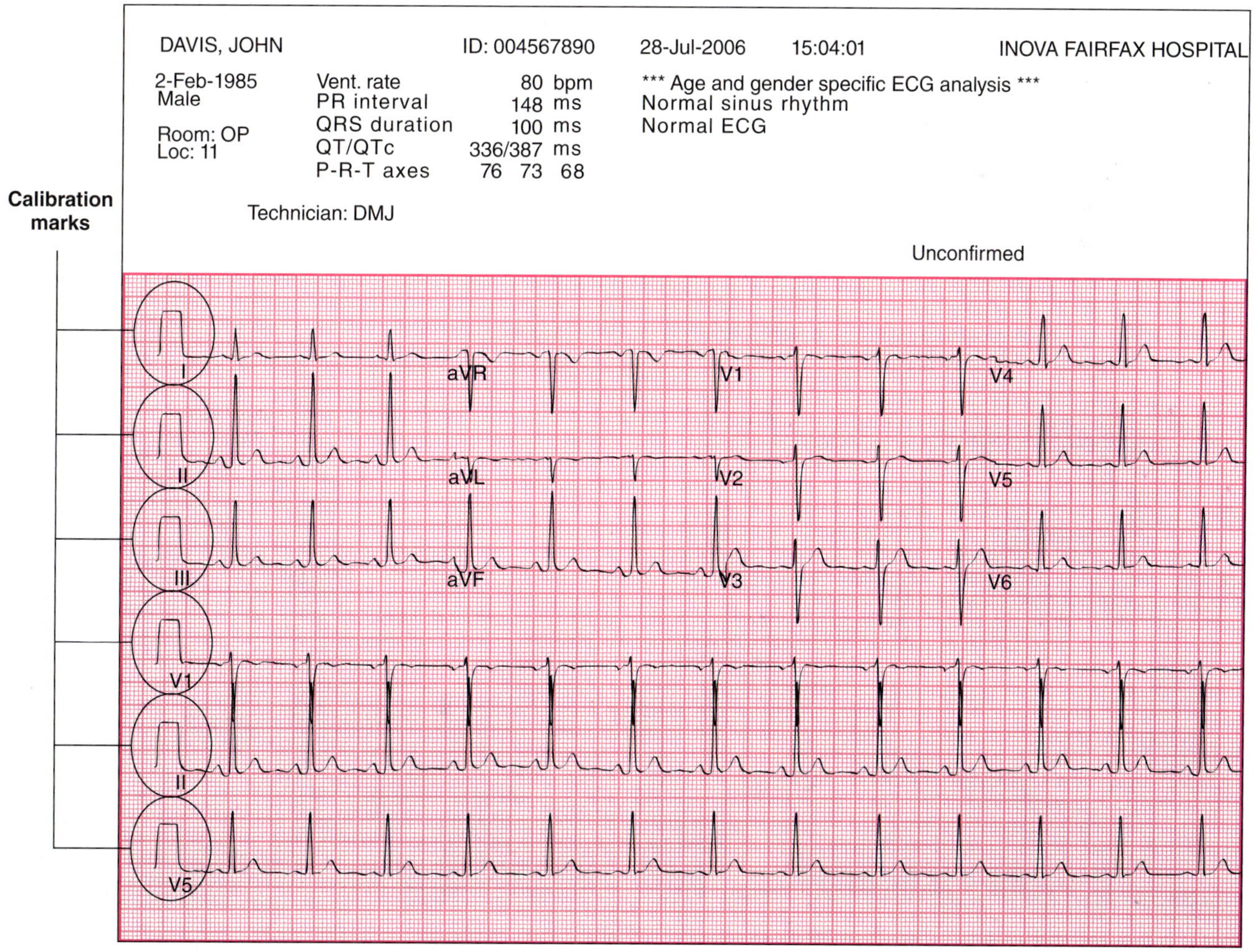

Patient Education & Communication

Know Your ECG Machine

Become familiar with the ECG machine you will be using before performing an ECG. Your uncertainty could cause anxiety or nervousness in the patient who is having the ECG performed.

Artifact Filter

hertz (Hz) A unit of frequency that indicates cycles or events per second.

artifact Unwanted marks on the ECG tracing caused by activity other than the heart's electrical activity.

The ECG machine you are using may have an artifact filter selection. The usual setting is between 40 and 150 **hertz (Hz)** (a unit of frequency that indicates cycles or events per second). Forty Hz is normally used to reduce **artifact** or abnormal marks on the ECG tracing due to muscle tremor and slight patient movement. We discuss artifact in more detail in the chapter *Performing an ECG*. Remember that the artifact filter will correct only the printed output. If the computer performs interpretation, it will interpret the results from the actual nonfiltered information from the patient, not what is printed or viewed on the screen. This could cause inaccurate interpretation by the computer, which is why it is essential that a physician as well as the computer interprets all ECGs. Some filtering of artifact will prohibit the view of pacemaker spikes. Pacemaker spikes are unique markings on an ECG that indicate a patient has an artificial pacemaker. It is important to know how to modify the filter to allow for pacemaker spikes to be seen.

LCD Display

There are various other controls on the ECG machine that the user can set or use to enter information. For example, the user can enter data about the patient to be included on the printout along with the ECG results. These data can also be entered electronically using a scanner on the patient's identification band (Figure 3-11). This information is entered into the LCD (liquid

Figure 3-11 *A.* The patient data can be entered and the ECG tracing viewed on the LCD display. *B.* Some machines include a bar code scanner to identify the patient and to automatically enter the patient information onto the tracing.

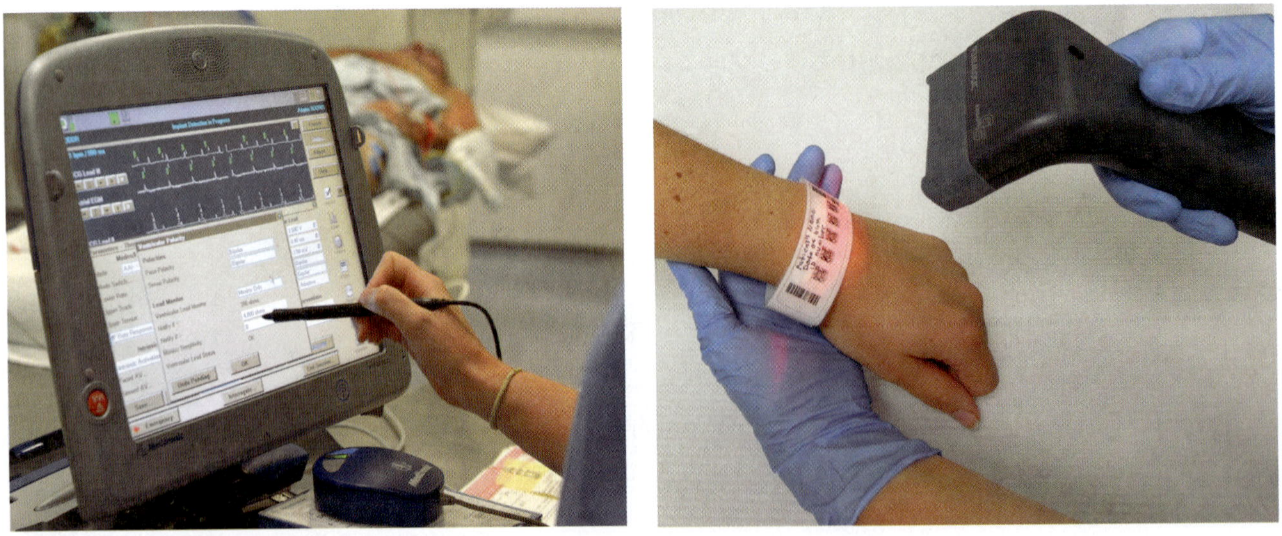

A. *B.*

crystal diode) display. This is the area of the machine where you can view the patient information you have entered. It is also where information from the ECG's computer is displayed. For example, some machines can detect if the arm leads or chest leads are reversed and display this information in the LCD panel.

Heart Rate Limits

If the ECG machine has computer interpretation, the user may be able to set the heart rate limits. In other words, the operator can set the heart rate that the machine will interpret as too slow—**bradycardia**—or too fast—**tachycardia.** If the heart rate is above or below the number set, the machine will indicate this by sounding an alarm and marking on the tracing.

bradycardia A slow heart rate, usually less than 60 beats per minute.

tachycardia A fast heart rate, usually greater than 100 beats per minute.

Lead Selector

Most 12-lead ECG machines record each of the leads automatically. However, a lead selector can be used to run each lead individually in case one or more leads need to be repeated.

Troubleshooting

Changing the Gain

When the deflections on the ECG tracing are too short or too tall, you will need to correct the gain. Be certain the machine is standardized correctly, and then adjust the gain control if necessary.

If you are recording an ECG and the deflections or spikes of the tracing are not large enough, what should you do?

____

____

Checkpoint Questions (LO 3.3)

1. What are some reasons that you may change the speed of the ECG tracing?

____

____

2. Name the major controls of the ECG machine.

____

____

3.4 Electrodes

Electrodes are sensors that are placed on a person's skin to pick up the electrical activity of the heart and conduct it to the ECG machine. Electrodes come in a variety of types and are disposable.

Figure 3-12 *A.* Disposable electrodes come in various shapes and sizes. Electrolyte gel or paste is not necessary because it is already contained on these electrodes. *B.* Standard resting tab electrodes are inexpensive, disposable, and easy to use for a routine ECG.

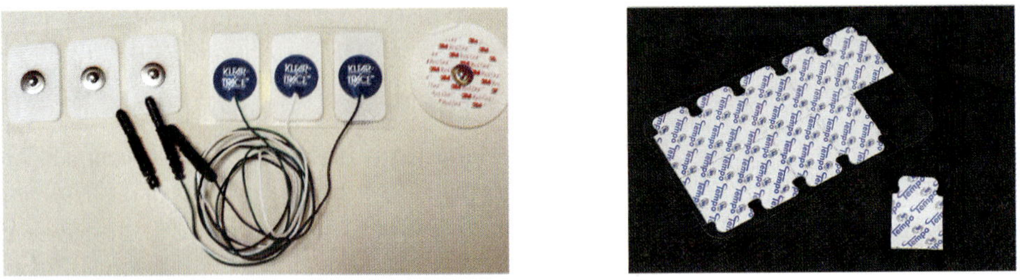

A. *B.*

Disposable electrodes are used because they reduce the possibility of cross-contamination and can be simply removed and discarded for easier cleanup (Figure 3-12). The self-adhesive types stick easily to the patient's body. The gel is already applied so the electrodes will properly conduct the electrical impulses.

Each disposable electrode is normally used for only one ECG. The only exception occurs when a second ECG is performed on the same patient immediately after the first and the electrodes have not been disturbed. For example, if you are transferring a patient from an outpatient facility to a hospital, you should leave the electrodes in place for the emergency medical personnel. They will be recording one or more ECGs on the way to the hospital. However, if the electrodes stay on the patient's skin any longer than two sequential readings, the gel will dry out, resulting in inaccurate ECG tracings.

For hospitalized patients, longer-lasting silver electrodes are available. These electrodes are used for patients who require multiple and frequent ECGs (serial ECGs). When serial ECGs are required, it is important to ensure the same lead placement for each. A slight change often causes a change in the tracing. The silver electrodes are kept on the patient and checked daily.

No matter what type of electrodes are used, they must be handled and stored correctly. If a package contains more electrodes than needed, the remaining electrodes must be kept in a sealed plastic bag so the gel will not dry out. Always check the expiration date on the package before use. Make sure the electrode gel has not dried out on any electrode. Even new electrodes should be checked before placement. Additionally, you should never mix two different types of electrodes. This could cause an inaccurate tracing, which could result in incorrect treatment for the patient.

Checkpoint Question (LO 3.4)

1. Which type of electrode is used when monitoring a patient who will be having serial ECGs done?

____

____

3.5 ECG Graph Paper

The ECG machine records an image of the heart's electrical activity onto a graph on the screen or paper. This image is the ECG waveform, or a series of waves and complexes recorded from the activity in the heart. The graph provides increments to measure the electrical activity produced on the tracing. Understanding the ECG graph intervals and what they represent is essential to interpreting the ECG.

The two most commonly used types of graph paper are standard grid and dot matrix (Figure 3-13). Both are heat- and pressure-sensitive. Because the paper is pressure-sensitive, you should handle it carefully to avoid marking it. Marks on the paper could make the tracing difficult to read or cause the tracing to be read inaccurately. In addition, certain substances, such as alcohol, plastic, sunlight, and x-ray film, can erase the tracing. Once the ECG is completed, it should be stored away from these substances. Some companies offer recording paper that requires no special handling or storage. This paper guarantees that the tracing will last for up to 50 years.

Dot matrix paper has some advantages over standard grid paper. Dot matrix reports require less ink, are easier to read, and produce sharper photocopies, yet dot matrix paper is much less commonly used. One advantage of standard grid paper is that it is slightly less expensive (Figure 3-14).

Troubleshooting

Handle the ECG Report with Care

Handle and store the ECG report with care. It can be damaged easily; and, if damaged, it cannot be interpreted by the physician.

The physician places a stack of charts on top of an ECG report you just placed on his desk. What should you do?

____

____

Figure 3-13 Choose the right size and type of graph paper for the ECG machine you will be using.

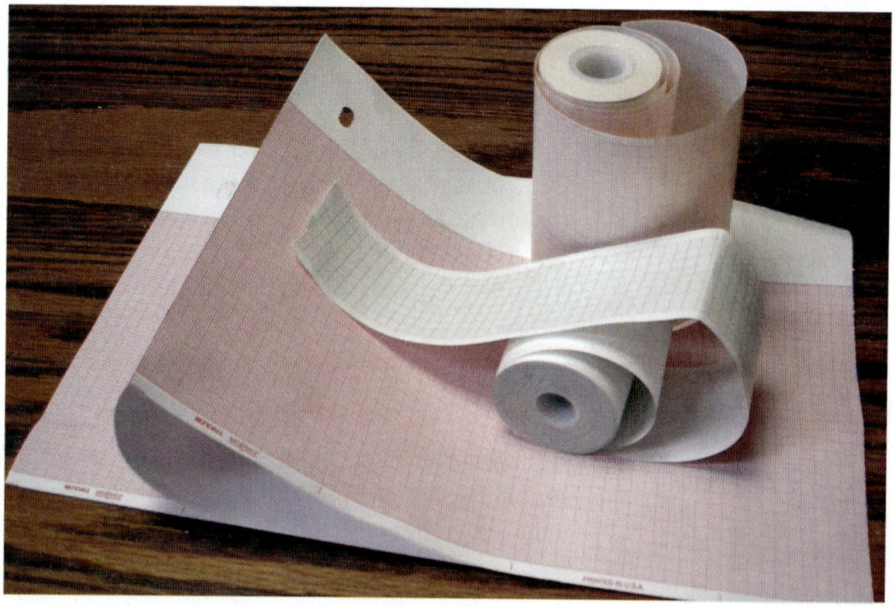

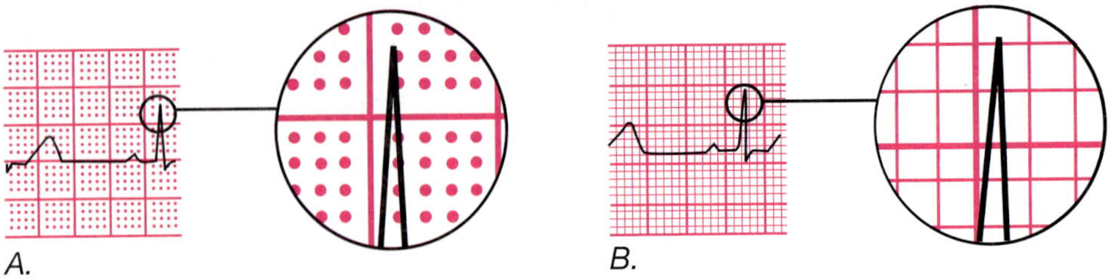

Figure 3-14 Comparison of ECG graph paper: dot matrix paper (*A*) requires less ink, is easier to read, and produces sharper photocopies, whereas standard grid paper (*B*) is slightly less expensive.

Figure 3-15 While performing an ECG, a thick red line at the bottom of the graph paper indicates that the paper needs to be changed.

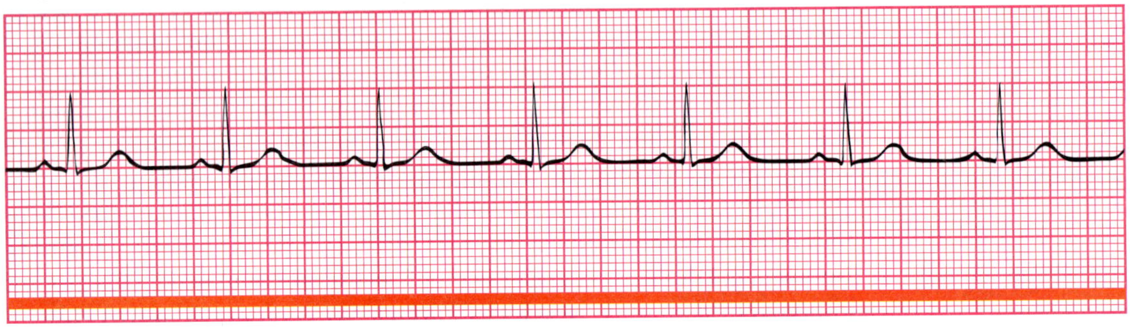

Prior to performing an ECG, make sure the machine has enough paper to record the results. Each machine has a paper loading procedure that you should become familiar with. Many of the machines warn you when the paper is nearly gone by making a red mark across the bottom of the tracing (Figure 3-15). Read the manufacturer's directions for specific instructions on how to change the ECG machine paper. Keep a supply of paper on the ECG cart in case you run out of paper in the patient's room or examination room.

Measurements

The ECG graph paper consists of precisely spaced horizontal and vertical lines. The horizontal increments represent time, measured in millimeters (mm). The vertical increments represent voltage, indicated in millivolts (mV). The heavy lines form boxes that are 5 mm by 5 mm in size. At the standard paper speed of 25 mm/sec, the paper grid can be translated into specific numerical values. The smallest box on the graph paper is 1 mm square and represents 0.04 second in time and 0.1 mV in voltage. One second equals 25 mm, or five heavy lines. Therefore, each vertical heavy line represents 0.20 second. Two large boxes represent 10 mm, which equals 1 centimeter (cm) for vertical measurement. ECG machines must be calibrated so that 1 cm = 1 mV. Each horizontal heavy line represents 5 mm or 0.5 mV (Figure 3-16). A calibration mark should always be verified on the left-hand side of the ECG before printing.

Law & Ethics

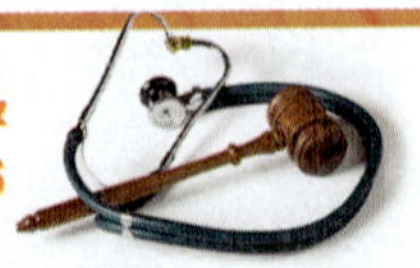

Maintaining Patient Records

Handling the ECG paper and report correctly is essential because the ECG report is part of a patient's medical records and must be maintained for at least seven years.

Figure 3-16 The ECG paper allows measurement of both time and voltage. Note that each small box is either 0.1 mV in voltage or 0.04 second in time.

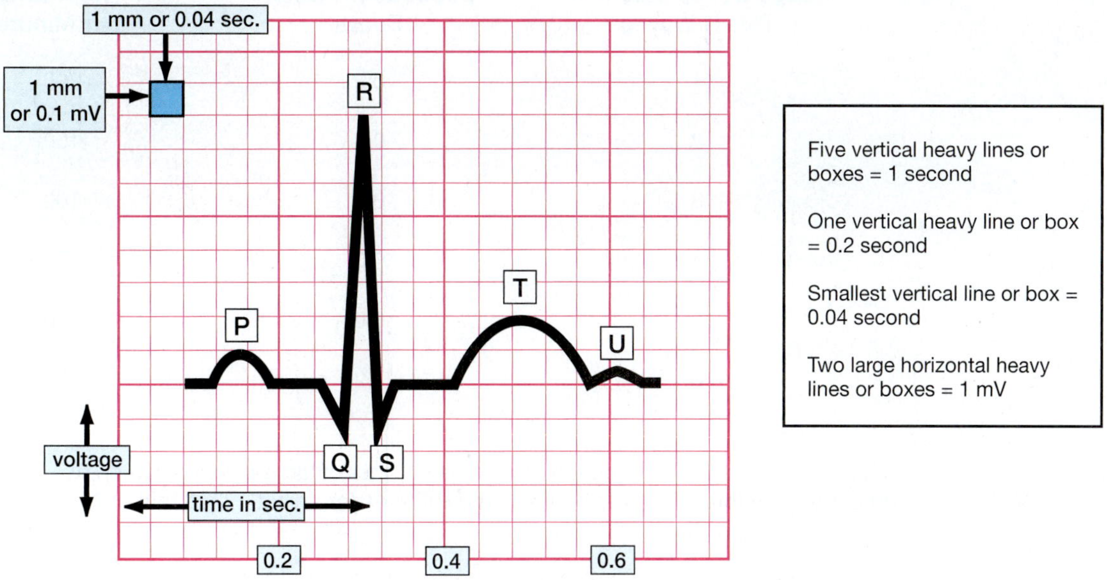

Checkpoint Question (LO 3.5)

1. When the paper speed is 25 mm/sec, how many small boxes represent 1 minute?

____

____

3.6 Calculating Heart Rate

A quick look at the ECG tracing can give you an idea of the heart rate. The more space between the QRS complexes, the slower the heart rate. The less space between the QRS complexes, the faster the heart rate. A more accurate approximation can be done using a variety of methods:

1. The R-R method: useful for approximation of heart rate when the rhythm is regular
2. The 1500 method: the most accurate for use with regular rhythms
3. The 6-second method: the only technique available to use for irregular rhythms, but it can also be used for regular rhythms

The R-R Method

When you are running the ECG at 25 mm/sec, there are 300 large boxes in a 1-minute strip. This method is sometimes called the *300 method.* You need to first determine the number of large boxes between two R waves on the ECG tracing. Divide this number into 300. For example, if there were five boxes between the R waves, the heart rate would be 300 divided by 5, which equals

TABLE 3-2 Calculating Heart Rates by Measuring the R-R Interval

Large Boxes between Two R Waves	Seconds between Beats	Heart Rate per Minute
1	0.2	300
2	0.4	150
3	0.6	100
4	0.8	75
5	1.0	60
6	1.2	50

Figure 3-17 To estimate the heart rate with the R-R method, count the number of large boxes between two R waves and divide into 300. In this figure there are four full boxes between the R waves for an estimated rate of 75.

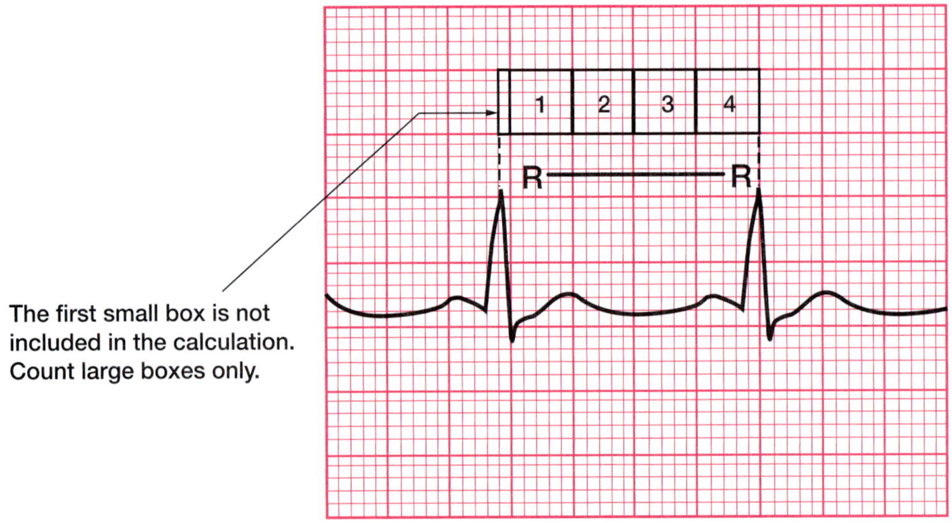

60 beats per minute. Table 3-2 provides the approximate heart rates based on this method of calculation. Figure 3-17 illustrates the process for calculating heart rates using the R-R wave method. This technique is the least accurate method because incomplete boxes are not counted or included in the calculation.

The 1500 Method

The most accurate method for determining the rate of a regular rhythm is the 1500 method, named such because in a 1-minute interval there are 1,500 small squares. To use this method, count the number of small squares between two consecutive R waves and then divide that number into 1,500. For example, if you count 25 small squares between two R waves, you will divide that into 1,500 (1,500 ÷ 25 = 60). The heart rate would be 60 beats per minute (Figure 3-18). *This technique allows you to measure to a minimum distance of 0.5 mm (one-half small box).* Because the calculation is based on the number of small squares, it has by far the smallest margin for heart rate error. *Note:* When using the 1500 technique, round to the nearest whole number. Round down if the fractional beat is less than 0.5, or round up if it is 0.5 or more. For example, 86.4 = 86 and 76.7 = 77.

Figure 3-18 Using the 1500 method, count the number of small boxes between two R waves and divide into 1,500. In this example, there are 38 small boxes. 1,500 ÷ 38 = 39.47, which rounds down to 39 beats per minute.

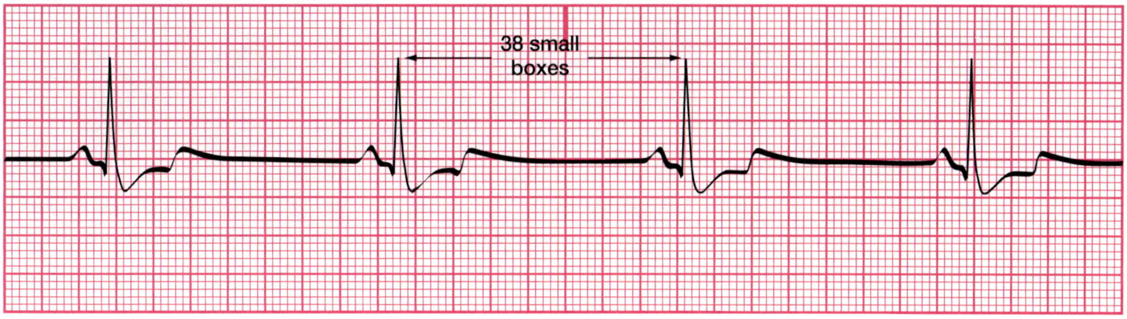

The 6-Second Method

The third method (*and the only one to be used for approximating irregular heart rhythms*) is called the *6-second method.* First, identify a 6-second section of the tracing. The ECG paper is usually marked with a vertical line at 3-second intervals on the top or bottom of the strip. You will need to view two sections or 30 boxes. Second, count the number of complete complexes seen in one 6-second interval. Each complex must include the P, QRS, and T waves. The complex should not be counted unless it is complete. Third, multiply the number of complexes by 10 to determine the estimated heart rate (Figure 3-19 and "Troubleshooting—Counting the Heart Rate").

Figure 3-19 To estimate the heart rate with the 6-second method, locate a 6-second section of the ECG rhythm strip (each small black line or heavy red mark at the top of the strip indicates 15 boxes or three seconds), count the number of complete complexes in this section, then multiply the number of complexes by 10. In this figure, eight complete complexes equal an estimated heart rate of 70. Complex number 8 cannot be counted because it is not completely within the 6-second strip.

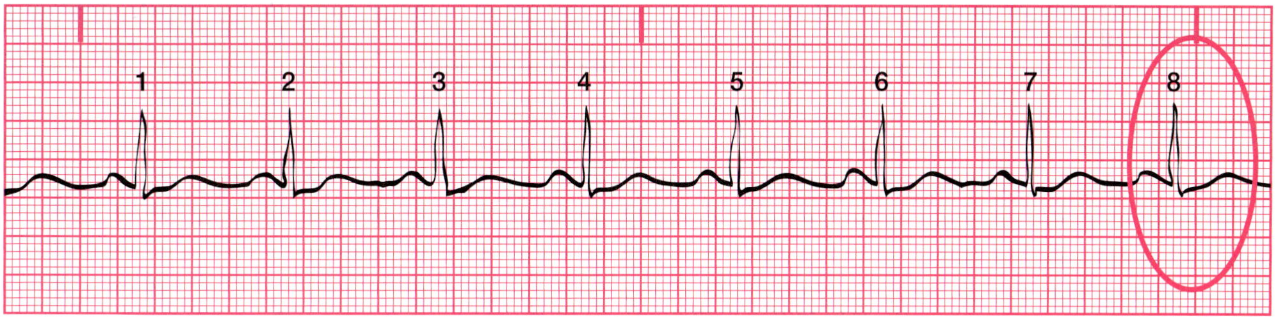

Troubleshooting

Counting the Heart Rate

When calculating the heart rate by counting the complexes in a 6-second interval, count the complete complexes only. If there is a portion of a complex at each end of the 6-second section you are using, find another section on the tracing to view. Never count incomplete complexes; this will make your results inaccurate.

(Continued)

(Troubleshooting, continued)

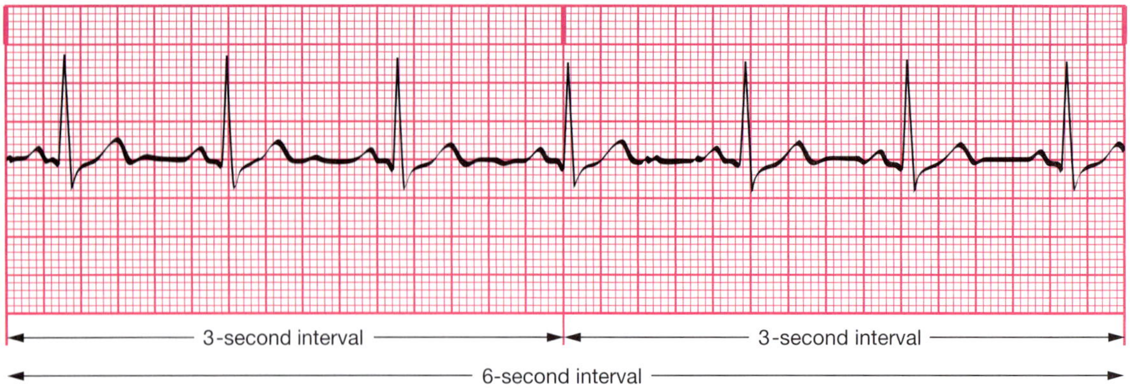

Multiply the number of complete complexes by 10

What is the number of complexes in the above 6-second interval? What is the heart rate?

____

____

Checkpoint Questions (LO 3.6)

1. Calculate the heart rate for this ECG strip using the 1500 method.

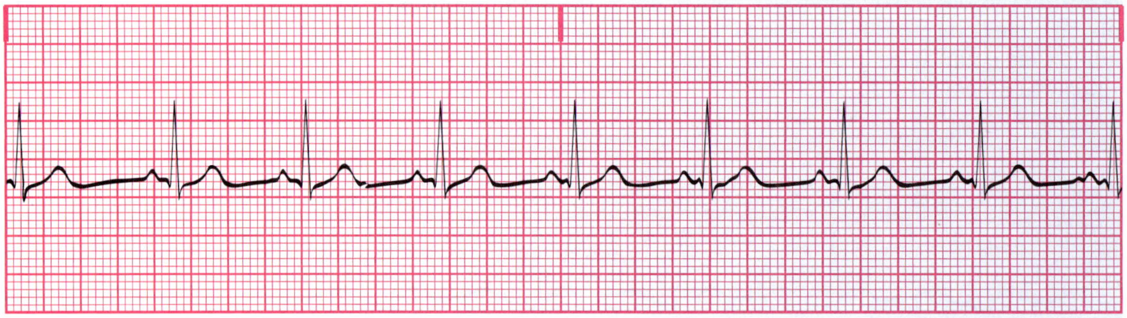

____

2. Estimate the heart rate for this ECG strip.

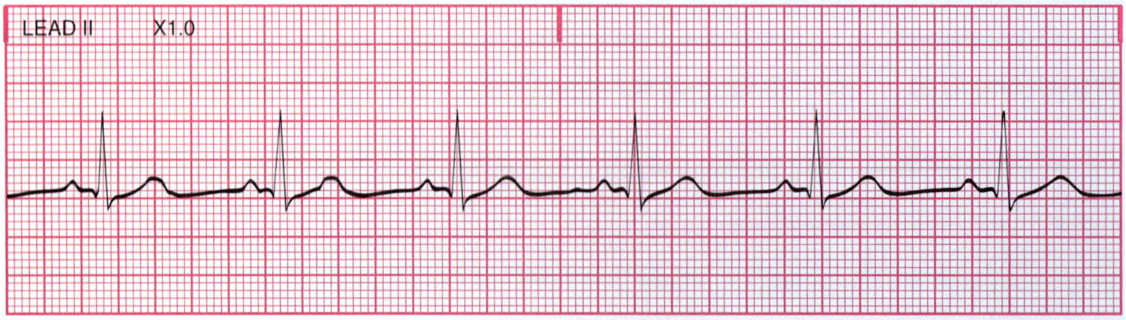

____

Chapter Summary

Learning Outcomes	Summary	Pages
3.1 Explain the three types of leads and how each is recorded.	Three types of leads are used to produce the ECG: limb, augmented, and chest leads. Limb leads are bipolar, meaning they measure electricity in two directions. Augmented leads are unipolar because they measure toward one electrode on the body. Chest leads record activity between six points on the chest and within the heart.	54–59
3.2 Identify the functions of common ECG machines.	The ECG machine has three basic functions: input, signal processing, and output display.	59–63
3.3 Explain how each ECG machine control is used.	The controls for the ECG machine include the speed, gain, artifact filter, LCD display, heart rate limits, standardization, and the lead selector.	64–67
3.4 Recognize common electrodes.	Various types of disposable electrodes are used, depending on the equipment and type of ECG being recorded.	67–68
3.5 Describe the ECG graph paper.	ECG graph paper has boxes that are 5 mm by 5 mm and are divided into smaller boxes that measure 1 mm by 1 mm. Each small box indicates 0.04 second in time horizontally and 0.1 mV in voltage vertically.	69–71
3.6 Calculate heart rates using an ECG tracing.	There are three common ways to calculate the heart rate, including the R-R (300) method, the 1500 method, and the 6-second method.	71–74

Chapter Review

Matching I

Match the lead names on the left with their lead types on the right. (LO 3.1)

_______ **1.** V1
_______ **2.** aVR
_______ **3.** lead I
_______ **4.** lead II
_______ **5.** aVL
_______ **6.** V3
_______ **7.** V4
_______ **8.** V6
_______ **9.** aVF
_______ **10.** lead III
_______ **11.** V2
_______ **12.** V5

a. limb lead
b. augmented lead
c. precordial lead

Matching II

Match the ECG terms on the left with their definitions on the right.

_______ **13.** single-channel (LO 3.2)
_______ **14.** speed (LO 3.3)
_______ **15.** input (LO 3.3)
_______ **16.** gain (LO 3.3)
_______ **17.** lead (LO 3.1)
_______ **18.** multichannel (LO 3.2)
_______ **19.** mV (LO 3.5)
_______ **20.** mm (LO 3.5)
_______ **21.** signal processing (LO 3.2)
_______ **22.** electrode (LO 3.4)
_______ **23.** output display (LO 3.3)

a. disposable sensors that detect the electrical activity of the heart
b. changes the height (size) of the ECG tracing
c. data that are entered into an ECG machine
d. indicates time on the ECG tracing
e. conductor wire attached to the ECG machine
f. ability to record more than one lead tracing at a time
g. indicates voltage on the ECG tracing
h. displays the tracing for the electrical activity of the heart
i. amplifies the electrical impulse and converts to mechanical action
j. records one lead tracing at a time
k. controls how fast the machine records during an ECG tracing

Multiple Choice

Circle the correct answer.

24. ECG machines have three basic functions. They are (LO 3.2)

- **a.** input, signal processing, and output display.
- **b.** input, standardization, and output display.
- **c.** multichannel, single-channel, and signal processing.
- **d.** standardization, input display, and output display.

25. To perform an ECG with accuracy, the best source to obtain specific information about the machine is (LO 3.2)

- **a.** the policy and procedure manual.
- **b.** the manufacturer's directions.
- **c.** your supervisor.
- **d.** your textbook.

26. The most commonly used electrodes are _____ and are used _____. (LO 3.4)

- **a.** disposable, more than once
- **b.** reusable, more than once
- **c.** disposable, once
- **d.** reusable, once

27. "Bipolar leads" means that (LO 3.1)

- **a.** one electrode is placed on the chest and the machine arbitrarily places one behind the person.
- **b.** both positive and negative electrodes are placed on the patient's body.
- **c.** Einthoven's triangle is not used.
- **d.** one of the leg limbs is used while the machine augments the rhythm.

28. What is the purpose of the LCD display? (LO 3.3)

- **a.** To allow entry and display of patient information
- **b.** To show the results of the ECG
- **c.** To sound alarms and errors
- **d.** To assist the patient to understand the procedure

29. The term *multichannel ECG* indicates that (LO 3.2)

- **a.** you enter all the data into the machine prior to running a tracing.
- **b.** three or more leads are recorded at one time.
- **c.** you do not have to mount each lead separately.
- **d.** all of the answers are correct.

30. What is the standard paper speed for an ECG machine? (LO 3.3)

- **a.** 25 mm/sec
- **b.** 50 mm/sec
- **c.** 0.25 mm/sec
- **d.** 0.50 mm/sec

31. Which of the following is *not* a type of lead? (LO 3.1)

- **a.** Limb
- **b.** Augmented
- **c.** Input
- **d.** Precordial

32. An artifact filter helps obtain a clear ECG tracing by (LO 3.3)
  a. maintaining artifact or abnormal marks on the ECG tracing.
  b. always ensuring accurate readings by the computer.
  c. always recognizing that the patient has a pacemaker.
  d. all of the answers are correct.

33. Computerized interpretation (LO 3.3)
  a. can be used for actual diagnostic interpretation.
  b. never has to be validated by a physician.
  c. must always be validated by a physician.
  d. none of the answers are correct.

34. The horizontal reading on the ECG paper represents _____, and the vertical readings represent _____. (LO 3.5)
  a. voltage, time
  b. time, height
  c. time, voltage
  d. voltage, millivolts

35. Which lead tracing must be augmented by the ECG machine to be able to see the different ECG waveforms? (LO 3.1)
  a. Lead I
  b. Lead II
  c. Lead V6
  d. Lead aVF

36. The Einthoven triangle is formed by using which of the following placement sites? (LO 3.1)
  a. Right arm, left arm, left leg
  b. Right arm, left leg, right leg
  c. Right arm, middle of chest, left leg
  d. None of the answers are correct

Matching III

Match the line sizes on the left with their times on the tracings at 25 mm/sec paper speed on the right. *Note:* A heavy line or box is 5 small boxes. (LO 3.5)

_______ 37. five heavy lines or boxes
_______ 38. one vertical heavy line or box
_______ 39. smallest vertical line or box

a. 1 second
b. 0.04 second
c. 0.2 second

Matching IV

Match the lead wires on the left with the most common colors on the right. (LO 3.1)

_______ 40. left leg (LL)
_______ 41. right arm (RA)
_______ 42. right leg (RL)
_______ 43. left arm (LA)

a. green
b. white
c. black
d. red

Label the Parts

44. Label the lead tracings that produce the Einthoven triangle by writing the identifying letters in the appropriate boxes. (LO 3.1)

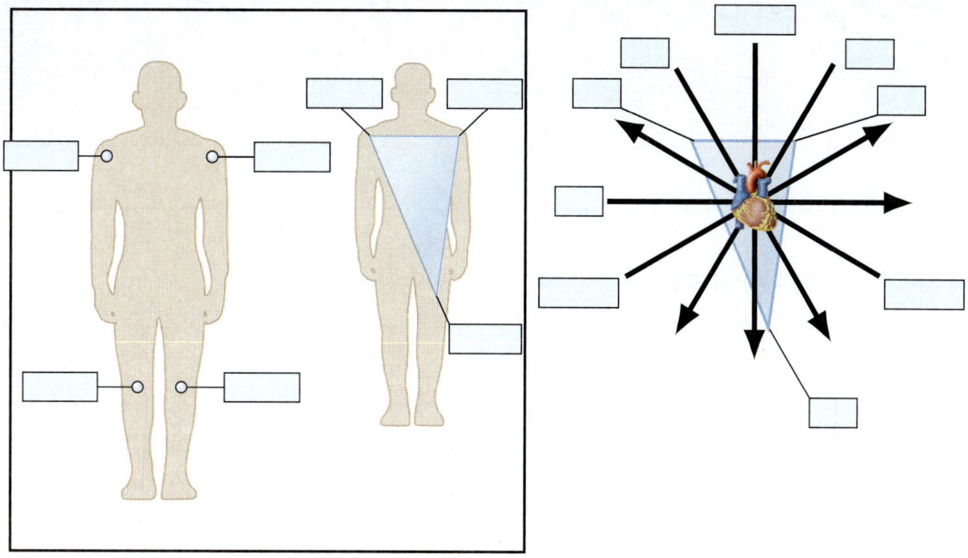

45. Label the measurements by writing them in the appropriate boxes. (LO 3.5)

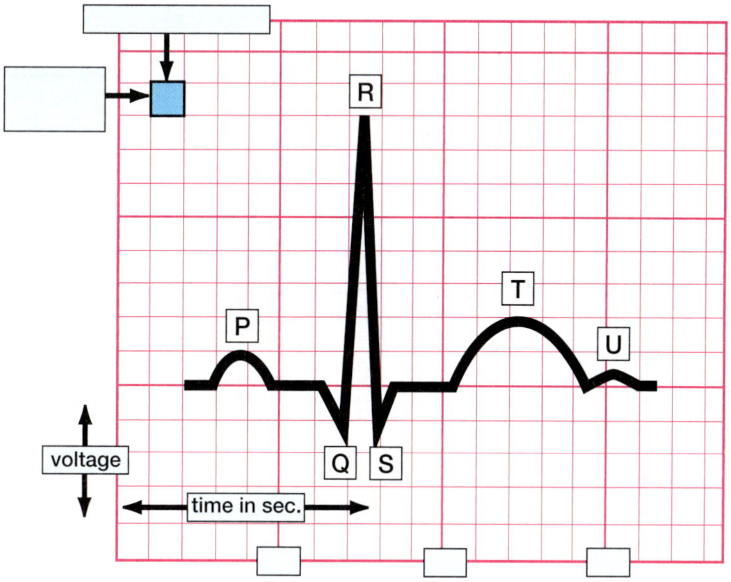

46–47. Estimate the heart rate using the R-R wave method. (LO 3.6)

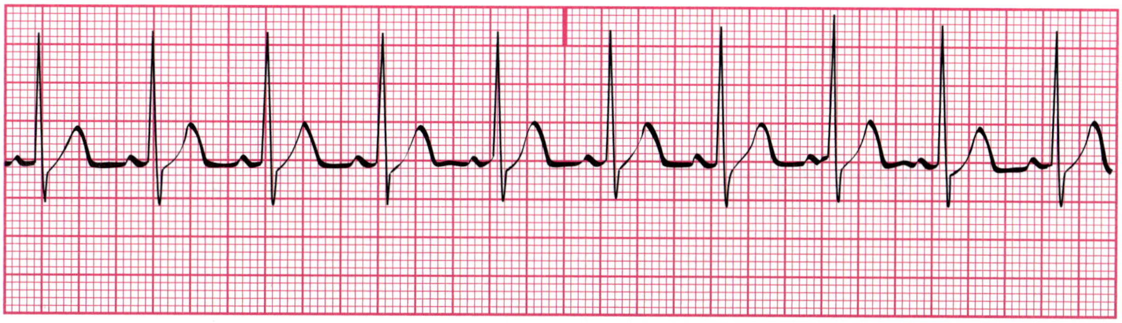

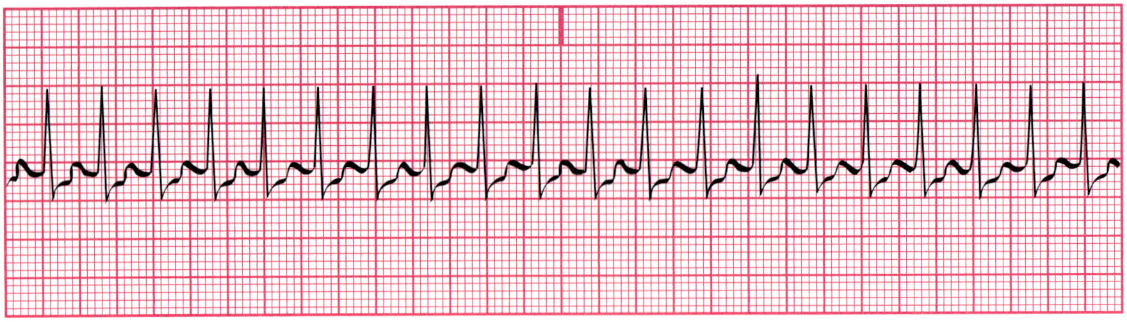

48–49. Estimate the heart rate using the 6-second method. (LO 3.6)

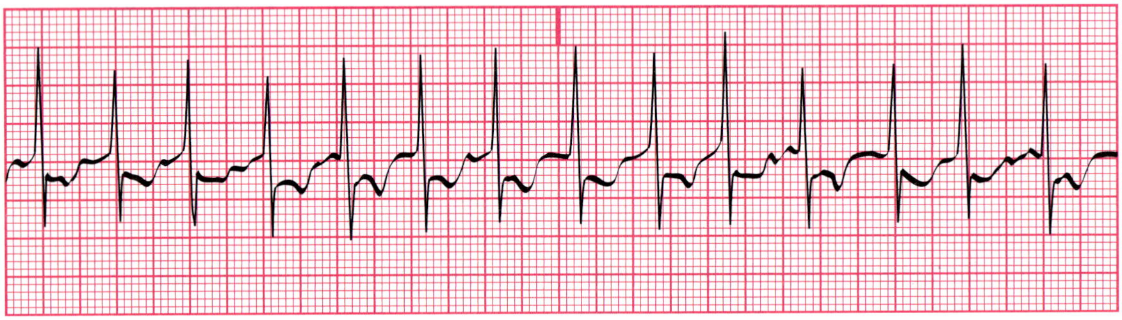

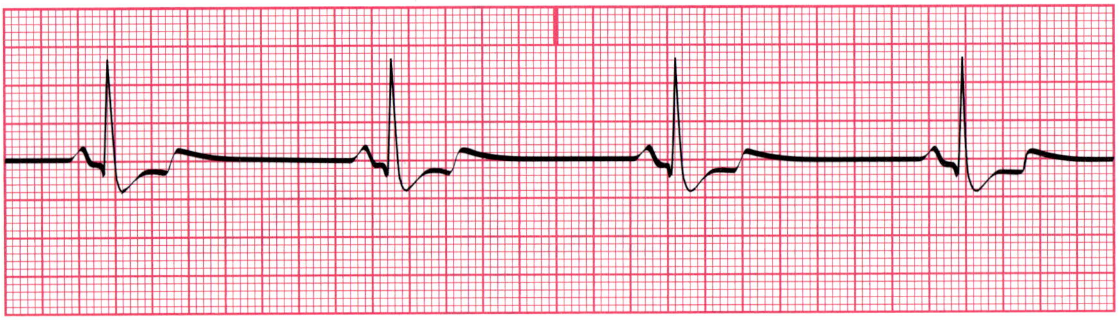

50–51. Determine the heart rate using the 1500 method. (LO 3.6)

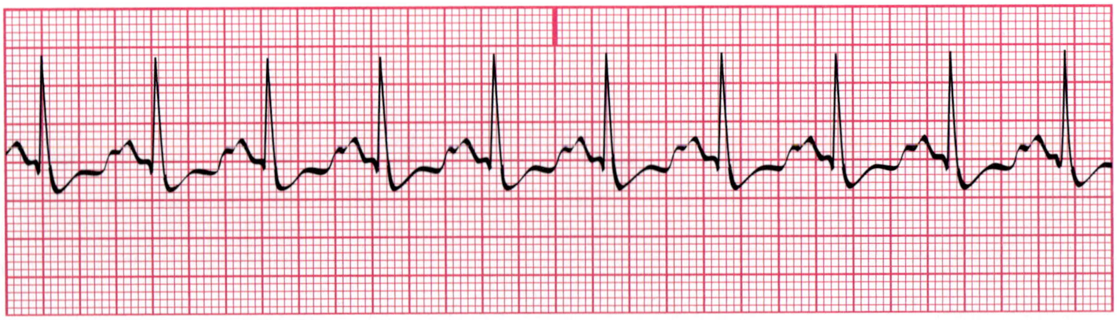

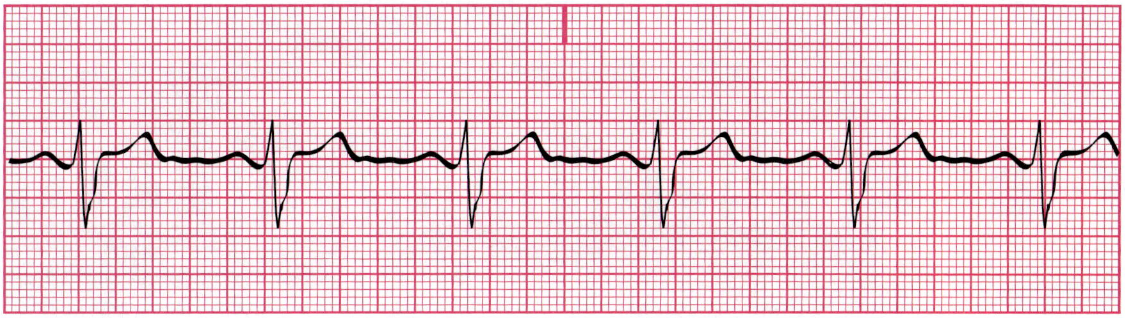

____

Critical Thinking Application *What Should You Do?*

Read the following situations, and use your critical thinking skills to determine how you would handle each. Write your answer in detail in the space provided.

52. When you start to perform an ECG on a patient, you notice a red line along the bottom of the ECG paper. What should you do? (LO 3.5)

____

____

53. When preparing to do an ECG, you find an open package of disposable electrodes on top of the ECG cart. Would you use these electrodes? Why or why not? (LO 3.4)

____

____

54. You are preparing to attach the electrodes and lead wires for a 12-lead ECG. You are unable to read the letters on each of the lead wires. You place the electrodes and lead wires, but when you run the tracing it looks like a bunch of scratches. What do you think the problem is and how would you solve it? (LO 3.1)

____

____

55. When performing a 12-lead ECG, you notice that the tracing line is very thick and hard to view. In addition, one of the leads does not record properly. What would you do? (LO 3.3)

____

____

connect® Now that you have completed the material in the chapter text, go to Connect and complete any chapter activities you have not yet done.

4 Performing an ECG

Learning Outcomes

4.1 Carry out preparation of the patient, room, and equipment for an ECG.

4.2 Describe the communication needed during the ECG procedure, including the actions to take if a patient refuses to allow an ECG to be performed.

4.3 Identify the anatomical landmarks that are used to apply the ECG chest electrodes to the correct locations.

4.4 Demonstrate the procedure for applying the electrodes and lead wires for a 12-lead ECG and cardiac monitoring.

4.5 Identify at least three ways to prevent infection and provide for safety during the ECG procedure.

4.6 Describe the procedure for recording a 12-lead ECG.

4.7 Identify types of artifact and how to prevent or correct them.

4.8 Describe how to report the ECG results.

4.9 Identify the steps for cleaning and caring for the ECG equipment.

4.10 Explain variations for a pediatric ECG procedure.

4.11 Distinguish between a routine ECG and cardiac monitoring.

4.12 Summarize special patient circumstances when performing an ECG.

4.13 Recall the steps for handling an emergency during the ECG.

Key Terms

alternating current (AC) interference
angle of Louis
anterior axillary line
dextrocardia
intercostal space (ICS)
midaxillary line
midclavicular line
midscapular line
paraspinous line
posterior axillary line
seizure
somatic tremor
suprasternal notch
wandering baseline

4.1 Preparation for the ECG Procedure

Now that you understand how the ECG is used, the anatomy of the heart, and the electrocardiograph, the next step is to record an ECG. The ECG experience should be pleasant for the patient and not produce anxiety. The ECG procedure must be done correctly, and the tracing must be accurate.

Prior to performing the ECG, you will need to prepare the room. Certain conditions in the room where the ECG is to be performed should be considered. For example, electrical currents in the room can interfere with the tracing. If possible, choose a room away from other electrical equipment and x-ray machines. Turn off any nonessential electrical equipment that is in the room during the tracing. The ECG machine should be placed away from other sources of electrical currents, such as wires or cords.

An ECG must be ordered by a physician or other authorized personnel, and an order form must be completed prior to the procedure. This form may be called a *requisition* or *consult* and should be placed in the patient's record. It should include why the ECG was ordered and the following identifying information:

- Patient name, identification number or medical record number, and birth date
- Location, date, and time of recording
- Patient age, sex, race, and cardiac and other medications the patient is currently taking
- Weight and height
- Any special condition or position of the patient during the recording

If this information is not included on the requisition or consult, you should ask the patient or find the information in the patient's record.

Most facilities now have computerized systems. The ECG order is frequently entered through this system. Entering the patient's identifying information into the computer will produce the order form and generate patient charges. Without a computer system, the information should be handwritten on the order form, consult, or requisition, whichever your facility uses.

Patient Education & Communication

Cardiac Medications

Certain cardiac medications can change the ECG tracing. Prior to the ECG procedure, determine if your patient is on any cardiac medications and, if so, inform the physician and write the names of the medications on the ECG report. See the appendix *Cardiovascular Medications* for examples of common cardiac medications.

The patient's identifying information should also be entered through the LCD panel on the ECG machine prior to the recording. If the ECG machine does not allow you to enter the information or there isn't time due to an emergency situation, you should write it on the completed ECG. Most importantly, all information should be written or entered accurately no matter what type of ECG machine or order system you are using.

Before beginning the procedure, make sure the ECG machine has a good supply of paper loaded in it. If a red line appeared across the bottom

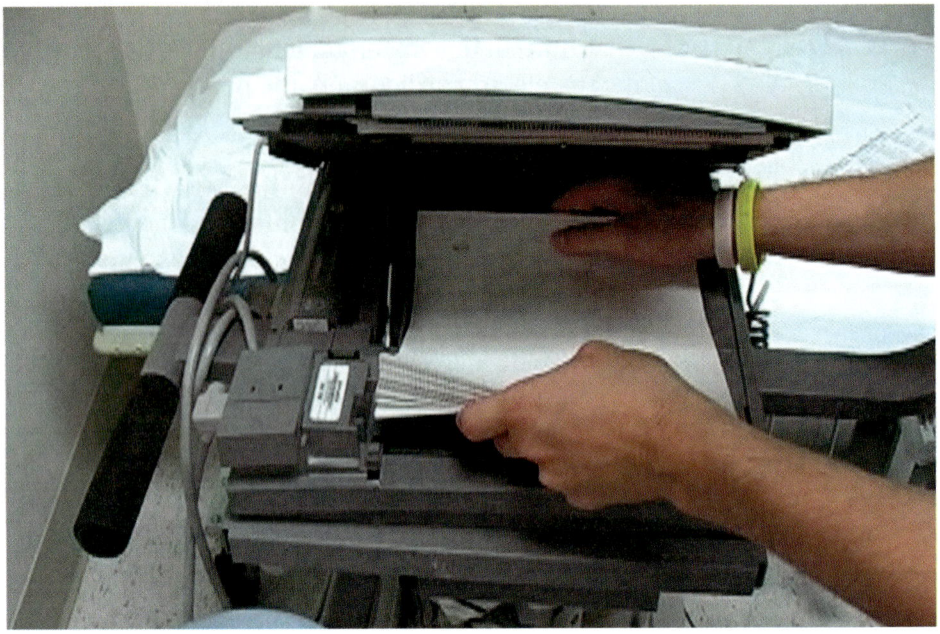

Figure 4-1 Make sure the ECG paper is properly loaded and aligned before recording an ECG.

of the last tracing, you should replace the paper in the ECG machine before beginning. This should be done prior to taking the ECG machine to the room where the patient is located. Review the operator's manual or consult your supervisor if you are unsure how to insert the new ream of paper. Most ECG machines have a release button or lever that opens the ECG equipment for the paper to be inserted. Place the paper inside the machine correctly. Thread it through the roller to the outside of the machine and align it properly. Close the paper-loading compartment, and run the machine to check for proper functioning and alignment (Figure 4-1).

Checkpoint Questions (LO 4.1)

1. Name four important aspects of preparing for the ECG procedure.

____

____

2. What information must be included on the ECG requisition?

____

____

4.2 Communicating with the Patient

Prior to performing any procedure, always ensure that you are performing the procedure on the correct patient. Correctly identifying the patient is the first step in ensuring that you are providing patient safety. The Joint Commission (TJC) has stated that every patient must be identified by two forms of identification. Introduce yourself by stating your name and job title. Ask the patient to state his or her name. Check the name on the patient identification band or patient's chart to verify the information. To ensure that it is the correct patient, ask the patient to state his or her birth date. Often patients have similar names, but their birth dates and medical record numbers will distinguish the correct patient. If the patient's information is incorrect, verify with your immediate supervisor for the next steps.

After you verify that you have the correct patient, explain what you are about to do. State, "I am going to perform an electrocardiogram on you today. Have you ever had an ECG done before?" Stating both ECG and electrocardiogram helps the patient relate that they are the same. If the patient has not had an ECG, explain the procedure in more detail. Assure the patient that the procedure is harmless and painless. Avoid using words that may frighten the patient such as *electricity* or *wires*. Patients, particularly children, who have not had an ECG before may be afraid of the machine and wires. The patient should be relaxed and comfortable. Maintaining a calm, competent manner and answering the patient's questions will help the patient relax.

Law & Ethics

Legal Record

The ECG is part of the medical record. Enter the patient information thoroughly and accurately. Remember, the patient's medical record can be used as part of a medical professional liability case.

If the patient refuses an ECG, determine the cause of the refusal. Some people may have fear or concern about the procedure. Provide any information or reassurance the patient may need. Frequently, patients see the wires and think the machine will shock them. Be sure you explain carefully that you are only going to measure the electricity that is already inside their body. If the patient still refuses, notify your supervisor and/or the ordering physician; the patient's reason for refusal must be documented.

In preparing for an ECG, provide the patient with privacy by pulling a curtain around the bed or closing the examination room door. Because many patients are fearful and/or feel they lack privacy, inform them that closing the door or curtain is for their privacy. The patient should remove any clothing above the waist. Provide the patient with a drape, such as a sheet or blanket. The patient may also wear a hospital-type gown with the opening in the front. The patient should remove any jewelry or items that would interfere with the electrode placement or touch the electrodes. This may include necklaces, watches, bracelets, belt buckles, or ankle bracelets. In addition, ask the patient to turn off and remove all electronic devices. These include things such as cell phones, PDAs, and MP3 players.

Patient Education & Communication

Explain the Procedure

Remember, even if a patient is not able to respond, he or she may still hear you. Always explain the procedure before beginning the ECG.

4.4 Applying the Electrodes and Leads

The limb electrodes are placed on the forearms or upper arms and the inside of the lower legs. You should pick a fleshy area with the least amount of hair. If placement of the arm leads on the patient's forearm is not possible due to injury, amputation, IV placement, casts, or other reason, you should choose a different site. The alternate site of placement for arm leads is on the deltoids (shoulders). The leads should be placed on the same site on each arm so that the placements are mirror images of each other. For example, if a patient has a cast or an IV on the left forearm, you will need to move *both* left and right electrodes to the shoulders.

When placement of the leg leads on the patient's lower legs or ankles is not possible, the alternate site for placement is on the upper legs. They should be placed as close to the trunk as possible. This may be necessary when the patient is an amputee or has an injury or bandage on one of the lower legs. The leads should be placed at the same site on each leg: If you place one lead above the knee on the left, then the right leg lead should also be placed above the knee. Attach the limb leads first because the ECG machine will not run without the limb leads being attached. However, the ECG machine will run if the limb leads are attached and the chest leads are not. This is important in the event that a patient is having a cardiac crisis. A tracing from the frontal plain is better than nothing. The physician could be looking at this tracing while you connect the precordial leads and run the full 12-lead ECG.

Before applying the electrodes on the chest, make sure the skin at the sites is clean and dry. Remove any lotion or oil from the skin with alcohol wipes or soap and water. You may use electrolyte pads to prep the skin. If the patient has a great deal of chest hair, you may shave small areas of the chest so the electrodes will adhere to the skin properly. However, the preferred method is to clip the hair instead of shaving. This prevents the patient from scratching the electrode site as the hair grows in and reduces the risk of infection as a result of small microcuts that may be caused by a razor blade. Table 4-1 summarizes the procedure for applying chest leads correctly.

Start by applying the V1 electrode. First locate the angle of Louis; then locate the second rib, which is adjacent to this landmark. Each intercostal space is felt between the ribs with the corresponding intercostal space below the rib location. The fourth intercostal space is the dent you feel between the fourth and fifth ribs. Chest lead V1 is placed at the right sternal border at this location. V2 should be placed at the fourth intercostal space on the left sternal border. Skip V3 and place V4 next. V4 is placed at the fifth intercostal space

TABLE 4-1 Applying Leads Correctly

- Choose a flat, nonmuscular area.
- Use the forearms and ankles for the limb leads if at all possible.
- Alternate sites include the upper arms near the shoulders (deltoids) and upper legs.
- Prep the skin with an electrolyte pad, if available.
- When necessary, cleanse the electrode sites with an alcohol pad, mild soap and water, or electrolyte pad.
- Dry the skin completely before applying the electrodes.
- If the patient is diaphoretic (sweaty), consider using antiperspirant, tincture of benzoin, or mastisol to help pads remain adhered to the patient's skin.
- Clip hair, instead of shaving. Use tape to remove cut hairs.
- Shave the hair from the site only if necessary, such as during an emergency.

TABLE 4-2 Chest Lead Placement

Lead Name	Lead Placement
V1	Fourth intercostal space, right sternal border
V2	Fourth intercostal space, left sternal border
V3	Halfway between V2 and V4
V4	Fifth intercostal space at the midclavicular line
V5	At the anterior axillary line on the same horizontal level as V4
V6	At the midaxillary line on the same horizontal level as V4

on the left midclavicular line. Locate the site of the intersection between the fifth intercostal space and the midclavicular line. In young people, this site is directly below the nipple. Now place V3 midway between V2 and V4. Continuing in the fifth intercostal space on the same horizontal level as V4, place V5 at the anterior axillary line. Place V6 at the midaxillary line on the same horizontal line as V4 (Table 4-2 and Figure 4-3). (Another method of placement for V5 and V6 is to place V6 first, then place V5 midway between V4 and V6.) The anatomical landmarks should always be located when placing chest electrodes. Do not place them visually.

The procedure is the same when placing the chest electrodes on a female. If the patient has large breasts, you can ask the patient to move her own breasts (if able); or, using the back of your hand, simply lift the left breast and place the electrodes in the closest position possible. The breast may sit on top of the electrode, but the electrode cannot sit on top of the breast. Leads V3, V4, and V5 will be the most affected by breast tissue. Electrodes should be placed as close as possible to the proper placement without placing the electrodes directly on the breast tissue because breast tissue is a poor conductor of electricity. In the event of large breasts, V3 may not be perfectly in line, but should be as close as possible to the midpoint halfway between V2 and V4. Make sure that all nonstandard electrode placements are documented. Note where the sensors were placed and why.

Figure 4-3 Chest lead placement.

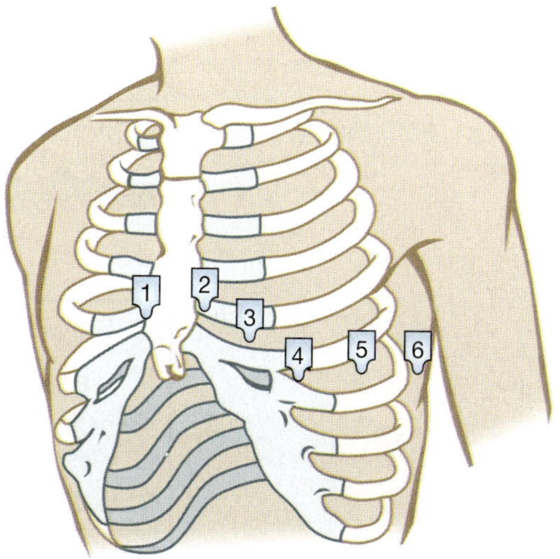

Troubleshooting

The Midclavicular Line

When locating the midclavicular line for chest lead placement, keep in mind that the midclavicular line does not always run directly through the nipple line. This is most often the case with obese patients or females with large breasts.

When applying the V4 electrode to a patient who weighs 326 pounds, you have difficulty finding the midclavicular line. What should you do?

____

____

After all of the electrodes have been properly positioned, attach the lead cable wires. Identify the correct cable for each electrode based on color and letter abbreviations. For example, the chest leads are marked V1 to V6 (Figure 4-4). The correct cable must be attached to the corresponding electrode to ensure an accurate tracing. When using electrodes with tabs on which alligator-type clips are used, chest and arm electrodes are placed with the tabs pointing downward toward the feet; the lower extremity electrodes are placed with the tabs pointing toward the head. Utilizing this technique reduces tension on the electrodes and provides a "cleaner," artifact-free tracing. Ultimately, refer to the manufacturer's directions in the operator's manual for the optimum placement technique recommended for your equipment. In all cases, the electrodes should be secure and the lead wires should be supported.

The ECG lead wire cables should follow the contours of the body when attached to the ECG electrodes. Avoid crossing or looping the wires outside

Figure 4-4 Color and letter coding identify the lead wires for an ECG machine.

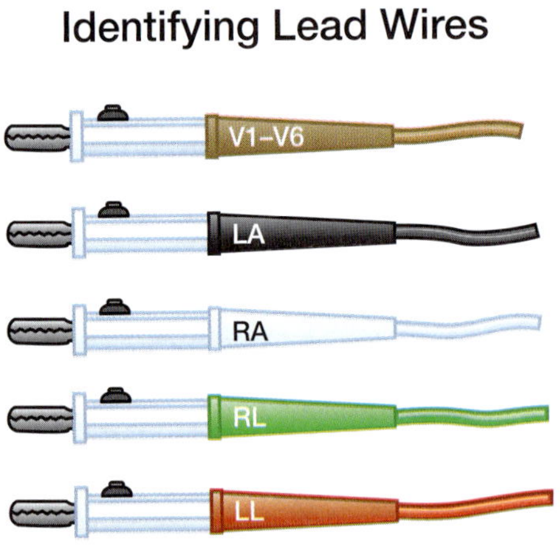

RA = right arm	White
LA = left arm	Black
RL = right leg	Green
LL = left leg	Red
V1 to V6 = chest leads	Brown*

*Chest lead label V1 to V6 are not always brown.

Figure 4-5 Correct (*A*) and incorrect (*B*) lead cable placement. Avoid looping the wires outside the body and check each wire once it is connected to ensure that there is no tension on the electrodes or leads.

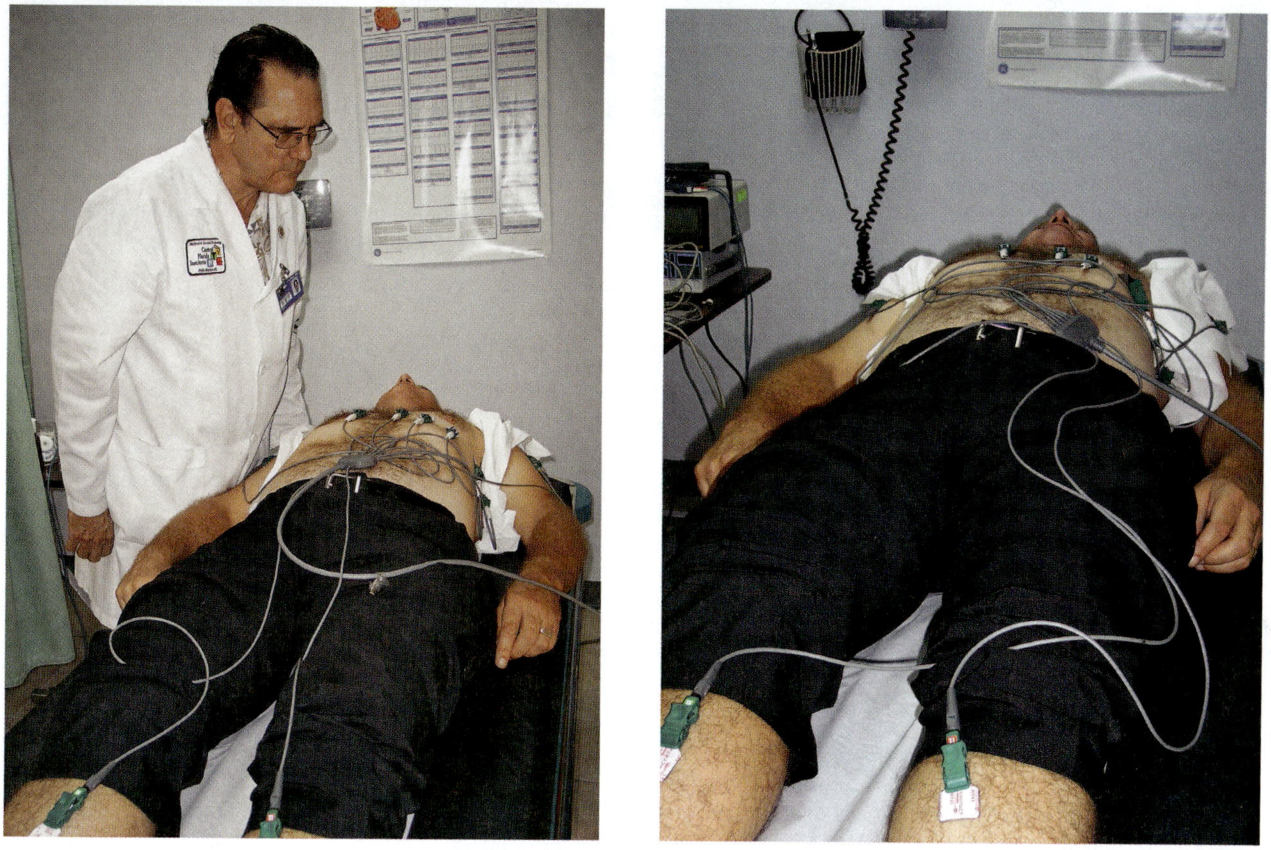

A. *B.*

of the body, and check each wire once it is connected to ensure that there is no tension on the electrodes or leads. Individual loops may be used to take up slack and prevent looping outside the body, thus reducing tension on the electrode (Figure 4-5).

Checkpoint Questions (LO 4.4)

1. How can you be certain you are attaching the lead wires to the electrodes properly?

____

____

2. Why should you place the limb electrodes before the chest electrodes?

____

____

4.5 Safety and Infection Control

When performing an ECG, you must practice universal or standard precautions at all times. These precautions are followed in all situations in which job exposure to blood or body fluids is likely. Wash your hands carefully before and after each procedure to prevent transfer of microorganisms. Wear gloves if there is a risk of exposure to the patient's blood or other body fluids.

TABLE 4-3 Infection Control Guidelines for Isolation of Hospitalized Patients

In addition to standard precautions, follow these guidelines and the policy of your place of employment to prevent the spread of infections.

Airborne Precautions

For patients known or suspected to be infected with microorganisms transmitted by minute airborne droplets:

- Use a private room that has monitored negative air.
- Keep the room door closed and the patient in the room.
- Wear special HEPA N-95, N-99, or N-100 masks for respiratory protection when entering the room of a patient with known or suspected infectious pulmonary tuberculosis.
- Do not enter the room of a patient known or suspected to have rubeola or varicella if you are susceptible; if you must enter the room, wear respiratory protection.
- Limit the movement and transport of patients from the room to essential purposes only.
- Place a surgical mask on the patient if transport or movement is necessary.

Droplet Precautions

For patients known or suspected to be infected with microorganisms transmitted by droplets that can be generated by the patient during coughing, sneezing, talking, or the performance of procedures:

- Place patient in a private room (special air handling and ventilation are not necessary and the door may remain open).
- Wear a mask when working within 3 feet of the patient.
- Limit the movement and transport of the patient from the room to essential purposes only.
- Use a mask on the patient if transport or movement is necessary.

Contact Precautions

Contact precautions are used for patients known or suspected to be infected or colonized with microorganisms that can be transmitted by direct or indirect contact. *Direct contact* includes hand or skin-to-skin contact that occurs when performing patient care that requires touching the patient's dry skin; *indirect contact* includes touching environmental surfaces or patient-care items in the patient's environment. For these patients:

- Place patients in a private room.
- Wear gloves according to standard precautions.
- Wear gloves when entering the room and while providing patient care.
- Change gloves after having contact with infective material that may contain high concentrations of microorganisms, such as feces and wound drainage.
- Remove gloves before leaving the patient's room.
- Wash hands immediately.
- Do not touch potentially contaminated environmental surfaces or items in the patient's room after glove removal.
- All equipment must be disinfected after leaving the patient's room. The 12-lead ECG machine must be wiped down immediately.

In the hospital, you will need to follow additional precautions for patients in isolation. Depending on the type of isolation, masks, eye protection, and gowns may be necessary, in addition to gloves, when entering the room. Follow the facility's policy and the guidelines provided in Table 4-3. You should know standard precautions related to all hospitalized patients and maintain them throughout the procedure. As a rule, it is better to wear gloves even if it is not necessary. Do not forget to wash your hands or perform hand hygiene before putting on the gloves and after removing them. See the appendix *Standard and Isolation Precautions* for more information.

General safety guidelines and safety measures specific to the ECG procedure must also be practiced. As described earlier in the chapter, before beginning the procedure you must identify, verify, and ensure that you are performing the procedure on the correct patient. Then you should raise the

Patient Education & Communication

Relocating Electrodes

If you place the electrodes in an alternate location for any reason, including amputation or bandages, be sure to document this on the 12-lead ECG recording.

Safety & Infection Control

Isolation Precautions

Isolation precautions include specific guidelines for caring for patients in isolation. Three types of isolation have been identified by the Centers for Disease Control and Prevention: airborne, droplet, and contact. See the appendix *Standard and Isolation Precautions* for detailed information about following these standards.

side rail on the unattended side of the patient's bed or exam table. If the patient is on an exam table, have him or her lie down and pull the extension out for his or her legs and feet. If the patient is on a gurney or hospital bed, remember to employ proper body mechanics by raising the bed to a comfortable working level and to raise the side rail on the opposite side of the bed for safety. As you may recall from the chapter *Electrocardiograpy,* good body mechanics includes using movements that maintain proper posture and avoid muscle and bone injuries.

Prior to performing the ECG, check to be sure that the grounding prong is securely attached to the plug. Plug the machine in securely. Ensure that the bed or exam table is not touching the wall or any electrical equipment. Be sure that the patient is not touching the bed or exam table frame or safety rail. Always check the insulation on the lead wires for cracks before each use. Ensure that all electronic devices the patient may have are turned off and removed from the patient (Table 4-4).

TABLE 4-4 Maintaining Safety During an ECG

- Check that the grounding prong is securely attached to the plug.
- Plug in the machine securely, making sure the cord is not separating from the receptacle.
- Ensure that the power cord insulation is intact.
- Remove the plug by pulling it out by the prong connection, not by pulling on the electrical cord.
- Raise the bed to a working height and return it to low position when completed.
- Keep the side rail up on the opposite side of the bed or exam table.
- Perform hand hygiene and wear gloves or other personal protective equipment as required.
- Use proper body mechanics at all times:
  - Keep feet apart and knees bent when lifting or moving a patient.
  - Have the patient assist, if able, or obtain assistance when necessary.
  - Face in the direction you are working, avoid twisting and reaching, and lift with your legs.

Prepare the patient for the procedure by first ensuring privacy and providing for the patient's safety and comfort during the ECG. The patient's door or curtain should be closed, and the patient's clothing appropriately removed and the patient draped for privacy. Assist the patient to dress and undress as needed to provide for comfort and safety. Once the procedure is complete, you should clean the lead wires, leads, and machine. If you performed an ECG on a patient in isolation or with a contagious disease, you will need to clean the equipment properly to prevent the spread of infection. Observe the guidelines at your place of employment and the manufacturer's directions for the correct cleaning technique. Once you have completed the entire procedure, including cleanup, you should wash your hands. Remember to thank the patient and ask if he or she needs any further assistance.

Safety & Infection Control

Practice proper body mechanics at all times to protect yourself from injuries when moving or lifting patients or other large or awkward items.

Checkpoint Questions (LO 4.5)

1. Name at least three things to do to ensure safety during an ECG.

____

____

2. Name three types of isolation precautions and describe the PPE required for each.

____

____

4.6 Operating the ECG Machine

Before operating the ECG machine, make sure you have done the following:

- Identified and communicated with the patient
- Prepared the patient and the room
- Provided for patient privacy
- Provided for safety and infection control
- Located and checked the equipment for functioning
- Loaded the ECG graph paper, if necessary
- Attached the electrodes and leads

Now you should be ready to operate the ECG machine. For an automatic ECG, simply press the Run or Auto button. Check the LCD display for errors. If the ECG machine provides an interpretation, it will print out along with the tracing. This process takes only about 15 to 20 seconds.

For a manual ECG machine, make sure the equipment is standardized and set to lead I. You may need to run a few complexes (complete ECG waveforms) and then insert a standardization mark. The mark should be set between the T wave of one complex and the P wave of the next. Follow specific directions provided in the operator's manual or according to your institution's policy and procedure.

Checkpoint Questions (LO 4.6)

1. What must be done before you run the actual ECG tracing?

____

____

2. Describe how you run the ECG machine to create the lead tracings.

____

____

4.7 Checking the ECG Tracing

Certain problems can occur when obtaining an ECG tracing. General troubleshooting guidelines should be followed to avoid these problems (Table 4-5). The most frequent problem is unwanted marks on the ECG. These marks are called *artifact.* The marks are not caused by the heart activity; they are caused by some other source of movement or electrical activity. When an ECG tracing has these unwanted marks, it may be difficult or impossible to read. You are responsible for producing a correct tracing without artifact. In order to do this, you must first recognize artifact and then be able to eliminate it. The three most common causes of artifact are somatic tremor, wandering baseline, and alternating current interference. See Table 4-6 for ways to correct these causes of artifact.

Somatic Tremor

somatic tremor Voluntary or involuntary muscle movement; also known as body tremor.

Sometimes a patient's muscles will move, either voluntarily or involuntarily, which can produce **somatic tremor,** also known as body tremor. Movement of the muscles of the body is controlled by electrical voltages. These voltages are erratic, unlike the cardiac voltage, which is consistent. Somatic tremor appears as small erratic spikes on the ECG tracing (Figure 4-6).

Voluntary muscle movements can be due to tension, fear, gum chewing, talking, uncomfortable position, or pain. They may also be due to shivering or tense muscles. You should identify the correct cause before proceeding with the ECG. Knowing the cause will help you eliminate the artifact. Warm or reassure the patient if he or she is cold or frightened. Encourage slow, deep breaths to help calm the patient. Remind the patient to refrain from moving or talking.

TABLE 4-5 Troubleshooting Techniques During an ECG

- Perform good skin preparation.
- Use new (unused) electrodes and clean clips.
- Make sure personal electronic devices are turned off and removed from the patient.
- Ensure that the bed or examination table is not touching the wall or any electrical equipment.
- Ensure that the patient is not touching the frame, side rail, or any metal part of the bed or examination table.
- Always check the insulation on the lead wires for cracks before use.
- Ensure that there is no stress on the lead wires or electrodes.

TABLE 4-6 Correcting Artifact

Type of Artifact	Cause	Correction
Somatic tremor	Involuntary muscle movement: shivering, muscle tension, pain, fear	Reassure the patient, warm the patient, and encourage him or her to take slow, deep breaths.
	Voluntary movement: talking, chewing gum	Remind the patient not to make any movement during the procedure.
	Movement due to neuromuscular disorder such as Parkinson's disease	Have the patient put his or her hands, palms down, under the buttocks.
Wandering baseline	Improperly applied electrodes or poor skin preparation	Apply electrodes securely, make sure that the entire surface is in contact with the patient's skin.
	Pulling on electrodes from unsupported lead wires	Remove tension from lead wires.
	Oil, lotion, dirt, or hair on the skin under the electrodes	Clean the skin with alcohol and gauze or an alcohol prep pad.
	Old, corroded, or dirty electrodes or clips; too little or dried-out electrode gel	Use new disposable electrodes and store unused ones in a sealed plastic bag; if using gel, apply plenty of new solution to electrodes.
Alternating current (AC) interference	Improper grounding	Ensure that the plug has three prongs and is plugged into a grounded electrical outlet.
	Other electrical equipment	Wait until any other procedure is done, if possible, and unplug equipment.
	Lead wires crossed and not pointed toward the hands and feet	Reposition the lead wires to ensure that they follow limbs and are pointed in the proper direction.
	Electrical wiring in the walls or ceiling	Move the patient's bed away from the wall (use a 45-degree angle if necessary).
Interrupted baseline	Corroded or dirty leads	Clean the leads after each use.
	Damaged cable	Inspect cables and connections before each use.

Troubleshooting

Multiple ECGs

If your hospitalized patient requires daily ECGs for comparison by the physician, the ECG tracing may look different if the electrodes are placed in different sites on the chest and limbs. Each time you record an ECG on the patient, place the leads on the same site or as close as possible to the placement from the previous ECG. Some facilities will permit placing small marks on the patient to ensure that electrode placement will be consistent for multiple (serial) ECGs.

You are doing your third ECG on a patient in three days. Where should the electrodes be placed?

____

____

Figure 4-6 Somatic tremor appears as small erratic spikes on the ECG tracing.

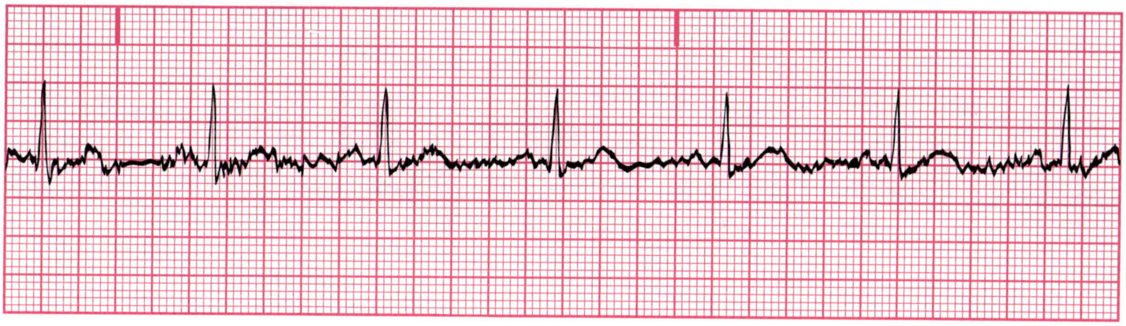

Sometimes involuntary muscle movements are due to Parkinson's disease or other neuromuscular disorders. These are more difficult to control. Have patients who suffer from neuromuscular disorders put their hands, palms down, under their buttocks. This will decrease the tremor and improve the tracing. If a patient has this type of tremor, make a note of it on the ECG tracing.

Wandering Baseline (Baseline Shift)

wandering baseline
Artifact in which the tracing drifts away from the center of the graph paper. Also known as baseline shift.

Wandering baseline, or baseline shift, occurs when the tracing drifts away from the center of the graph paper (Figure 4-7). Baseline shift can have many causes. Typically, it is due to improper electrode application such as the following:

- Too loose or incorrect electrode application
- Tension or pulling on electrode lead wires
- Too little electrode gel or solution
- Old or dried-out electrode gel or solution
- Corroded or dirty electrodes
- Oil, lotion, dirt, or hair under the electrodes
- Poor or no skin preparation

To avoid problems with wandering baseline, apply the electrodes securely and make sure they are not too loose or too tight. Be certain that the entire surface is in contact with the patient's skin. Check the lead wires and remove any tension from them. Use fresh electrode gel or new disposable electrodes. Make sure that previously opened electrodes have been stored in a plastic bag or container. Clean the reusable leads after each use. Clean the patient's skin carefully before applying electrodes.

Figure 4-7 Wandering baseline occurs when the baseline of the ECG tracing drifts away from the center of the ECG graph paper.

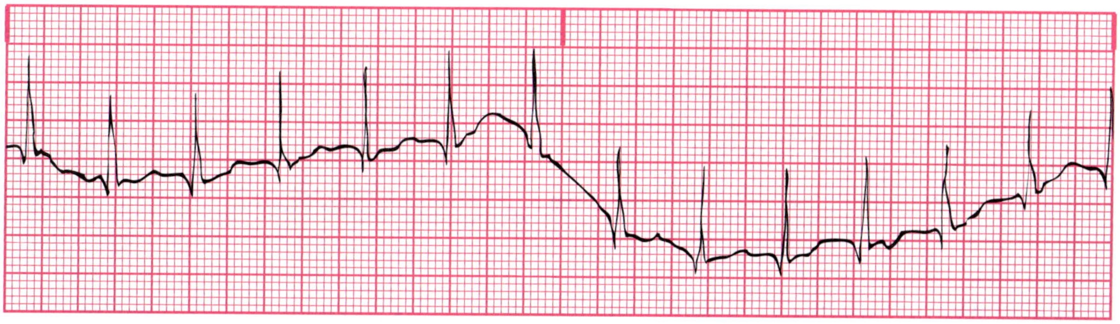

Figure 4-8 Alternating current (AC) interference appears as uniform small spikes on the ECG tracing.

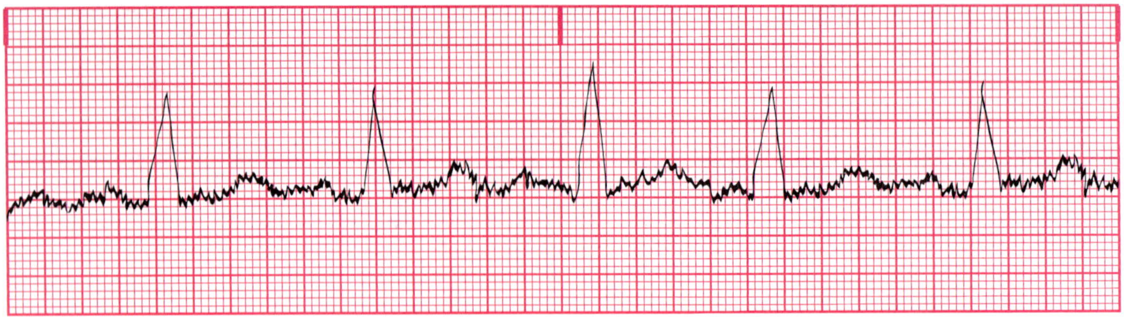

Alternating Current (AC) Interference

alternating current (AC) interference Unwanted markings on the ECG caused by other electrical current sources.

Alternating current is normally present in all electrical equipment and wiring in the walls. Sometimes the wires can radiate or leak a small amount of energy into the immediate surrounding area. When a patient is present in this area, the patient's body may pick up some of the current. This current is then registered on the ECG and is called **alternating current (AC) interference.** AC interference appears as uniform small spikes on the ECG tracing (Figure 4-8).

Many different things can cause AC interference artifact. These include improper grounding, other electrical equipment, or, on rare occasions, lead wires crossed. Eliminating the cause and using proper technique can prevent AC interference artifact. Eliminating sources of electrical current, ensuring proper grounding of the machine, and attaching the lead wires correctly can reduce AC interference.

The cause of AC interference is sometimes difficult to determine. You may still have AC interference even after you have checked that the machine is properly grounded, the lead wires are correct, and other equipment is turned off. In order to find the source, time permitting, you can try this technique. Run leads I, II, and III and look for interference. Evaluate each strip for interference to determine the direction or source of interference (Table 4-7). For example, if you have the most interference in leads II and III, the source is probably near or on the left leg. You may need to rotate the bed or exam table at a 45-degree angle away from the source. Also, do not forget the proper placement of the lead cables. They should follow the body contours and be lying flat against the skin. In addition, the power cord should not touch the bed or exam table frame. This is another possible source of electrical interference.

Artifact can also be caused by other sources. High-tension wires and transformers on a power pole and diathermy machines that use high-frequency currents to provide heat for heat treatments can cause AC

TABLE 4-7 Troubleshooting AC Interference

Leads with Most AC Interference Noted	Source of Interference or Direction
Leads I and II	Right arm
Leads I and III	Left arm
Leads II and III	Left leg

interference. Electrocautery, IV pumps, feeding tubes, and x-ray machines can also interfere if they are in the room or an adjacent room. Even the electrical wires in the walls, ceiling, and floor, although they are not visible, can cause artifact. Most ECG machines have a battery that allows you to unplug the machine from the electrical outlet and still perform the ECG. Unplugging the machine eliminates any AC interference that may be produced from the electrical outlet.

Troubleshooting

Handling a Flat-Line Tracing

If a flat line without deflections occurs during the tracing, it could be asystole (absence of a heartbeat). Remain calm and check the patient first because the patient is your number one concern. If the patient is able to respond, check the electrodes, lead wires, and cables.

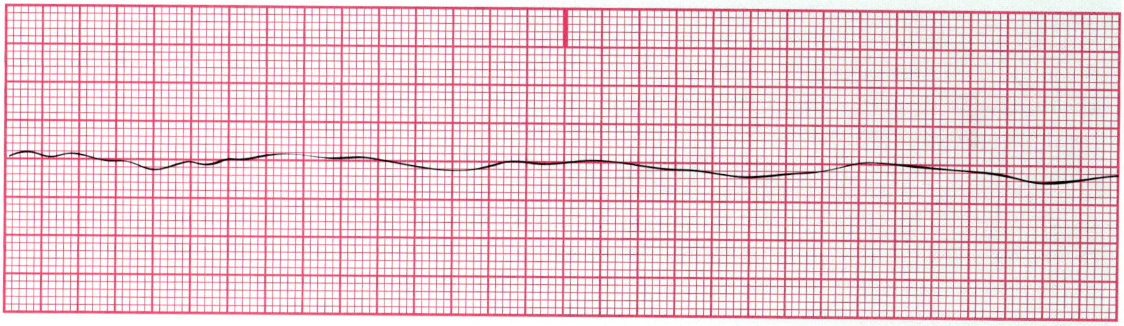

The patient's ECG tracing looks like the one pictured here. What should you do?

____

Other Problems

There are some additional problems you may encounter when obtaining an ECG. One example is an interrupted baseline on one or more leads. This appears as a flat line on the tracing. This could occur when a wire is not plugged in correctly or is loose. If a flat line occurs on more than one lead, it may be that the wires have been switched. Check your machine cables and connections. Ensure that the machine is set to obtain a tracing. Do not forget to check for loose or broken lead wires, which may also cause a break in the complexes or an interrupted baseline.

After troubleshooting any problem, if you cannot correct it, report it to your supervisor. If it is an AC interference problem, the biomedical engineering department, if available, may need to track down the source of the interference. It could also be that the machine requires service. In this case, the manufacturer should be called for information and assistance.

Checkpoint Questions (LO 4.7)

1. What is the most likely cause of the following artifact?

____

____

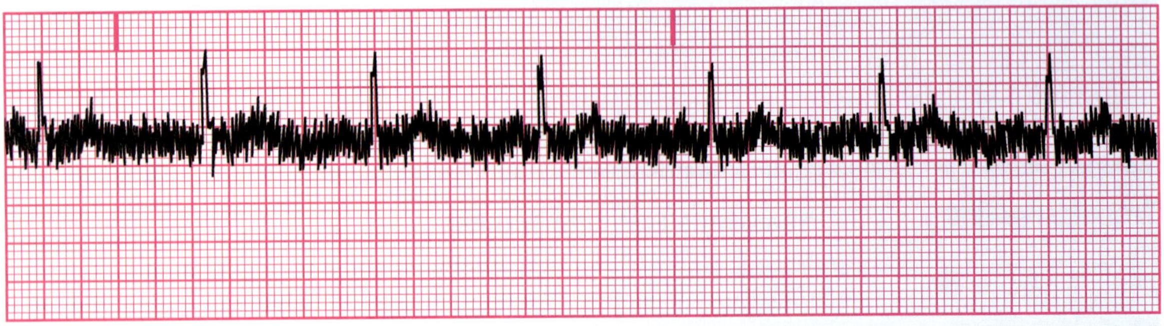

2. Name three causes of wandering baseline.

____

____

4.8 Reporting ECG Results

When you have completed an ECG, use the method your facility requires for reporting the results. Check your facility policy to be certain you are placing the completed ECG tracings in the appropriate place. In many situations, you will be required to make two copies, one to be placed on the patient's chart and the other to be read by the consulting physician. In the hospital, the second copy is often taken back to the ECG department or stored on the computer for evaluation in the ECG laboratory. The second copy may also be placed in a box at the nursing station where the patient is located. In an ambulatory care facility, it may be attached to the front of the chart and/or placed on the physician's desk.

Some facilities have a computer that can read the ECG electronically and store it in a central database for future reference. In addition, sometimes ECG tracings are faxed or electronically sent to other locations. These procedures require special equipment. You may be asked to perform either of these procedures. If so, you must be trained using your facility's equipment. If the ECG was ordered stat (immediately), you will need to give the results directly and immediately to your superior or the physician. If your supervisor is not available, ensure that the results are with the medical record, then find your supervisor or the ordering physician and notify him or her that the ECG has been completed. Remember, in a stat situation the patient may have a condition that needs immediate treatment, and no time should be wasted.

Billing is another issue to consider when reporting completion of an ECG. When you enter the data into the machine or on the designated form, they must be complete and accurate. If the patient is not charged for the procedure, this can have an adverse effect on the hospital's finances and subsequently on your job. Check the facility policy to be certain you have completed the necessary steps to ensure that the patient will be charged.

In many facilities, the information is entered into a computer to be sent to the billing department. You may need to enter the patient's diagnosis, which is provided by the physician and is found on the chart. Each diagnosis has a special diagnostic code, known as an ICD-10 code. In most cases, you will need to identify the correct ICD-10 code when entering the information for the billing department. Using these codes helps ensure that the facility is reimbursed for the procedure.

Checkpoint Questions (LO 4.8)

1. How should you report a stat ECG?

____

____

2. Why is it critical to enter the correct and complete data into the computer when performing an ECG?

____

____

4.9 Equipment Maintenance

Care and maintenance of the ECG machine is your responsibility. Become familiar with the manufacturer's instructions for operation and maintenance of the ECG machine. The operator's manual for the machine you are using will include specific directions about routine care and maintenance. General day-to-day care and maintenance include cleaning the ECG machine and stocking the supplies, such as electrodes, skin preparation, paper, and cleaning supplies.

Safety & Infection Control

Maintaining the ECG Equipment

Cleaning the ECG machine and maintaining the supplies are necessary for safe and efficient ECG recording and accurate tracings.

Keep the ECG machine clean to prevent transmission of infection and to create a positive image of yourself and the facility where you are employed. Use a small amount of nonabrasive cleaner on the equipment case, cover, and control panel. Wipe the machine dry with a soft cloth. Follow the specific directions in the operator's manual for the disinfection procedure.

The cables and electrode clips should be disinfected frequently. Use a soft cloth moistened with disinfectant and wipe the entire cable and clip. You can also use packaged disinfectant wipes if they are available. To determine the type of disinfectant you should use, check the policy at the facility where you are working. Keep these available on the ECG cart. Do not place the cables or ECG machine in fluid or use heat sterilization. Do not use acetone, ether, or other harsh chemicals or solvents. Always follow the manufacturer's directions for best results.

Carefully maintain the alligator clips used to attach the lead wires to the electrodes. Check them to ensure that the pins fit snugly on the electrode. Check for small amounts of electrolyte paste or gel that may cling to the clips. These bits of paste may prevent good contact with the electrodes (Figure 4-9).

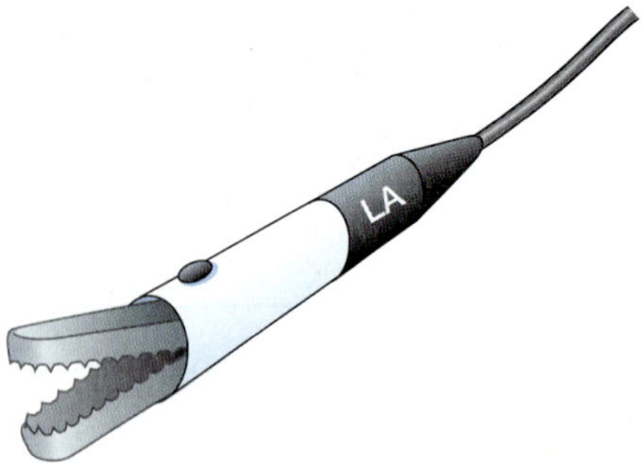

Figure 4-9 This alligator-type clip is frequently used to attach lead wires to the electrodes. Wipe the clips clean after use to prevent electrolyte gel or paste from getting stuck between the teeth of the clip.

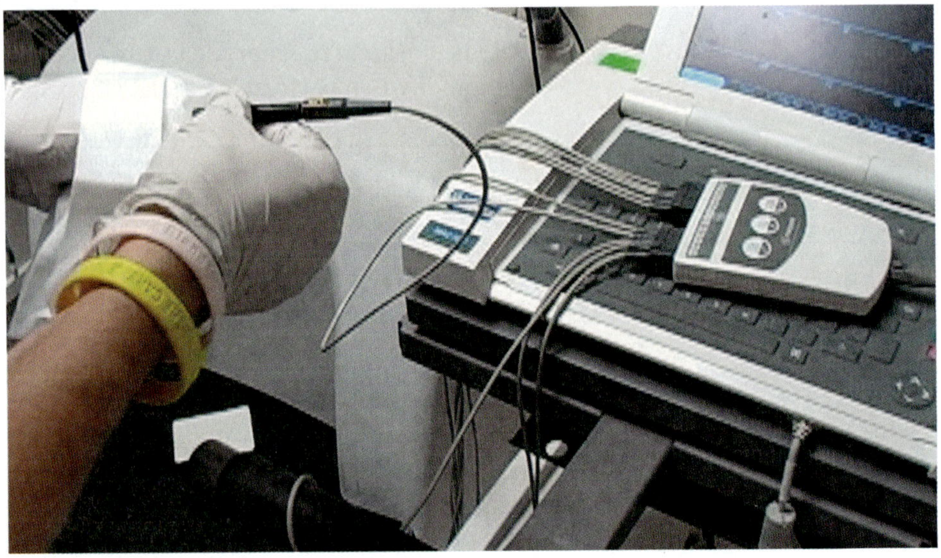

Figure 4-10 Before storing, clean each lead wire and clip with disinfectant. For safety, inspect each wire for cracks or fraying.

Wipe down the patient cables and lead wires with a damp cloth. Replace them neatly on the ECG machine for storage (Figure 4-10). Inspect them regularly for cracks or fraying. Replace any cables that are damaged. See Procedure Checklist 4-1 at the end of this chapter to practice recording an ECG.

Checkpoint Question (LO 4.9)

1. Why should you know how to troubleshoot and maintain the equipment for an ECG?

____

____

4.10 Pediatric ECG

When preparing a child for an ECG, it is important to give simple directions that he or she can understand. Identify yourself and explain what you are going to do. Allow the child to ask questions. Avoid technical words like *electrodes* and *electrocardiogram.* Use the word *stickers* to describe electrodes. If the child is fearful of the "stickers," allow him to place the stickers on a toy, doll, or parent. This will show the child that the procedure does not hurt. Explain that you are going to take a "picture" of the child's heart. Because children can usually identify with picture taking, this will help them understand that they need to be still during the "picture."

Figure 4-11 For infants and small children, you may need to place V3 on the right side of the chest to prevent crowding of the chest electrodes. This alternate method of placement is known as V3R and is sometimes used on adults as well.

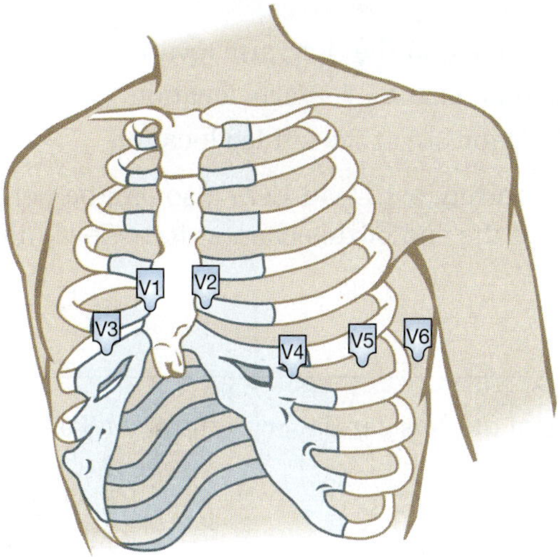

Always identify the child by name and check his or her identification wristband. If the parents are present, you may allow them to stay. For a small child or infant, the parent can assist by letting the child lie quietly in his or her arms. A fussy infant may be soothed using a pacifier. If you are unable to soothe an irritable infant, you may need to wait until he or she falls asleep. For older children, you can allow them to apply their own arm and leg electrodes. Adolescents may prefer to be alone with you during the procedure. Ask them if they would like their parent(s) to stay or leave.

When the ECG tracing is completed, talk about the procedure. Give verbal praise and be supportive. Reward the child with an age-appropriate item or activity such as stickers or a special trip to the playroom.

Smaller, pediatric electrodes are available and should be used for pediatric patients. In addition, for infants or children with very fast heart rates, you may find it necessary to adjust the paper speed to 50 mm/sec. This will allow the physician to view each of the deflections on the ECG tracing. If you make this adjustment, don't forget to note on the ECG recording when completed.

An ECG for a child is performed with the same lead placement as for an adult. The chest lead V6 must be placed exactly on the midaxillary line. Because of the small size of the chest, correct placement becomes even more important. Small differences in placement can make a difference in the ECG tracing. Because of crowding on the chest, it may be necessary to move the V3 lead to the right side of the chest. It should be placed on the right side in the same location as it normally would be on the left. This is known as a V3 right (V3R) (Figure 4-11).

Checkpoint Questions (LO 4.10)

1. Why do you frequently need to adjust the paper speed to 50 mm/sec for infants and small children?

____

____

2. When you change the paper speed to 50 mm/sec, what else should you do?

____

____

4.11 Cardiac Monitoring

Patients may require continuous cardiac monitoring at the scene of an emergency, in the hospital during or after surgery, or when they have cardiac, pulmonary, or electrolyte problems. In addition to the cables, monitor, and disposable supplies (electrodes), the monitoring systems used in a hospital may include devices that monitor the heart rate and rhythm, blood pressure, cardiac output, and arterial blood oxygen saturation.

During continuous cardiac monitoring, typically either lead II or a modified chest lead (MCL) is used because they provide the best ability to view the P wave. Exact placement of the electrodes affects the view of the heart and the resulting waveform. Three electrodes are placed, and the placement may vary depending on the system used.

- White cable with electrode (labeled RA) at the right arm location
- Black cable with electrode (labeled LA) at the left arm location
- Red cable with electrode (labeled F or LL) at the left leg location

During continuous cardiac monitoring, a 12-lead ECG also can be performed. See Procedure Checklist 4-2 at the end of this chapter to review and practice this procedure.

Checkpoint Question (LO 4.11)

1. What is the difference between continuous cardiac monitoring and a routine ECG?

____

____

4.12 Special Patient Considerations

Occasionally you will need to record lead tracings other than the basic 12. You may need to record a heart rhythm strip, which is a single strip showing only one lead tracing. The heart rhythm is usually produced in lead II and is about 10 seconds of running time. Many ECG machines will print this strip on the bottom of the 12-lead tracing or following the completion of the 12-lead recording. A rhythm strip is used to check for heart rhythm abnormalities. You may also be asked to provide a V4R (a tracing run with V4 placed on the right side of the chest) on an adult for cases of right ventricular infarction.

You may encounter other circumstances that require you to make modifications to the basic 12-lead procedure. When changes in the placement of leads is necessary for any reason, a note should be included on the tracing. Consider the following when placing leads and recording tracings in a patient's chart:

- V1 and V2 may have to be placed higher due to breast implants or patients with large breasts. See Figure 4-12.
- Do not place the electrode on a woman's breast. Move the breast with the back of your hand and place the electrode under it. If this is done, note on the ECG tracing that the electrodes (V3, V4, and V5) are placed lower than required.
- If a woman has had a mastectomy, be careful placing the electrodes—the skin may be fragile. Note that the patient had a mastectomy and which breast is affected on the ECG tracing: "(L), (R), or bilateral mastectomy."
- If the patient is an amputee, place the limb leads on the upper chest and lower abdomen instead of on the arms and legs. Make sure the leads are in the same place on each side of the body.

Figure 4-12 Leads V1 and V2 are placed higher on the chest for patients with large breasts.

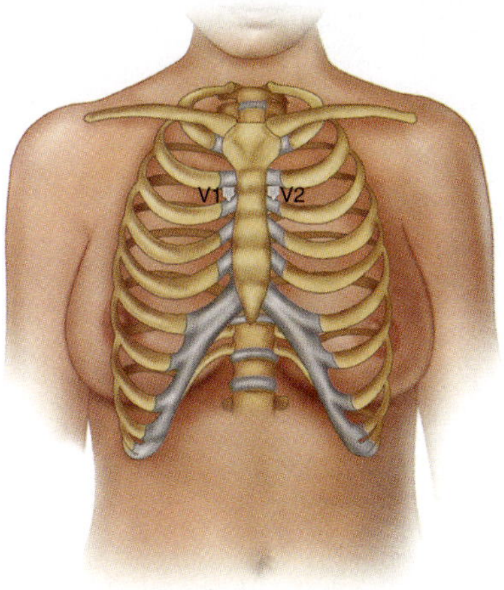

- Alternate locations may be necessary due to interference from burns, dressings, chest tubes, and so on. Remember to document if electrodes are moved to a different location and why.
- A pregnant woman should have the lower limb leads placed on the thighs, not the abdomen. Place the patient on her left side slightly, by using a small rolled towel under the right hip to reduce pressure on the inferior vena cava. Document on the ECG that the patient is pregnant and the number of months.
- Geriatric patients generally have thin skin, which is part of the normal aging process. Apply the electrodes carefully and remove gently to prevent damage to their skin. You may need to use adhesive remover to break the adhesive bond of the sensors. This significantly reduces the risk of tearing the skin. Geriatric patients may have some readings on the ECG tracing that are age-related and are considered normal.
- If the patient is unable to lie on his or her back, be sure to indicate on the tracing the position of the patient during the tracing.
- When someone is in a permanent fetal position with arms drawn tightly over the chest, you may need to place the electrodes on the back. They will need to be positioned over the heart on the left side of the back. Today's small, thin, disposable electrodes are easier to place under a patient's arms, so place on the back only if necessary.
- When the heart is on the right side of the chest rather than on the left, a condition known as **dextrocardia,** the physician will order a right-side 12-lead ECG (described below). This is the only case in which the aVR tracing will produce a positive deflection. On the ECG tracing report, you should indicate that you did a right-side ECG.

dextrocardia When the heart is on the opposite or right side of the chest.

You may be asked to perform a right-side or posterior ECG as ordered by the physician. These expanded data tracings enable the physician to detect problems with the right ventricle and posterior wall of the left ventricle.

The right-side 12-lead ECG has chest leads placed in a "mirror image" of the standard 12-lead ECG. They are placed at the same anatomic levels but on the opposite side of the chest. V1 is placed on the 4th intercostal space, left sternal margin; V2 is placed on the 4th intercostal space, right sternal margin; and so on, continuing to the patient's right. See Figure 4-13. The chest leads are commonly identified as V1R, V2R, V3R, V4R, V5R, and V6R. These additional leads are periodically requested by the physician after a standard 12-lead ECG has been obtained.

The *posterior 12-lead ECG* (or leads on the patient's back) focuses on the posterior aspect of the heart. As shown in Figure 4-14, the chest leads are identified as V7, V8, and V9 (posterior left chest) and V9R, V8R, and V7R (posterior right chest) and are placed as follows:

posterior axillary line Imaginary line on the back that runs vertically from the shoulder down on the outer edge of the rib cage.

midscapular line Imaginary line on the back that runs vertically through the center of the scapula.

- **V7** is located at the left **posterior axillary line** (an imaginary line on the back of the chest that runs vertically from the shoulder down on the outer edge of the rib cage) in a straight line from V6. You will reposition the V1 lead to this location.
- **V8** is located at the left **midscapular line** (an imaginary line on the back of the chest that runs vertically through the center of the scapula) in a

Figure 4-13 Use these lead placements for patients with dextrocardia, a condition in which the left ventricle, left atrium, and aortic arch are located on the right side of the chest.

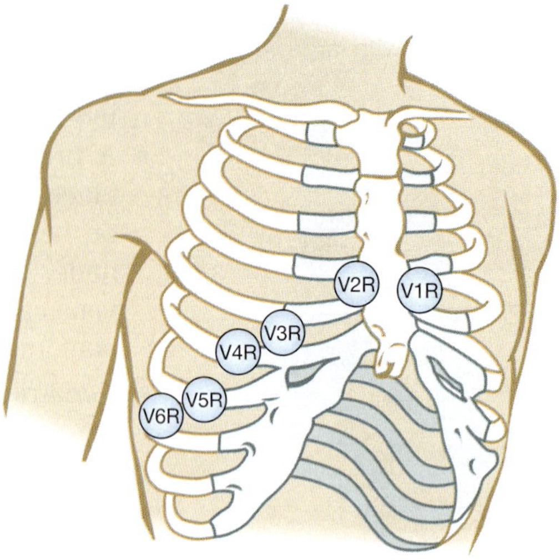

Figure 4-14 Posterior 12-lead locations. Cables V1 through V6 are placed going from the patient's posterior left in order to the patient's posterior right.

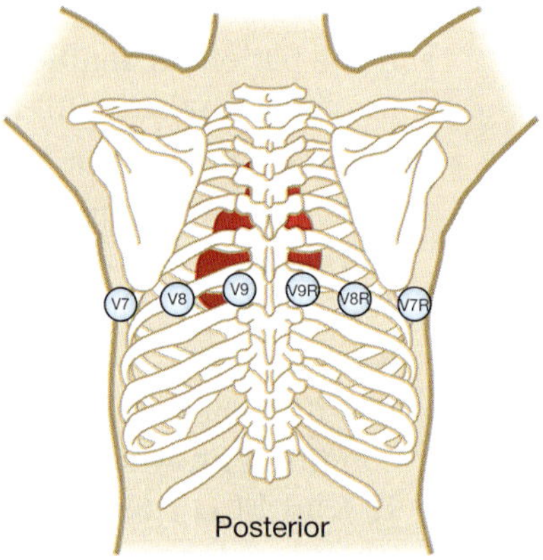

- V7: Left posterior axillary line, V6 level (Use Cable V1)
- V8: V8 (skip) place at midpoint on a horizontal line between V7 and V9 (Use Cable V2)
- V9: Left paraspinous border, V6 level (Use Cable V3)
- V9R: Right paraspinous border (Use Cable V4)
- V8R: V8R (skip) place at midpoint on a horizontal line between V7R and V9R (Use Cable V5)
- V7R: Right posterior axillary line (Use Cable V6)

straight line horizontally from V7; it will be placed halfway between V7 and V9. You will reposition the V2 lead to this location. Skip V8 until you have placed V9.

paraspinous line Imaginary line on the spine that runs vertically through the side of the spine.

- **V9** is located at the left **paraspinous line** (an imaginary line next to the spine that runs vertically along the side of the spine) in a straight line from the V7 lead. You will move the V3 lead to this location. (Go back and place V8 halfway between V7 and V9 in a straight line.)
- **V9R** is placed at the right paraspinous line in a straight line from the V9 lead. You will reposition the V4 lead to this location.

- **V8R** is located at the right midscapular line in a straight line from V7; it will be placed halfway between V7R and V9R. You will reposition the V5 lead to this location.
- **V7R** is located at the right posterior axillary line. You will reposition the V6 lead to this location (see Figure 4-14).

When you record any ECG tracing, it is critical that you indicate any modification in electrode placement. The position of the electrodes affects the ECG tracing because the electrodes are focused on a different aspect of the heart and could potentially provide the wrong information if not noted.

Some facilities have specialized equipment for these less common tracings, but it is not essential. You can obtain the ECG tracing by adding these leads with the standard 12-lead ECG machine. This procedure can be simple when you know where to place the electrodes. First, run a standard 12-lead ECG as described earlier. Second, using the precordial cables (V1–V6), place additional electrodes in the appropriate locations and run a second 12-lead ECG. It is important that you do not forget to write on the labels of the new leads.

Note: Limb lead cables and electrode locations do not change. Only the chest leads and electrodes are changed.

Checkpoint Questions (LO 4.12)

1. What should you remember when asked to record a right-side or posterior ECG?

____

____

2. What additional ECG procedure may the doctor order for a patient with dextrocardia? Why?

____

____

4.13 Handling Emergencies

Cardiac or Respiratory Arrest

During a cardiac or respiratory arrest, frequently called a Code Blue emergency, be ready to perform the tracing as quickly and efficiently as possible. An ECG is usually ordered "stat" in these situations. If possible, enter the patient's information into the ECG machine. Remain available but out of the way until the ECG is needed. You may need to take just the machine into the room and not the cart, if space is limited.

Because the patient's condition changes frequently during a Code Blue emergency, you may need to perform two ECGs in a row. Perform the first ECG and leave the electrodes in place in order to perform the second ECG quickly. Indicate on the tracing "repeat ECG—same lead placement." This will make the physician aware that the electrodes were not removed between tracings.

seizure An interruption of the electrical activity in the brain that causes involuntary muscle movement and sometimes unconsciousness.

Seizure

If a patient has a **seizure** during the ECG, stay with him or her. Protect the patient from injury. Do not try to restrain the patient. Call for help, and report the seizure. Once the seizure is over, perform the ECG again and write on the ECG strip "postseizure."

Checkpoint Question (LO 4.13)

1. What should you do if your patient has a seizure while you are starting to record an ECG?

____

____

Chapter Summary

Learning Outcomes	Summary	Pages
4.1 Carry out preparation of the patient, room, and equipment for an ECG.	The patient, the room, and the equipment must be properly prepared prior to performing an ECG.	83–84
4.2 Describe the communication needed during the ECG procedure, including the actions to take if a patient refuses to allow an ECG to be performed.	When a patient refuses an ECG, you should identify the cause, alleviate any fears, and, if the patient still refuses, notify your supervisor and document the refusal on the medical record.	84–86
4.3 Identify the anatomical landmarks that are used to apply the ECG chest electrodes to the correct locations.	In order to place the electrodes properly for an ECG, you must be able to locate anatomical landmarks, including the midclavicular line, anterior axillary line, intercostal spaces, suprasternal notch, and angle of Louis.	86–87
4.4 Demonstrate the procedure for applying the electrodes and lead wires for a 12-lead ECG and cardiac monitoring.	An ECG is performed using the ECG machine, lead wires, and electrodes. The patient must be identified correctly, the tracing must be correct, and safety must be maintained during the procedure.	88–91
4.5 Identify at least three ways to prevent infection and provide for safety during the ECG procedure.	To ensure safety and prevent infection during an ECG: • Follow standard precautions; most importantly, hand hygiene. • Follow isolation precautions and use personal protective equipment when necessary. • Check the plug and power cord. • Raise the bed and keep the side rail up. • Use two patient identifiers before the procedure.	91–94
4.6 Describe the procedure for recording a 12-lead ECG.	The ECG procedure includes identifying, communicating with, and preparing the patient; maintaining safety, privacy, and infection control; checking and preparing the room and equipment; attaching the electrodes and leads; and then operating the ECG machine and reporting the results.	94–95

(Continued)

Learning Outcomes	Summary	Pages
4.7 Identify types of artifact and how to prevent or correct them.	Three types of artifact include: • Somatic tremor caused by muscle movement • Wandering baseline, usually caused by improperly applied electrodes or poor skin prep • AC interference, caused by some type of electrical interference	95–100
4.8 Describe how to report the ECG results.	ECGs are recorded electronically and in paper fashion. Although they may be "read" by the machine, they must be provided promptly in a proper format to the practitioner who will be interpreting them.	100–101
4.9 Identify the steps for cleaning and caring for the ECG equipment.	Upon completion of an ECG, the equipment must be cleaned and stored properly according to your facility guidelines and the manufacturer's recommendations.	101–102
4.10 Explain variations for a pediatric ECG procedure.	During a pediatric ECG, the chest lead V3 may need to be placed on the right side of the chest due to the small size of the chest.	102–103
4.11 Distinguish between a routine ECG and cardiac monitoring.	Cardiac monitoring uses three leads with different placements.	103–104
4.12 Summarize special patient circumstances when performing an ECG.	Many special patient considerations can occur during an ECG, such as for female patients, pregnant patients, amputees, and geriatric patients.	104–107
4.13 Recall the steps for handling an emergency during the ECG.	During a cardiac or respiratory arrest, perform the ECG stat; in some cases, take just the machine into the room and be prepared to run two ECGs in a row. During a seizure, remain calm, do not restrain the patient, and call for help.	107–108

Chapter Review

Matching I

Match the landmarks on the left with their locations on the right. (LO 4.3)

_______ **1.** suprasternal notch

_______ **2.** fifth intercostal space

_______ **3.** manubrium

_______ **4.** right clavicle

a. extends from the sternum to the scapula
b. the space between the fifth and sixth ribs
c. the top of the sternum
d. the dip at the base of the neck just above where the clavicle attaches to the sternum

Match the leads on the left with their correct placement on the right. (LO 4.4)

_______ **5.** V1

_______ **6.** V2

_______ **7.** V3

_______ **8.** V4

_______ **9.** V5

_______ **10.** V6

a. fifth intercostal space, at the anterior axillary line
b. fourth intercostal space, left sternal border
c. fifth intercostal space at the midaxillary line
d. fifth intercostal space at the midclavicular line
e. fourth intercostal space, right sternal border
f. halfway between V2 and V4

Match the imaginary lines on the left with their locations on the right. (LO 4.3)

_______ **11.** midclavicular line

_______ **12.** midaxillary line

_______ **13.** anterior axillary line

a. front of the axilla
b. middle of the axilla
c. usually passes through the nipple line

Multiple Choice

Circle the correct answer.

14. For placement of the electrodes, how is the ICS located? (LO 4.3)
a. Locating the sternum and feeling for a dip at the edge
b. Finding the ribs near the nipple line
c. Locating the clavicle and feeling for a dent directly below it
d. Locating the space between the clavicle and V4

15. What would be the first and most appropriate thing to say if a patient refuses an ECG? (LO 4.2)
a. "Will you tell me why you don't wish to have an ECG done?"
b. "Don't worry; it takes only a few seconds."
c. "Your doctor has ordered this test, and it must be done."
d. "I will have to report your refusal to my supervisor."

16. When applying chest leads, V4 is placed (LO 4.4)
   a. midway between V3 and V5.
   b. at the fourth ICS, right sternal border.
   c. at the fifth ICS, left midclavicular line.
   d. at the fourth ICS, left sternal border.

17. When applying chest leads, V2 is placed (LO 4.4)
   a. midway between V3 and V5.
   b. at the fourth ICS, right sternal border.
   c. at the fifth ICS, left midclavicular line.
   d. at the fourth ICS, left sternal border.

18. To prevent disease transmission during an ECG, you should (LO 4.5)
   a. check the ground prong.
   b. wash your hands.
   c. raise the side rail.
   d. lower the bed.

19. Safety procedures specific to the ECG include which of the following? (LO 4.5)
   a. Wash hands; clean up all spills immediately.
   b. Lower bed; raise the side rail.
   c. Check the ground prong; give the patient the call signal.
   d. Check the lead wires, insulation, and ground prong.

20. Which of the following would *not* be done prior to performing an ECG? (LO 4.1)
   a. Receive and validate the order.
   b. Write ECG variations on tracing.
   c. Check and change paper if necessary.
   d. Enter patient data into the machine.

21. When applying chest leads, V1 is placed (LO 4.4)
   a. midway between V3 and V5.
   b. at the fourth ICS, right sternal border.
   c. at the fifth ICS, left midclavicular line.
   d. at the fourth ICS, left sternal border.

22. Marks on the ECG tracing caused by another source of activity are (LO 4.7)
   a. asystole.
   b. conduction marks.
   c. artifact.
   d. arrhythmias.

23. Somatic tremors are caused by (LO 4.7)
   a. electrical current leak.
   b. tracing drifts away from the center.
   c. muscle movement.
   d. contact with another electrical device.

24. You noticed a wandering baseline on the ECG tracing. What measure(s) should you take to correct the problem? (LO 4.7)
   a. Apply new electrodes.
   b. Reposition the electrodes.
   c. Ensure that the wires are not crossed.
   d. All of the answers are correct.

25. You notice that leads I and II have a lot of artifact while recording a 12-lead ECG. Which electrode is probably not placed appropriately? (LO 4.6)
   a. Right arm
   b. Left arm
   c. Left leg
   d. None of the answers are correct

26. Which of the following is *not* a specific type of isolation precaution implemented for hospitalized patients? (LO 4.5)
   a. AIDS precautions
   b. Droplet precautions
   c. Airborne precautions
   d. Contact precautions

27. Which of the following are ways to correct AC interference? (LO 4.7)
   a. Unplug electrical equipment; move bed away from wall.
   b. Apply electrodes securely; remove tension from lead wires.
   c. Have patient place hands under his or her buttocks; remind patient not to move.
   d. Replace loose electrodes; have the patient turn slightly to the side.

28. Which of the following are ways to correct somatic tremor? (LO 4.7)
   a. Unplug electrical equipment; move bed away from wall.
   b. Apply electrodes securely; remove tension from lead wires.
   c. Have patient place hands under his or her buttocks; remind patient not to move.
   d. Replace loose electrodes; have the patient turn slightly to the side.

29. Which of the following are ways to correct wandering baseline? (LO 4.7)
   a. Unplug electrical equipment; move bed away from wall.
   b. Apply electrodes securely; remove tension from lead wires.
   c. Have patient place hands under his or her buttocks; remind patient not to move.
   d. Replace loose electrodes; have the patient turn slightly to the side.

30. When applying chest leads, V6 is placed (LO 4.3)
   a. in line with V4 on the midaxillary line.
   b. at the fourth ICS, right sternal border.
   c. at the fifth ICS, left midclavicular line.
   d. at the fourth ICS, left sternal border.

31. If your patient has an amputated left lower leg, where should you place the electrodes? (LO 4.11)
   a. LL on left upper leg, RL on right lower leg
   b. LL on left lower abdomen, RL on right lower abdomen
   c. LL on left lower leg, RL on right upper leg
   d. LL on left lower abdomen, RL on right lower leg

32. When performing a 12-lead ECG on an infant or small child, do all of the following *except* (LO 4.10)
   a. speak in children's terms.
   b. use smaller ECG electrodes.
   c. perform a V3R tracing.
   d. use a special ECG machine.

33. Approach the patient from the _____ when performing an ECG. (LO 4.6)
   a. left side
   b. right side
   c. top
   d. bottom

True/False

Read each statement and determine if it is true or false. Circle the T or F. For false (F) statements, correct them on the lines provided.

T F 34. Natural skin oils, moisturizers, and perspiration can contribute to artifact on an ECG tracing. (LO 4.7)

____

T F 35. The letter *R* is placed after any tracing when the electrode is not in its usual position and has been placed on the right side of the patient's chest. (LO 4.11)

____

T F 36. Because an ECG is *not* an invasive procedure, it is not necessary to wear personal protective equipment (PPE) when performing this procedure under any circumstances. (LO 4.5)

____

Matching II

Match the terms on the left with their definitions on the right.

______ **37.** intercostal space (ICS) (LO 4.3)

______ **38.** midaxillary line (LO 4.3)

______ **39.** stat (LO 4.12)

______ **40.** anterior axillary line (LO 4.3)

______ **41.** artifact (LO 4.7)

______ **42.** seizure (LO 4.12)

______ **43.** midclavicular line (LO 4.3)

______ **44.** somatic tremor (LO 4.7)

______ **45.** angle of Louis (LO 4.3)

______ **46.** AC interference (LO 4.7)

______ **47.** wandering baseline (LO 4.7)

______ **48.** sternal border (LO 4.3)

______ **49.** dextrocardia (LO 4.11)

______ **50.** midscapular line (LO 4.3)

a. an interruption of the electrical activity of the brain that causes involuntary muscle movement and sometimes unconsciousness

b. a bony prominence located approximately 1 inch below the suprasternal notch, where the manubrium and the body of the sternum are joined

c. outer edge of the sternum

d. the space between two ribs

e. an imaginary line on the chest that runs vertically through the center of the clavicle

f. drifting of an ECG tracing away from the center of the paper; also called baseline shift

g. an imaginary vertical line that starts in the middle of the axillary region (armpit)

h. unwanted marks on the ECG caused by electrical activity from sources other than the heart

i. unwanted markings on the ECG tracing caused by other electrical sources

j. an imaginary vertical line on the back that starts in the middle of the scapula

k. immediately

l. voluntary or involuntary muscle movement; also known as body tremor

m. an imaginary vertical line starting at the edge of the chest where the axillary region begins

n. condition in which the heart is on the reverse side of the chest

Identification

51. (1.–9.) Identify the landmarks on the chest drawing by writing the names on the lines provided. (LO 4.3)

1. ____________________
2. ____________________
3. ____________________
4. ____________________
5. ____________________
6. ____________________
7. ____________________
8. ____________________
9. ____________________

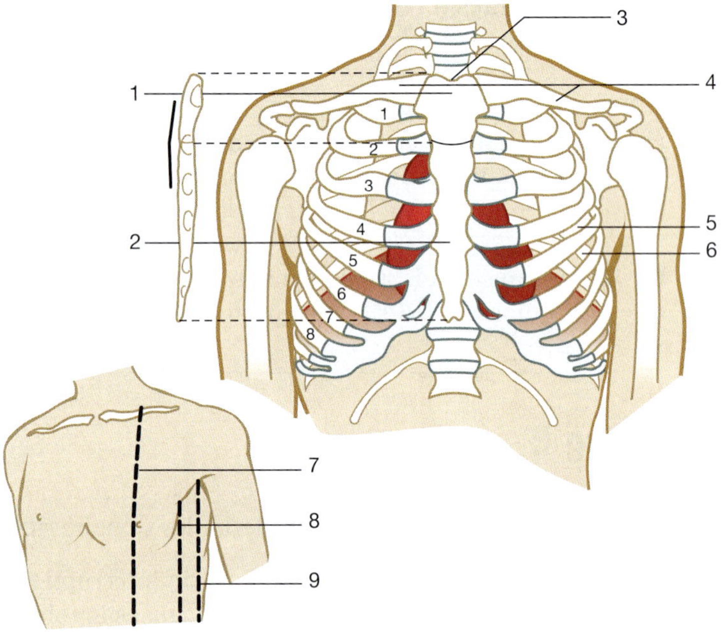

52. Identify each lead and describe its location for a 12-lead ECG by writing on the lines provided. (LO 4.4)

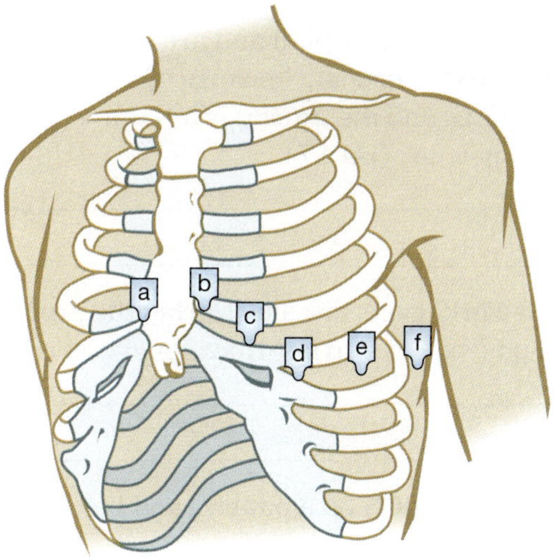

a. ______________________________

b. ______________________________

c. ______________________________

d. ______________________________

e. ______________________________

f. ______________________________

Critical Thinking Application *What Should You Do?*

Read the following situations, and use your critical thinking skills to determine how you would handle each. Write your answer in detail in the space provided.

53. You are working in a local hospital and are called to perform an ECG on a patient who is in a coma and was admitted to the hospital because of a myocardial infarction. You set up the machine and begin to run the ECG, and the tracing is a flat line. You know that a flat line is serious. What would be the first thing you do? (LO 4.7)

____

____

54. Your patient has Parkinson's disease. During the procedure, you notice a lot of artifact. What kind of artifact would you expect it to be? How could you reduce the artifact? (LO 4.7)

____

____

55. You are performing an ECG on a patient, and he or she begins to complain of chest pain. What should you do? (LO 4.12)

____

____

56. When you finish performing an ECG, the patient asks you for a copy. What do you do? (LO 4.8)

____

____

connect® Now that you have completed the material in the chapter text, go to Connect and complete any chapter activities you have not yet done.

Procedures

Use the following Procedure Checklists 4-1 and 4-2 to practice and perform the skills presented in this chapter. (LO 4.8 and 4.10)

PROCEDURE CHECKLIST 4-1

Recording an Electrocardiogram

	Practice		Practice		Test		Mastered	
Procedure Steps *(Rationale)*	**Yes**	**No**	**Yes**	**No**	**Yes**	**No**	**Date**	**Initials**
Preprocedure								
1. Receive and validate the order.								
2. Check the machine for proper functioning, including electrical cord, lead wires, and paper.								
3. Obtain the necessary supplies.								
4. Read the specific information from the manufacturer's instructions.								
5. Ensure that adequate paper is available.								
6. Change or add paper if necessary.								
7. Enter the data into the ECG machine if available.								
Procedure								
1. Identify the patient using two forms of identification.								
2. Explain the procedure.								
3. Wash hands.								
4. Position and prepare the patient. Ask the patient to turn off and remove electronics. (Prevents artifact)								
5. Provide for privacy and prevent exposure. (Provides comfort, alleviates stress)								
6. Ensure that the bed or exam table is not touching the wall. (Prevents artifact)								
7. Move the bed or exam table away from electrical equipment. (Prevents artifact)								
8. Ensure that the patient is not touching the headboard, footboard, or side rails. (Prevents artifact)								
9. Cleanse and prepare the skin as necessary.								
10. Apply electrodes to the limbs and chest.								

(Continued)

Procedure Steps *(Rationale)*	Practice Yes	Practice No	Practice Yes	Practice No	Test Yes	Test No	Mastered Date	Mastered Initials
Procedure (*continued*)								
11. Attach the lead wires, ensuring that no tension is on wires. Make a stress loop. (Prevents discomfort to the patient and helps prevent artifact)								
12. Enter the additional patient data in the LCD panel if necessary.								
13. Press the Run button.								
14. Check the tracing for quality. Observe for artifact.								
15. Run the additional ECG if necessary.								
16. Observe the LCD display for errors.								
17. Turn off the machine and unplug when completed.								
18. Remove the electrodes and clean the skin, if necessary.								
19. Assist the patient to a safe and comfortable position.								
Postprocedure								
1. Write on ECG tracing any variations in lead placement, reason for poor-quality tracing, or change in tracing speed. (Ensures accurate evaluation)								
2. Provide the results to the licensed practitioner.								
3. Place the completed ECG tracing in the appropriate area.								
4. Clean the leads.								
5. Drape the lead wires of the machine in an orderly fashion.								
6. Return the machine to the designated storage location.								

Comments: ______________________________

____

____

____

____

Signed

Evaluator: ______________________________

Student: ______________________________

PROCEDURE CHECKLIST 4-2

Continuous Cardiac Monitoring

Procedure Steps (*Rationale*)	Practice Yes	Practice No	Practice Yes	Practice No	Test Yes	Test No	Mastered Date	Mastered Initials
Preprocedure								
Gather the supplies and equipment: • Cardiac monitor (check monitor before applying to the patient) • Cable and lead wires • Electrodes • Skin prep supplies (i.e., alcohol, gauze pads, razor as necessary) • Gloves								
Procedure								
1. Identify the patient.								
2. Introduce yourself.								
3. Explain what you are going to do to the patient, and ask if the patient has any questions.								
4. Ask the patient to undress from the waist up (assist as necessary). Provide the patient with a gown or drape to use for privacy.								
5. Wash your hands and don medical exam gloves.								
6. Expose only the areas necessary to perform the procedure (maintain patient privacy).								
7. Select appropriate locations and prep the skin. (Brisk circular rub with dry gauze, rasp, or alcohol; let alcohol dry.) *Note:* Avoid bony prominences. • Right arm—just under the clavicle and medial to the right shoulder • Left arm—just under the clavicle and medial to the left shoulder • Left leg—upper abdomen at the margin where the abdomen and lowest rib meet								
8. Shave or clip hair if necessary (follow facility policy).								
9. Attach the electrodes to the ends of the cables.								
10. Place the white cable with electrode (labeled RA) on the right arm location.								
11. Place the black cable with electrode (labeled LA) on the left arm location.								

(*Continued*)

Procedure Steps (*Rationale*)	Practice Yes	Practice No	Practice Yes	Practice No	Test Yes	Test No	Mastered Date	Mastered Initials
Procedure (*continued*)								
12. Place the red cable with electrode (labeled F or LL) on the left leg location. *Note:* Remember to press around the outer edge of the electrode to ensure good adhesive contact with the skin. *Note:* Remember to press around the center of the electrode to ensure good gel-to-skin contact with conductive media (reduces artifact). *Note:* It may be necessary to make stress loops and tape them directly to the patient.								
13. Attach the cable clip to the sheet or patient gown to reduce tugging on electrodes (reduces artifact).								
14. Turn the cardiac monitor on and select lead II.								
15. Select the heart rate limits according to local policy.								
16. Observe the heart rate and rhythm—troubleshoot if artifact is noted.								
17. Print a rhythm strip for further analysis and reporting to licensed healthcare practitioner.								
Postprocedure								
1. Remove gloves and wash hands.								
2. Document the procedure.								

Comments: ______________________________

____

____

____

Signed

Evaluator: ______________________________

Student: ______________________________

Rhythm Strip Interpretation and Sinus Rhythms

5

Learning Outcomes

5.1 Explain the process of evaluating ECG tracings and determining the presence of dysrhythmias.

5.2 Describe the criteria used to classify dysrhythmias, including rhythm, rate, P wave morphology, PR interval measurement, and QRS duration measurement.

5.3 Identify normal sinus rhythm using the criteria for classification, and explain how the rhythm may affect the patient, including basic patient care and treatment.

5.4 Identify sinus bradycardia using the criteria for classification, and explain how the rhythm may affect the patient, including basic patient care and treatment.

5.5 Identify sinus tachycardia using the criteria for classification, and explain how the rhythm may affect the patient, including basic patient care and treatment.

5.6 Identify sinus dysrhythmia using the criteria for classification, and explain how the rhythm may affect the patient, including basic patient care and treatment.

5.7 Identify sinus arrest using the criteria for classification, and explain how the rhythm may affect the patient, including basic patient care and treatment.

Key Terms

asystole
bradycardia
cardiac output
hypotension
ischemia
J point
morphology
palpitations
stroke volume
syncope
tachycardia
vagal tone

5.1 Rhythm Interpretation

The ECG is an important tool used for the diagnosis and treatment of various cardiac and other related diseases. The recorded tracing of the ECG waveforms produced by the heart can reveal basic information about a patient's condition. The ability to evaluate various ECG waveforms is an

Figure 5-2 Measuring the P-P wave interval.

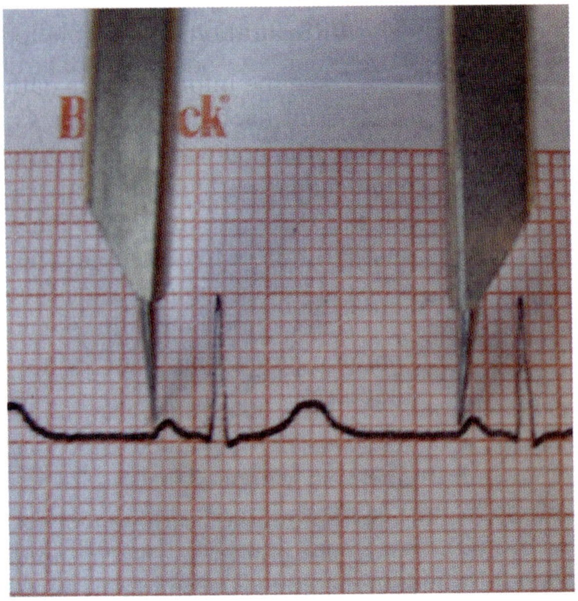

Figure 5-3 Waves, intervals, and segments.

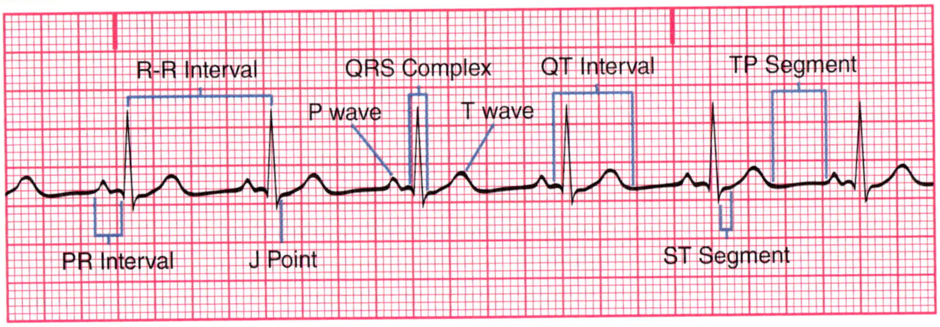

Next, determine the rhythm of the QRS complex. Because the QRS complex is a configuration of three waves, it is important to analyze this interval from the same wave in each of the QRS complexes. For example, it is often easiest to see the R wave of the QRS complex. Measuring the R-R wave interval is easy due to its upward deflection (Figure 5-3). Occasionally, the QRS complex does not exhibit an R wave, in which case you can use the point of the Q and S wave junction as an easy point of evaluation. Most importantly, you must measure the same part of the waveform for each QRS complex to determine the regularity of the ventricular depolarization. The first point of the caliper should be placed on the first QRS complex and the other point placed on the next QRS complex. The interval should be evaluated throughout at least a 6-second strip to determine the rhythm of the QRS complexes.

Step 2: Determining the Atrial and Ventricular Rates

The method used to calculate the heart rate is based on whether the rhythm is regular or irregular. The heart rate must be determined for both atria and ventricles. The atrial rate is determined by the P-P wave interval measurements, and the ventricular rate is determined by the R-R wave measurement. The atrial and ventricular rates are usually the same; sometimes, however, the rates may be different due to conditions occurring in the myocardium. It is important to note if the atrial rate is different from the ventricular rate because this will help narrow the selection of dysrhythmias. The methods used to differentiate the rates are described in the following sections.

Regular Rhythm

Once you have determined that the rhythm is regular, you can use this method to calculate the atrial and ventricular rates. The caliper interval of the P-P or R-R measurement is placed on the ECG paper to determine the number of small boxes or duration of time. (Remember that each small box is equal to 0.04 second.) Move the caliper interval to the top or the bottom of the page so that the number of boxes can be determined without interference from the ECG tracing. Once you have counted the small boxes, divide the number into 1,500 to calculate the atrial rate. The ventricular rate is determined in the same manner except you will need to count the number of boxes *between* the QRS complexes. Table 5-1 provides the heart rates based on the number of small boxes between the two P or two R waves. This method of calculation provides an accurate heart rate similar to measuring a person's pulse. The actual rate is extremely important when the heart rate is either abnormally fast or slow. These conditions are known as **tachycardia** (more than 100 beats per minute [*bpm*]) and **bradycardia** (less than 60 beats per minute).

tachycardia A fast heart rate, usually greater than 100 beats per minute

bradycardia A slow heart rate, usually less than 60 beats per minute.

Irregular Rhythm

When the rhythm is irregular, as determined in step 1, the interval between the P waves or the QRS complexes is not constant. To determine the heart rate for an irregular rhythm, use the 6-second method: multiply the number of P waves and QRS complexes in a 6-second strip by 10. This method is often used in emergencies to determine an estimated heart rate (pulse rate) for the patient.

Interpret-TIP

Many variables affect the QT interval, including heart rate, coronary heart disease, electrolyte imbalance, and antidysrhythmic medications. A shorter or longer than normal QT interval may indicate that the patient is at an increased risk for certain dysrhythmias and sudden death.

Step 3: Identifying the P Wave Morphology

Analyzing P waves and their relationship with the QRS complex is necessary to determine the type of dysrhythmia. The P wave reflects the atrial contraction and how the electrical current is moving through the atria. The relationship between the P wave and QRS complex provides information regarding the coordination between atrial and ventricular contractions. Several questions need to be answered when analyzing the P wave.

- *Are the shapes and waveforms all the same?* If they appear to be different, the current is moving through the atria using more than one pathway. Sometimes the P wave may not occur, or it may be buried within the QRS complex or the previous T wave.
- *Does each P wave have a QRS complex following it?* In normal conduction pathways, the QRS complex always follows the P wave. If there are additional P waves or QRS complexes present without a P wave, the normal conduction pathway may not have been used, and the atria and ventricles are not contracting together.

TABLE 5-1 Calculating Heart Rates with a Regular Rhythm

Small Boxes in P-P or R-R Interval	Heart Rate	Small Boxes in P-P or R-R Interval	Heart Rate	Small Boxes in P-P or R-R Interval	Heart Rate
4	375	20	75	36	42
5	300	21	71	37	40
6	250	22	68	38	39
7	214	23	65	39	38
8	188	24	62	40	38
9	167	25	60	41	37
10	150	26	58	42	36
11	136	27	55	43	35
12	125	28	54	44	34
13	115	29	52	45	33
14	107	30	50	46	33
15	100	31	48	47	32
16	94	32	47	48	31
17	88	33	45	49	31
18	83	34	44	50	30
19	79	35	43		

A rate calculator like the one shown below can also be used for regular rhythms. The start mark is placed at the first P wave or R wave, whichever you are using. Where the next consecutive P or R wave lines up is the approximate heart rate.

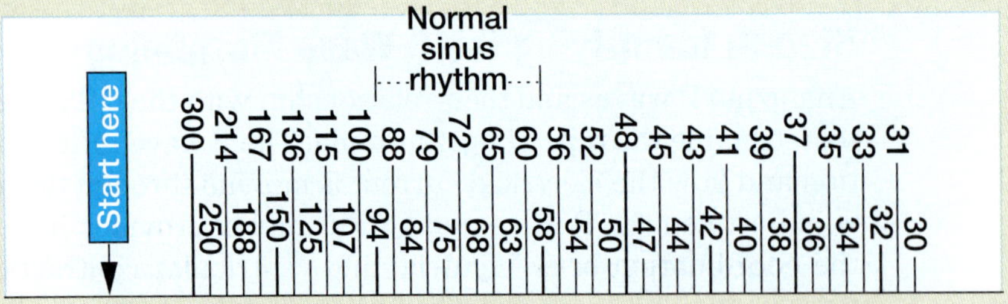

Step 4: Measuring the PR Interval

The PR interval measures the length of time it takes the electrical current to be initiated at the sinoatrial node and travel through the electrical current pathway to cause ventricular depolarization. The PR interval is determined by measuring from the beginning of the P wave to the beginning of the QRS complex. This is the first indication of ventricular depolarization. Not all tracings will show a Q wave. In the absence of a Q wave, the second caliper tip is placed at the beginning of the R wave. The normal range of the PR interval is 0.12 to 0.20 second (Figure 5-4).

Interpret-TIP

PR Interval

The smallest unit of measure for determining measurements is one-half of a small box. Remember, one small box represents 0.04 second. One half of 0.04 second is 0.02 second. When analyzing a rhythm tracing, you can measure to the nearest whole or one-half of a small box. Smaller measurements are not possible with the human eye; only a computer can read less than one-half of a box accurately. Therefore, the time interval you record should always be in multiples of 0.02 second.

PR intervals are also evaluated to ensure that the measurements are the same from one PR interval to the next. If the intervals have different measurements, either the electrical current is being delayed for some reason or it may be initiating from locations other than the sinoatrial node.

Step 5: Measuring the QRS Duration and Analyzing the Morphology

Measuring the QRS complex is essential in determining the duration of time it takes for the ventricles to depolarize or contract. This information is helpful in discriminating between different dysrhythmias. If the QRS complex is narrow, or within the normal limits of 0.06 to 0.10 second, current has traveled through the normal ventricular conduction pathways to activate the ventricles to contract. When the QRS complex is wide, 0.12 second or greater, the current is taking longer than normal to contract the ventricles.

J point A point on the QRS complex where the depolarization is completed and repolarization starts.

To measure the QRS duration and morphology, place the first caliper point where the QRS complex starts and the second point at the **J point** (Figure 5-5). The J point is located where the S wave stops and the ST segment is initiated. It marks the point at which ventricular depolarization is

Figure 5-4 The PR interval measured from the beginning of the P wave to the first indication of ventricular depolarization, which is usually the Q wave (downward portion) beginning of the QRS complex.

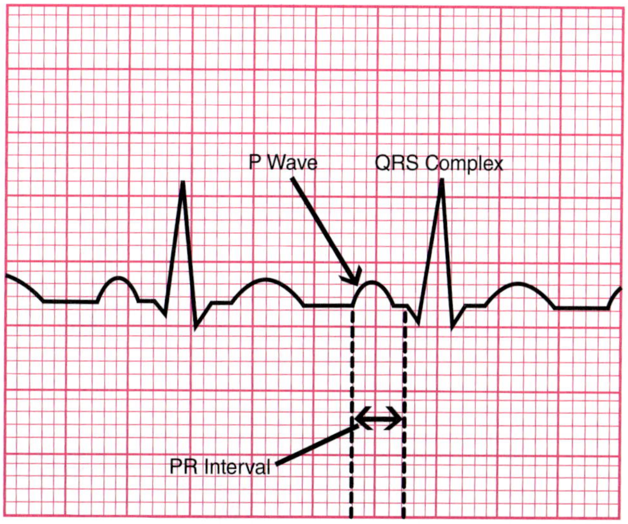

Interpret-TIP

QRS Measurement

Although a QRS measurement of 0.11 second is still considered within the normal range, this measurement can be provided only by an ECG machine. The human eye cannot discern less than 0.5 mm measurements.

completed and repolarization begins. It is important to carefully identify this ending point of the QRS complex because the ST segment may not be at the isoelectric line.

Several questions need to be answered when determining the QRS measurement and morphology (Figure 5-6). Specifics about how to answer these questions will be discussed when learning about abnormal rhythms.

- Are all the QRS complexes of equal length?
- What is the actual measurement, and is it within the normal limits?
- Do all QRS complexes look alike, and are the unusual QRS complexes associated with an ectopic or abnormal beat?

Figure 5-5 The J point is where the S wave stops and the ST segment starts.

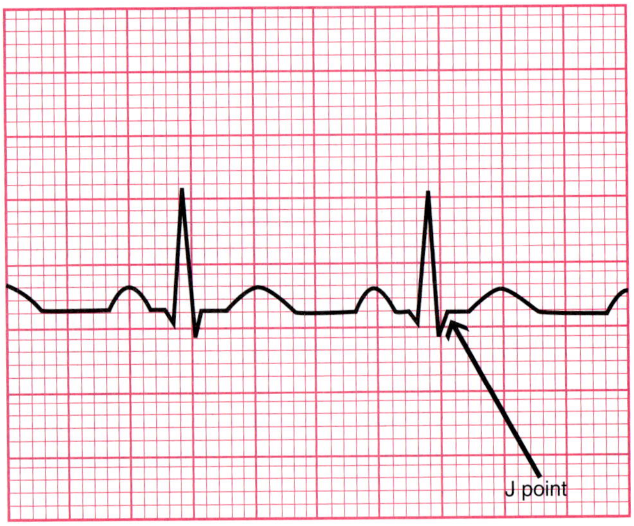

Figure 5-6 Measure the QRS duration from the beginning of the QRS complex to the J point.

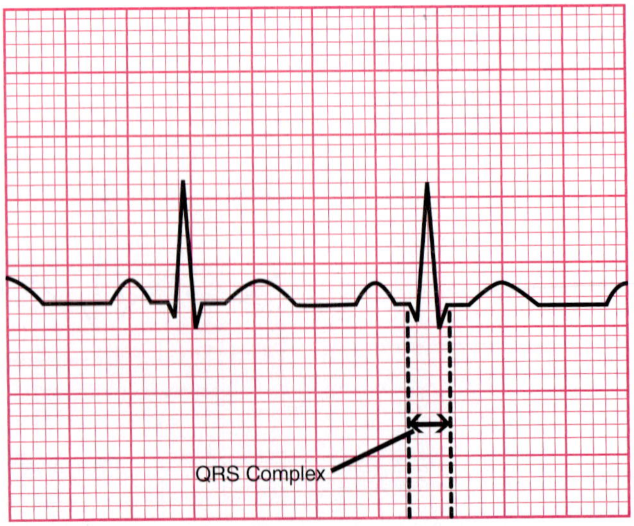

After you have completed these five steps of identifying the components of the rhythm, you will then compare the information to the specific criteria for classifying each of the dysrhythmias. The rest of this chapter explains the specific criteria for classification that will help you identify the various ECG rhythms.

Checkpoint Questions (LO 5.2)

1. Name the five components that must be evaluated on a rhythm strip.

____

____

2. A regular rhythm has 19 small boxes between two consecutive P waves. What is the heart rate?

____

____

3. After you measure the QRS duration and morphology, what other questions need to be answered?

____

____

5.3 Rhythms Originating from the Sinus Node

The sinoatrial (SA) node is the normal or primary pacemaker of the heart. It generates an electrical impulse that travels through the normal conduction pathway to cause the myocardium to depolarize. Electrical current starts at the sinoatrial node, travels the normal conduction pathway to the atrioventrical node, and continues through the bundle of His and bundle branches to the ventricles. Because the rhythm starts at the sinoatrial node, it is called *sinus rhythm*. The electrical current is produced at the sinus node at a rate of 60 to 100 beats per minute. The types of sinus rhythms are distinguished by heart rate and pattern and include sinus rhythm, sinus bradycardia, sinus tachycardia, and sinus dysrhythmia.

Normal sinus rhythm reflects a normally functioning conduction system (Figure 5-7). The electrical current is following the normal conduction pathway without interference from other body systems or disease processes.

Figure 5-7 Normal sinus rhythm.

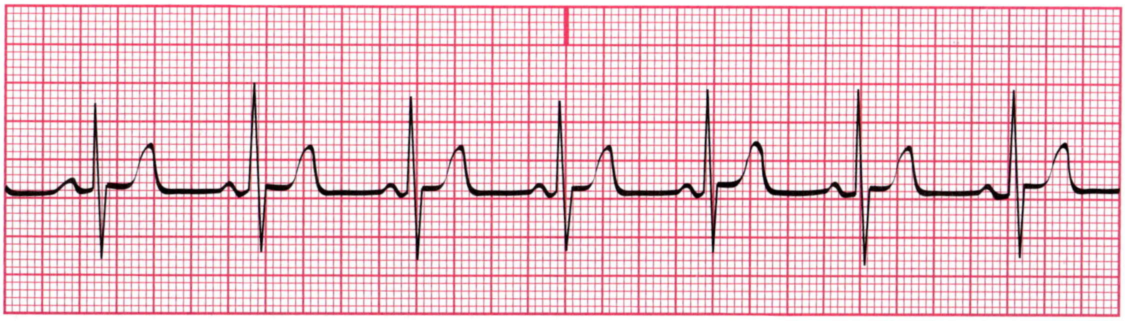

Criteria for Classification

- ***Rhythm:*** The intervals between the two P and two R waves occur in a consistent pattern.
- ***Rate:*** Both the atrial and the ventricular rates are between 60 and 100 beats per minute.
- ***P wave morphology:*** The P waves have the same shape and are usually upright in deflection on the rhythm strip. A P wave appears in front of every QRS complex.
- ***PR interval:*** The PR interval measurement is between the normal limits of 0.12 and 0.20 second. Each PR interval has the same appearance, without any variations.
- ***QRS duration and morphology:*** The QRS duration measurement is between 0.06 and 0.10 second, which is within normal limits. Each QRS duration and its morphology are the same, without any variations from QRS complex to complex.

Interpret-TIP

Normal Sinus Rhythm

Sinus rhythm is the only rhythm for which all five steps are within normal limits.

How the Patient Is Affected and What You Should Know

cardiac output The volume of blood the heart pumps each minute.

stroke volume The volume of blood ejected by one or both ventricles with each contraction.

Sinus rhythm is the desired rhythm. Patients with this rhythm should have normal **cardiac output.** Normal cardiac output means that the heart is beating adequately, pumping enough blood to the body's vital organs to maintain normal function. Signs and symptoms of adequate cardiac output include an alert and oriented patient with no difficulty breathing, no chest pain or pressure, and a stable blood pressure. Recall that the formula for determining cardiac output (CO) is heart rate (HR) × stroke volume (SV): HR × SV = CO. **Stroke volume** represents the volume of blood ejected by one ventricle during one contraction. The average ventricle ejects 70 mL of blood with each contraction.

Because this is a normal rhythm, no intervention is necessary. If the patient's rhythm returns to sinus rhythm from another dysrhythmia, it is always important to make sure that the patient is not experiencing problems with low cardiac output, which indicates that the heart is not pumping adequately (Table 5-2). Anytime a patient displays symptoms of low cardiac output, a licensed practitioner needs to be informed for further assessment.

Troubleshooting

Report the Patient Condition and the Tracing

The patient you are monitoring is very pale and appears to be breathing very fast. His monitor indicates a sinus rhythm. What should you do?

____

____

TABLE 5-2 **Signs and Symptoms of Decreased Cardiac Output**

Be aware of these signs and symptoms associated with decreased cardiac output during ECG monitoring.

Neurological	Cardiac	Respiratory	Urinary	Peripheral
• Change in mental status • Light-headedness • Dizziness • Confusion • Loss of consciousness	• Chest pain • Palpitation • Chest discomfort • Enlarged cardiac size • Congestive heart failure	• Difficulty breathing • Shortness of breath • Frothy sputum • Fluid present in lungs • Lung congestion	• Decreased urinary output of less than 30 mL in one hour	• Hypotension • Pale skin • Skin cool and clammy to the touch

Check Point Question (LO 5.3)

1. Using the criteria for classification, select the rhythm that most closely resembles normal sinus rhythm.

A.

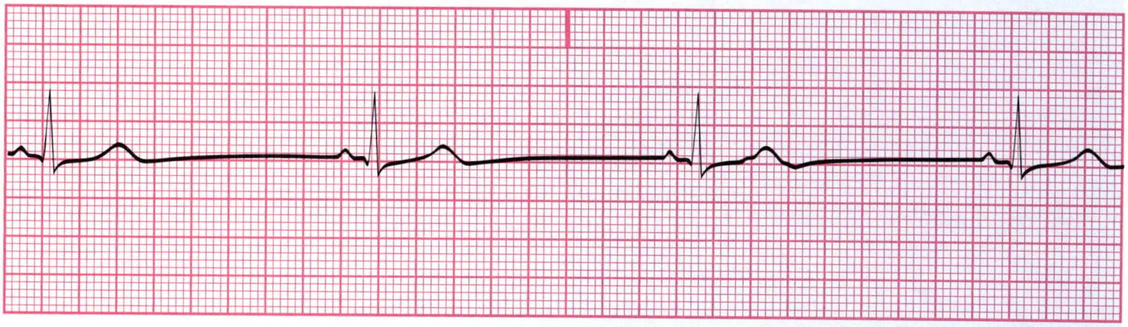

B.

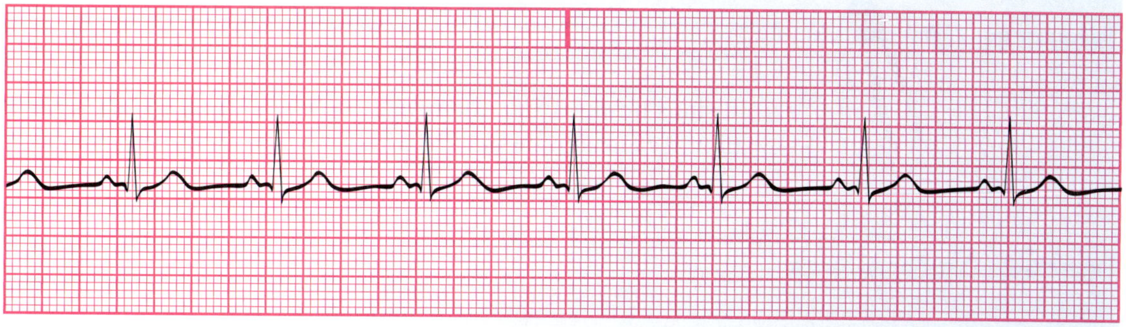

Which distinguishing feature(s) led you to make the selection?

____

____

____

Law & Ethics

Documenting the ECG Rhythm and Tracing

The ECG rhythm, which is considered a legal document, must be included in the patient's medical record. The patient's name, date, and time plus the initials of the person performing the ECG must be identified on each rhythm strip. Documentation of the ECG rhythm and the patient's condition help support the reason for the medical treatment.

5.4 Sinus Bradycardia

Sinus bradycardia is a sinus rhythm of less than 60 beats per minute (Figure 5-8). Sinus bradycardia originates from the SA node and travels the normal conduction pathway. The only difference between this rhythm and sinus rhythm is that the rate is less than the normal inherent rate of the SA node.

Criteria for Classification

- ***Rhythm:*** The R-R interval and P-P interval occur on a regular and constant basis.
- ***Rate:*** The atrial and ventricular rates are equal and less than 60 beats per minute.
- ***P wave morphology:*** The shape of each P wave is upright and uniform. There is a P wave in front of each QRS complex. No additional P waves or QRS complexes are noted.
- ***PR interval:*** The PR interval measurement is between the normal limits of 0.12 and 0.20 second. All PR intervals are the same.
- ***QRS duration and morphology:*** The QRS duration measurement is between the normal limits of 0.06 and 0.10 second. Each QRS duration and its morphology are the same, without any variations from QRS complex to complex.

Interpret-TIP

Sinus Bradycardia

In sinus bradycardia, the heart rate is less than 60 beats per minute, and all other measurements are within normal limits.

Figure 5-8 Sinus bradycardia.

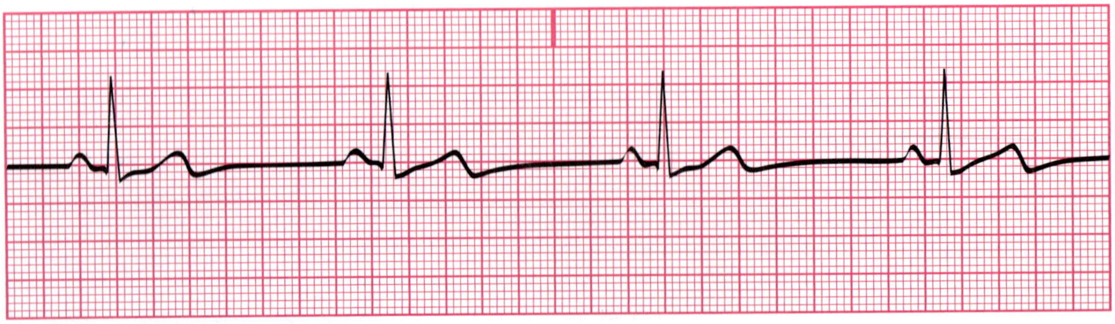

How the Patient Is Affected and What You Should Know

The patient who exhibits sinus bradycardia may or may not experience signs and symptoms of low cardiac output. For example, athletes may have sinus bradycardia normally. However, when administering an ECG to a patient with a slow heart rate, it is important to observe for the symptoms of low cardiac output (see Table 5-2). Remember that although the patient may look all right, he or she can quickly experience difficulties with low cardiac output. When you observe symptoms of low cardiac output, report any findings to a licensed practitioner immediately. This rhythm may require drug administration or application of a pacemaker.

Check Point Question (LO 5.4)

1. Using the criteria for classification, select the rhythm that most closely resembles sinus bradycardia rhythm.

A.

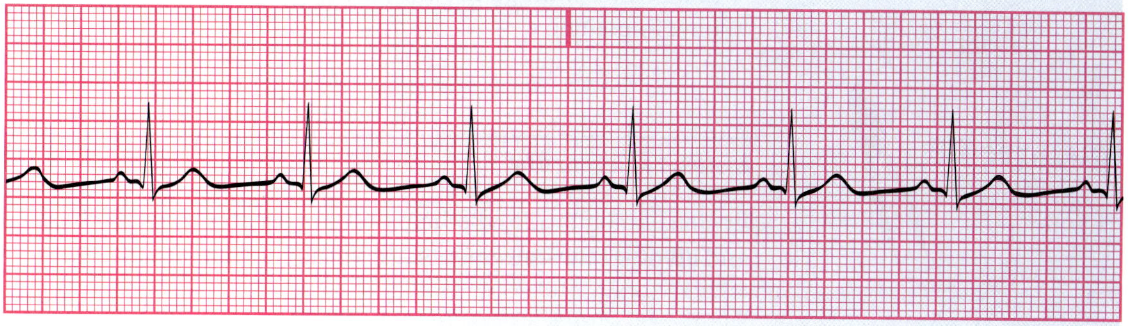

B.

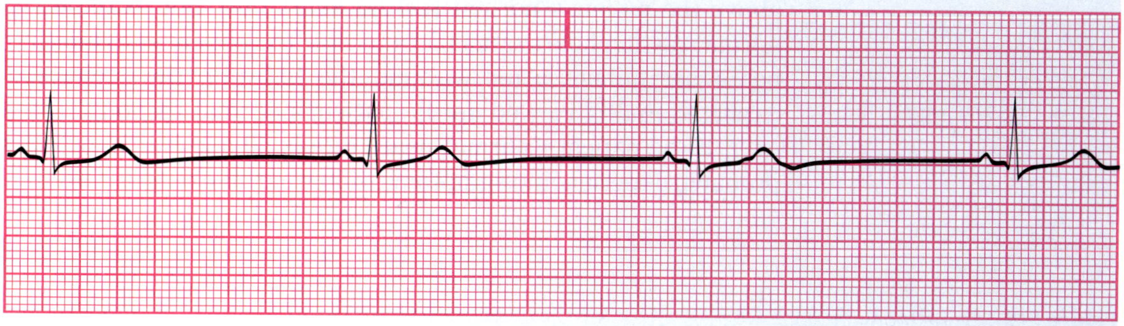

Which distinguishing feature(s) led you to make the selection?

____

____

____

5.5 Sinus Tachycardia

Sinus tachycardia is a condition in which the SA node fires and the electrical impulse travels through the normal conduction pathway, but the rate of impulse firing is faster than 100 beats per minute (Figure 5-9).

Criteria for Classification

- ***Rhythm:*** The R-R interval and P-P interval are equal and constant.
- ***Rate:*** The atrial and ventricular rates are the same, between 100 and 150 beats per minute.
- ***P wave morphology:*** The P waves have the same shape and usually are upright in deflection on the rhythm strip. There is a P wave in front of every QRS complex.
- ***PR interval:*** The PR interval measurement is between the normal limits of 0.12 and 0.20 second. Each PR interval is the same, without any variations.
- ***QRS duration and morphology:*** The QRS duration measurement is between the normal limits of 0.06 and 0.10 second. Each QRS duration and its morphology are the same, without any variations from QRS complex to complex.

Interpret-TIP

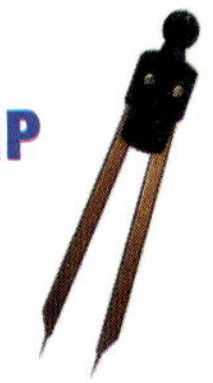

Sinus Tachycardia

In sinus tachycardia, the heart rate is greater than 100 beats per minute, and all other measurements are within normal limits.

How the Patient Is Affected and What You Should Know

The effect of this rhythm on the patient depends on the rate of tachycardia above the patient's normal resting heart rate. For example, if the patient's normal resting heart rate is 90 and now the patient is exhibiting a rate of 108 beats per minute after walking the hallway, the tachycardia would be expected and is viewed as the patient's normal response to exercise. However, if the patient's normal heart rate is 60 and it is now 140, the patient is probably experiencing symptoms of low cardiac output. Often the patient will

Figure 5-9 Sinus tachycardia.

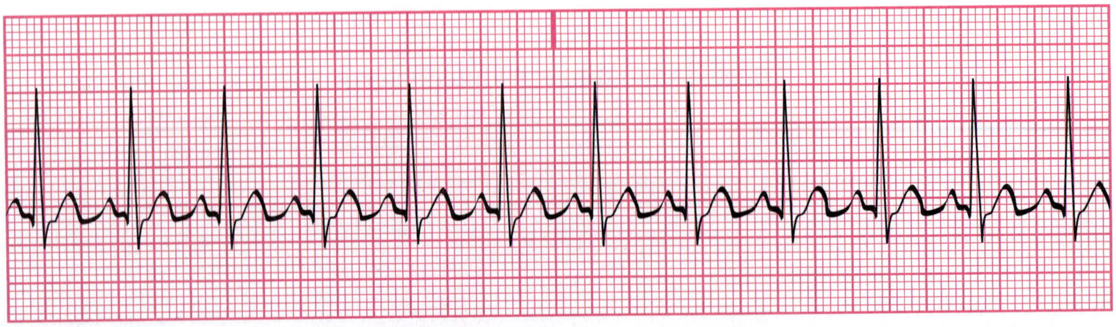

palpitations Fast heartbeat sensation felt by the patient, which may or may not be associated with complaints of chest pain.

complain of **palpitations** or "heart fluttering" with faster rates. If the patient has had a recent myocardial infarction, sinus tachycardia is considered to be more serious or even life threatening.

When caring for a patient who is experiencing sinus tachycardia, first observe for signs and symptoms of low cardiac output. If evidence of low cardiac output is observed, a licensed practitioner should be notified immediately. Medication may need to be administered by a licensed practitioner.

Check Point Question (LO 5.5)

1. Using the criteria for classification, select the rhythm that most closely resembles sinus tachycardia rhythm.

A.

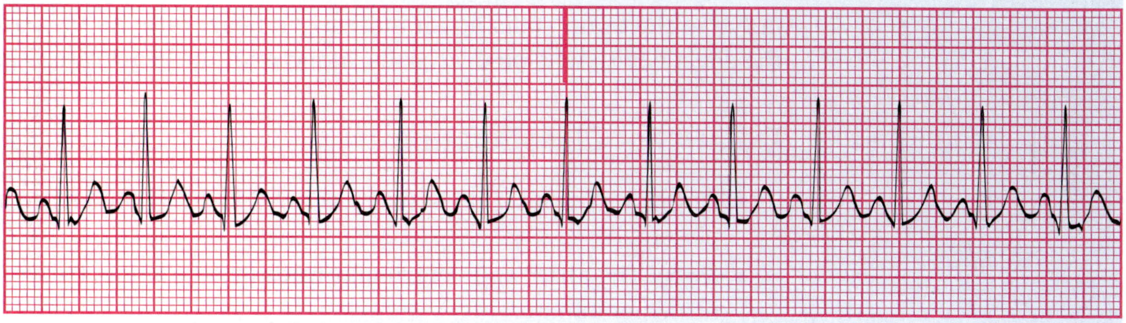

B.

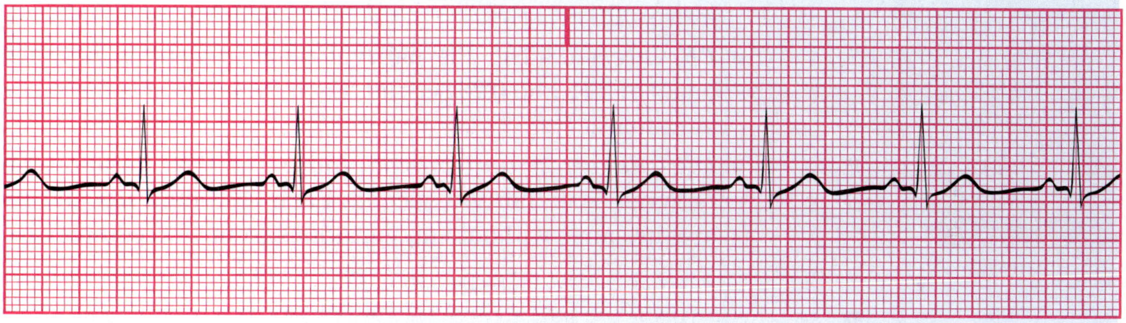

Which distinguishing feature(s) led you to make the selection?

____

____

____

5.6 Sinus Dysrhythmia

vagal tone A condition in which tension on the vagus nerve causes variation in the heart rate.

Sinus dysrhythmia is a condition in which the heart rate remains within normal limits but is influenced by the respiratory cycle and variations of **vagal tone.** *Vagal* refers to the action of the vagus nerve, a nerve that relays information between the brain and the internal organs, in this case the heart. *Tone,* in this context, refers to tension. For instance, when a patient inhales air, the pressure (tension) inside the chest cavity increases, causing pressure on the heart. The pressure on the heart sends information through the vagus

Figure 5-10 Sinus dysrhythmia.

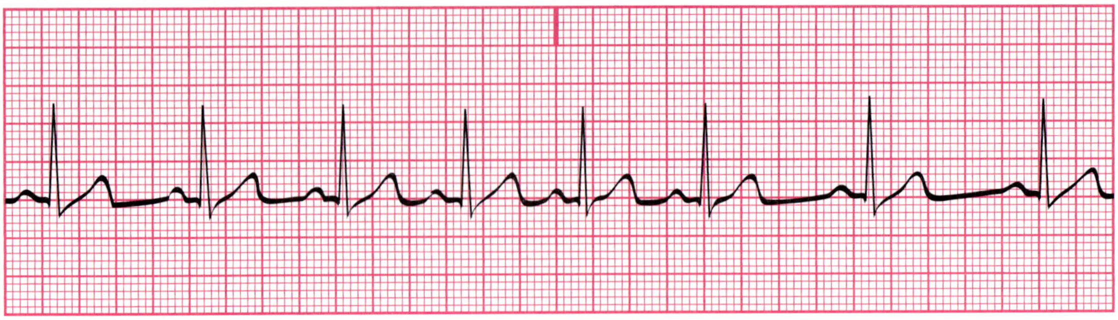

nerve to the brain, causing an increase in heart rate. As the patient exhales, the chest cavity tension decreases, along with the heart rate (Figure 5-10).

Criteria for Classification

- ***Rhythm:*** The interval between the P-P and R-R waves occur at irregular periods.
- ***Rate:*** The atrial and ventricular rates are the same, between 60 and 100 beats per minute.
- ***P wave morphology:*** The P waves have the same shape and usually are upright in deflection on the rhythm strip. There is a P wave in front of every QRS complex.
- ***PR interval:*** The PR interval measurement is between the normal limits of 0.12 and 0.20 second. Each PR interval is the same, without any variations.
- ***QRS duration and morphology:*** The QRS duration measurement is between 0.06 and 0.10 second. Each QRS duration and its morphology are the same, without any variations from QRS complex to complex.

Interpret-TIP

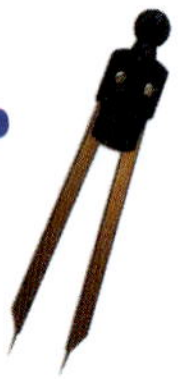

Sinus Dysrhythmia

In sinus dysrhythmia, the P-P and R-R intervals progressively widen, then narrow, following the patient's breathing pattern.

How the Patient Is Affected and What You Should Know

Patients usually show no clinical signs or symptoms with sinus dysrhythmia. If the irregularity is severe enough to decrease the heart rate to 40 to 50 beats per minute, the patient may complain of palpitations or dizziness. This depends on how slowly the heartbeats when the SA node is suppressed by the respiratory or vagal influences. You should notify the physician or other licensed practitioner when the heart rate slows below 50 or the patient complains of dizziness or palpitations. A copy of the rhythm strip should be mounted on the patient's medical record for documentation.

Check Point Question (LO 5.6)

1. Using the criteria for classification, select the rhythm that most closely resembles sinus dysrhythmia.

A.

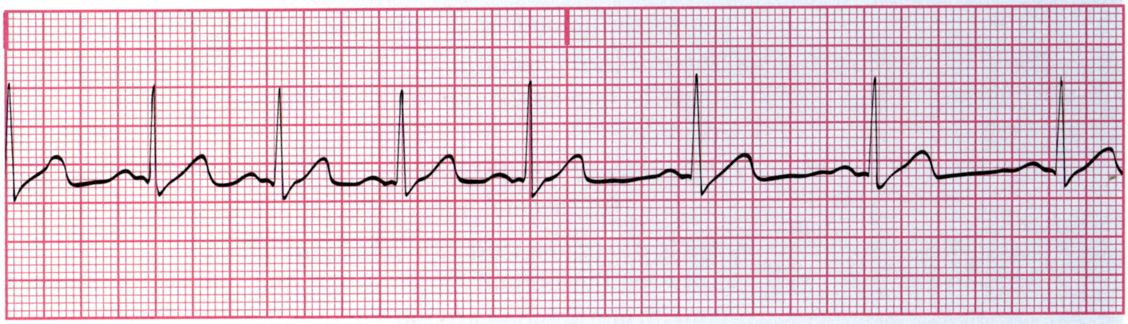

B.

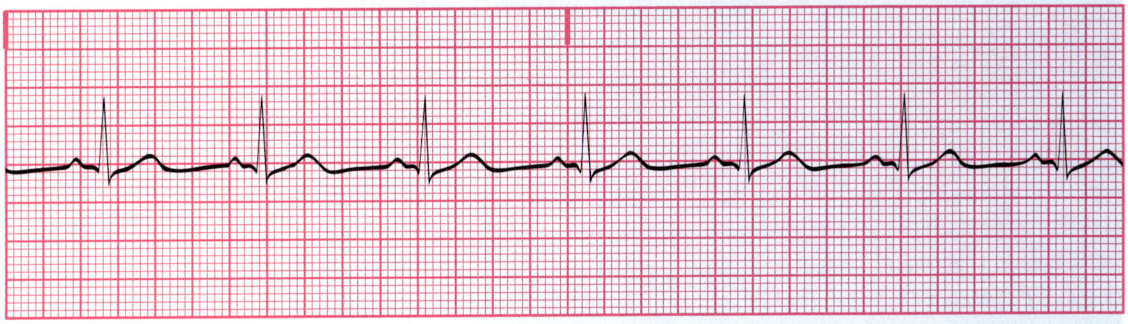

Which distinguishing feature(s) led you to make the selection?

____

____

____

5.7 Sinus Arrest

Sinus arrest, sometimes referred to as *sinus pause,* occurs when the SA node stops firing, causing a pause in electrical activity. During the pause, no electrical impulse is initiated or sent through the normal conduction system to cause either an atrial or a ventricular contraction (Figure 5-11).

Figure 5-11 Sinus arrest.

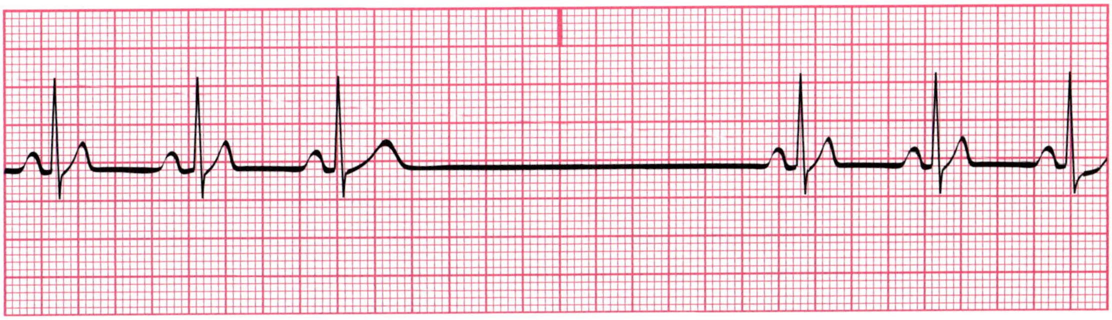

Criteria for Classification

- ***Rhythm:*** The cardiac complexes are regular before and after the sinus arrest period, but this rhythm is considered irregular due to the absence of electrical activity during the pause.
- ***Rate:*** The atrial and ventricular rates are the same. The rate varies, depending on the amount of electrical activity occurring from the sinoatrial node.
- ***P wave morphology:*** The P waves have the same shape and are upright in deflection on the rhythm strip. There is a P wave in front of every QRS complex.
- ***PR interval:*** The PR interval measurement is between the normal limits of 0.12 and 0.20 second. Each PR interval is the same, without any variations.
- ***QRS duration and morphology:*** The QRS duration measurement is between the normal limits of 0.06 and 0.10 second. Each QRS duration and its morphology are the same, without any variations from QRS complex to complex.
- ***Length of pause:*** The length of pause needs to be measured to determine how long the heart had no rhythm. To measure, place the calipers on the R-R interval around the pause. Once the time frame is determined, calculate the length of time for the pause by multiplying the number of boxes by 0.04 second. The frequency of pauses is also noted because the more frequent the pauses, the more urgent the situation.

ischemia Occurs when there is a sudden loss or reduction in blood supply (oxygen) to a region of the heart tissue. This occurs due to the presence of atherosclerotic plaque, blood clot, emboli, or even vascular spasm (Prinzmetal's angina).

It should be noted that the arrest period may be terminated by an escaped beat from one of the subsidiary pacemakers when the heart rate is less than 60 beats per minute. In this instance, there would be a junctional or ventricular escape beat, then resumption of the usual electrical activity.

Note: When sinus arrest reaches or exceeds 6 seconds, it is considered a medical emergency. Emergency procedures (Code Blue) must be initiated.

Interpret-TIP

Sinus Arrest

You will observe regularly occurring PQRSTs both before and after the arrest period. No electrical activity occurs during the arrest period.

How the Patient Is Affected and What You Should Know

The seriousness of sinus arrest depends on the length of the pause. The patient will experience signs and symptoms of decreased cardiac output if the pause is 2 seconds long and occurs on a frequent basis. The pauses may also cause periods of **ischemia** (when cells are deprived of oxygen), **hypotension** (low blood pressure), dizziness, and **syncope** (loss of consciousness).

hypotension A lower than normal blood pressure that can cause reduction of blood flow to vital organs.

syncope Loss of consciousness (fainting).

The patient may initially appear to be asymptomatic (without symptoms) and then develop signs and symptoms of low cardiac output. Therefore, it is important to observe the patient frequently for signs and symptoms of low cardiac output. Notify a licensed practitioner of these signs or symptoms, and provide information about the frequency and length of pauses. The patient will require immediate treatment. If sinus arrest reaches 6 seconds, this is considered a medical emergency and requires Code Blue procedures.

Troubleshooting

Sinus Arrest

asystole When no rhythm or electrical current is traveling through the cardiac conduction system.

A patient is in sinus arrest that lasts longer than 6 seconds. This indicates that no electrical current is traveling through the cardiac conduction system and is known as **asystole.** What should you do?

____

____

Check Point Question (LO 5.7)

1. Using the criteria for classification, select the rhythm that most closely resembles sinus arrest.

A.

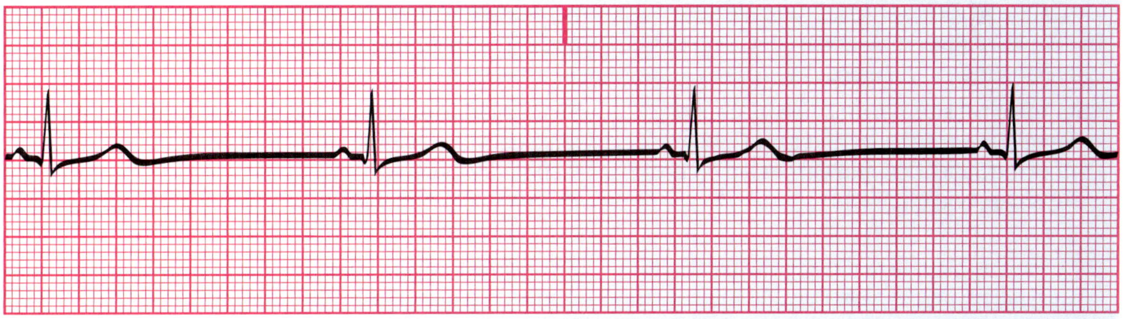

B.

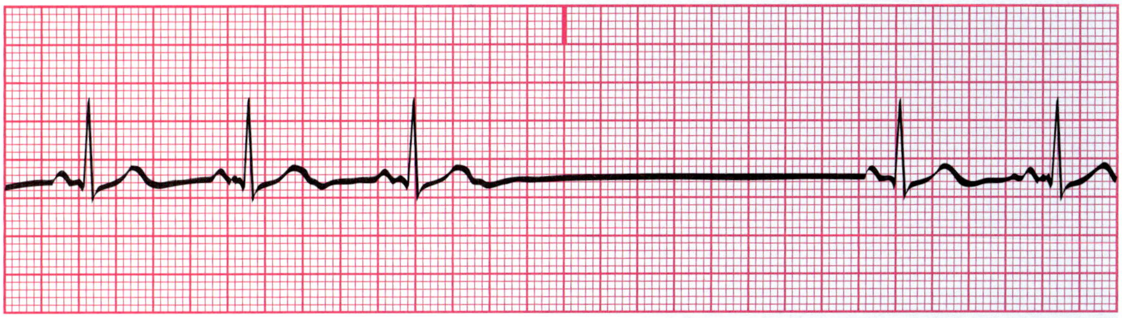

Which distinguishing feature(s) led you to make the selection?

____

____

____

Chapter Summary

Learning Outcomes	Summary	Pages
5.1 Explain the process of evaluating ECG tracings and determining the presence of dysrhythmias.	Evaluating an ECG requires basic knowledge of the waves, segments, and intervals of the tracing and the rate, rhythm, and regularity of the heartbeat.	121–122
5.2 Describe the criteria used to classify the dysrhythmias, including rhythm, rate, P wave morphology, PR interval measurement, and QRS duration measurement.	The process of evaluating an ECG tracing includes determining the ECG rhythm or regularity, determining the atrial and ventricular rates, identifying the P wave morphology, measuring the PR interval, measuring the QRS duration, and analyzing the morphology.	122–129
5.3 Identify normal sinus rhythm using the criteria for classification, and explain how the rhythm may affect the patient, including basic patient care and treatment.	Normal sinus rhythm is the result of a normally functioning electrical conduction system and requires no specialized patient care or treatment.	129–132
5.4 Identify sinus bradycardia using the criteria for classification, and explain how the rhythm may affect the patient, including basic patient care and treatment.	Sinus bradycardia is a rhythm of less than 60 beats per minute, with electrical activity originating in the SA node. The other four criteria are within normal limits.	132–133
5.5 Identify sinus tachycardia using the criteria for classification, and explain how the rhythm may affect the patient, including basic patient care and treatment.	Sinus tachycardia is a rhythm of greater than 100 beats per minute, with electrical activity originating in the SA node. The other four criteria are within normal limits.	134–135
5.6 Identify sinus dysrhythmia using the criteria for classification, and explain how the rhythm may affect the patient, including basic patient care and treatment.	Sinus dysrhythmia is a condition in which the heart rate remains within normal limits but is influenced by the respiratory cycle and variations of vagal tone, causing the rhythm to be irregular. The other four criteria are within normal limits.	135–137
5.7 Identify sinus arrest using the criteria for classification, and explain how the rhythm may affect the patient, including basic patient care and treatment.	Sinus arrest occurs when the SA node stops firing; this creates a pause in electrical activity, causing the rhythm to be irregular. The length of the pause may cause the heart rate to be less than 60 beats per minute. Otherwise, the other criteria are within normal limits.	137–139

Chapter Review

Matching

Match the terms related to rhythm strip interpretation on the left with their definitions on the right.

_______ **1.** heart rate less than 60 bpm (LO 5.2)

_______ **2.** the amount of blood being pumped by the heart (LO 5.3)

_______ **3.** low blood pressure (LO 5.6)

_______ **4.** lack of blood supply (LO 5.6)

_______ **5.** depolarization is completed and repolarization starts (LO 5.2)

_______ **6.** fast heartbeats felt by the patient (LO 5.4)

_______ **7.** loss of consciousness (fainting) (LO 5.6)

_______ **8.** heart rate greater than 100 bpm (LO 5.2)

_______ **9.** tension on a nerve, causing changes in heart rate (LO 5.6)

a. vagal tone
b. bradycardia
c. tachycardia
d. cardiac output
e. hypotension
f. palpitations
g. J point
h. syncope
i. ischemia

Multiple Choice

Circle the correct answer.

10. What is the rate of a normal sinus rhythm? (LO 5.3)
- **a.** 60 to 100 beats per minute
- **b.** 50 to 90 beats per minute
- **c.** 100 to 150 beats per minute
- **d.** 60 to 80 beats per minute

11. Which sinus rhythm has a rate that is consistently less than 60 beats per minute? (LO 5.4)
- **a.** Sinus tachycardia
- **b.** Sinus bradycardia
- **c.** Sinus dysrythmia
- **d.** Sinus arrest

12. Which question does *not* need to be answered when determining the QRS measurement? (LO 5.2)
   a. Are all the QRS complexes of equal length?
   b. What is the actual QRS measurement, and is it within the normal limits?
   c. Do all QRS complexes look alike?
   d. Is the R-R pattern regular?

13. Which sinus rhythm has a rate of more than 100 beats per minute? (LO 5.5)
   a. Sinus tachycardia
   b. Sinus bradycardia
   c. Sinus dysrhythmia
   d. Sinus arrest

14. Which rhythm shows an irregularity during inspiration and expiration? (LO 5.6)
   a. Sinus tachycardia
   b. Sinus bradycardia
   c. Sinus dysrhythmia
   d. Sinus arrest

15. The normal PR interval is (LO 5.2)
   a. 0.04 to 0.10 second.
   b. 0.12 to 0.20 second.
   c. 0.22 to 0.26 second.
   d. 0.28 to 0.32 second.

16. If a QRS complex measures 0.12 second or wider, it most likely indicates (LO 5.2)
   a. normal ventricular conduction.
   b. delayed ventricular conduction.
   c. increased delay at the AV node.
   d. myocardial infarction.

17. Which of the following is a common sign of low cardiac output? (LO 5.3)
   a. High blood pressure
   b. Alert and oriented
   c. Increased perfusion of vital organs
   d. Low blood pressure

Fill in the Blank

18. Sinus tachycardia may be a normal finding in a patient as a result of ______________________. (LO 5.5)

19. When sinus arrest continues for 6 seconds or more, it is considered ______________________. (LO 5.7)

20. The rhythm originating in the sinoatrial node that is considered normal is ______________________. (LO 5.3)

21. Two rhythms originating in the sinoatrial node that change the heart rate are ______________________ and ______________________. (LO 5.4, 5.5)

22. The rhythm originating in the sinoatrial node that is affected by vagal tone is ______________________. (LO 5.6)

Critical Thinking Application *Rhythm Identification*

Review the dysrhythmias pictured here and, using the criteria for classification provided in the chapter as clues, identify each rhythm and explain what criteria you used to make your decision. (LO 5.3 to 5.7)

23.

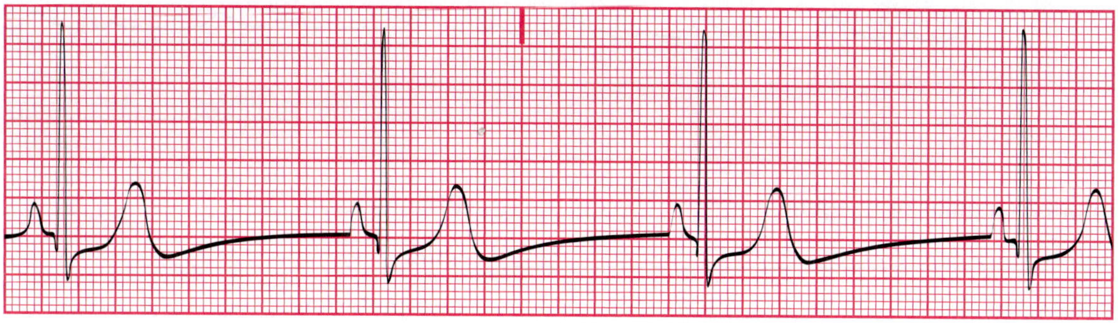

Rhythm (regular or irregular): ____________ PR interval: ____________

Rate: ____________ QRS: ____________

P wave: ____________ Interpretation: ____________

24.

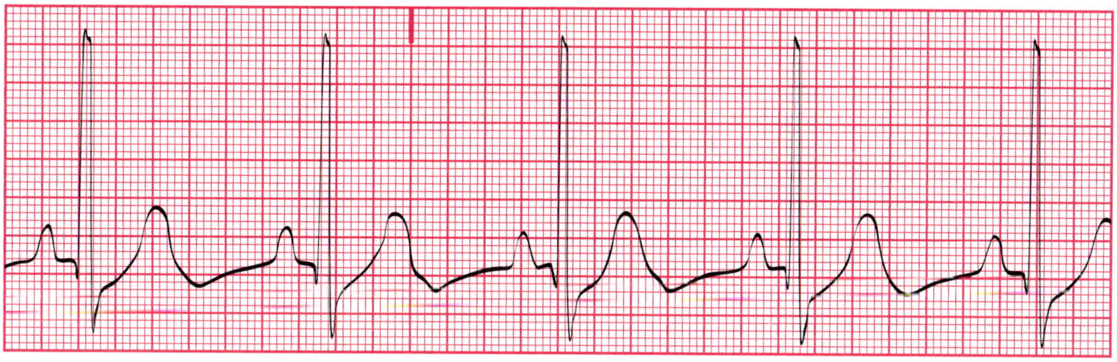

Rhythm (regular or irregular): ____________ PR interval: ____________

Rate: ____________ QRS: ____________

P wave: ____________ Interpretation: ____________

25.

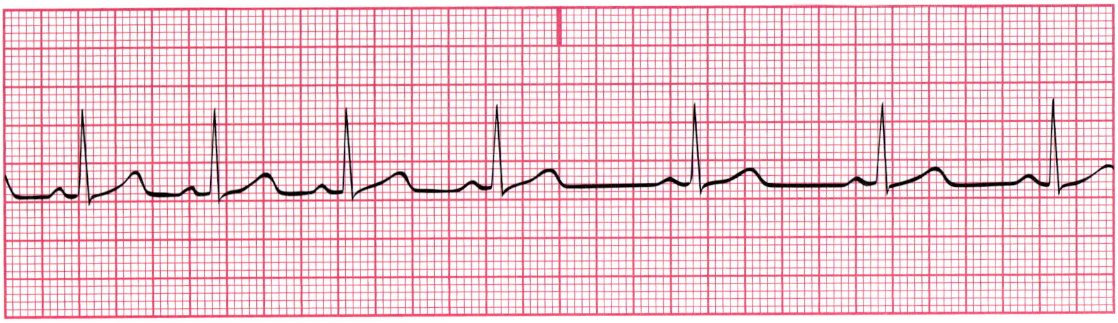

Rhythm (regular or irregular): ______________________ PR interval: ______________________

Rate: ______________________ QRS: ______________________

P wave: ______________________ Interpretation: ______________________

26.

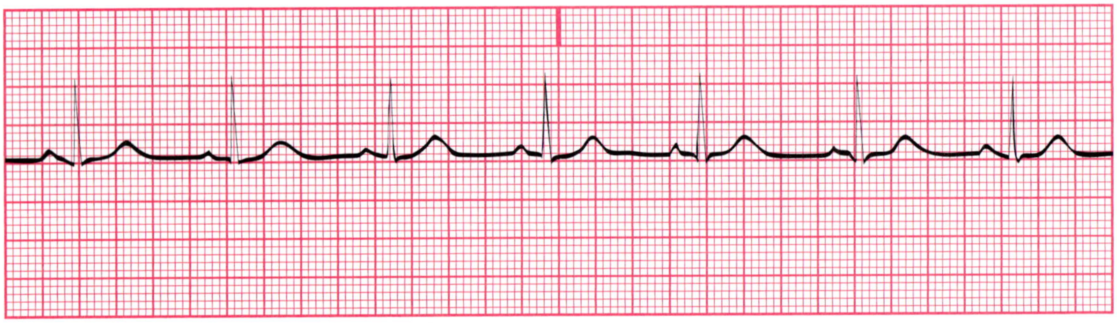

Rhythm (regular or irregular): ______________________ PR interval: ______________________

Rate: ______________________ QRS: ______________________

P wave: ______________________ Interpretation: ______________________

27.

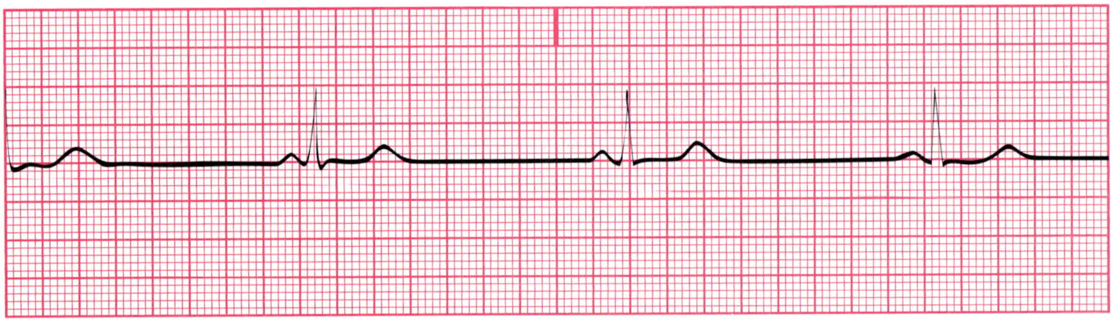

Rhythm (regular or irregular): ______________________ PR interval: ______________________

Rate: ______________________ QRS: ______________________

P wave: ______________________ Interpretation: ______________________

28.

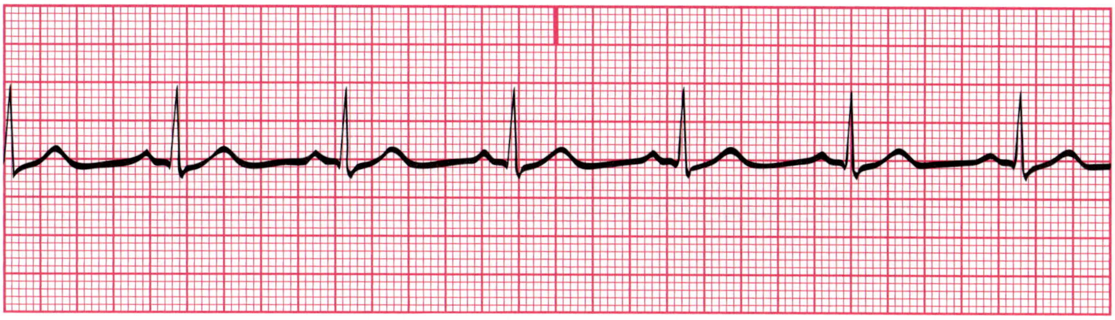

Rhythm (regular or irregular): ____________ PR interval: ____________

Rate: ____________ QRS: ____________

P wave: ____________ Interpretation: ____________

29.

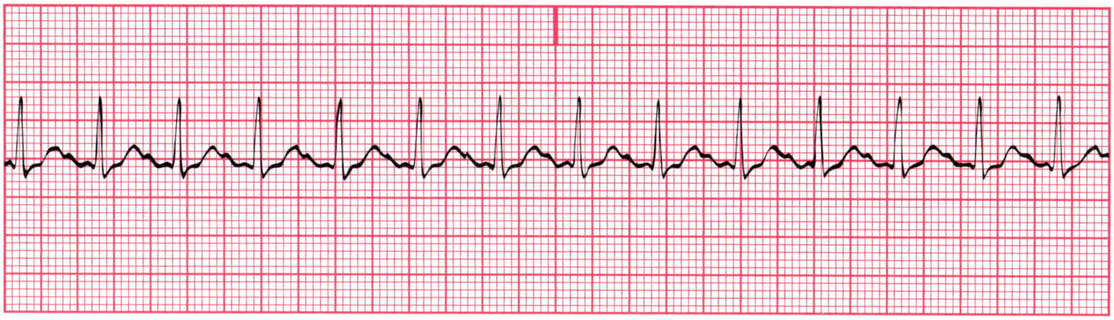

Rhythm (regular or irregular): ____________ PR interval: ____________

Rate: ____________ QRS: ____________

P wave: ____________ Interpretation: ____________

30.

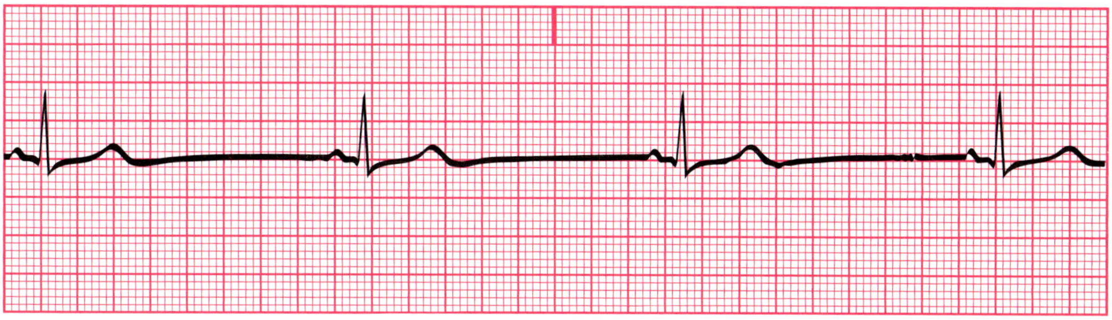

Rhythm (regular or irregular): ____________ PR interval: ____________

Rate: ____________ QRS: ____________

P wave: ____________ Interpretation: ____________

31.

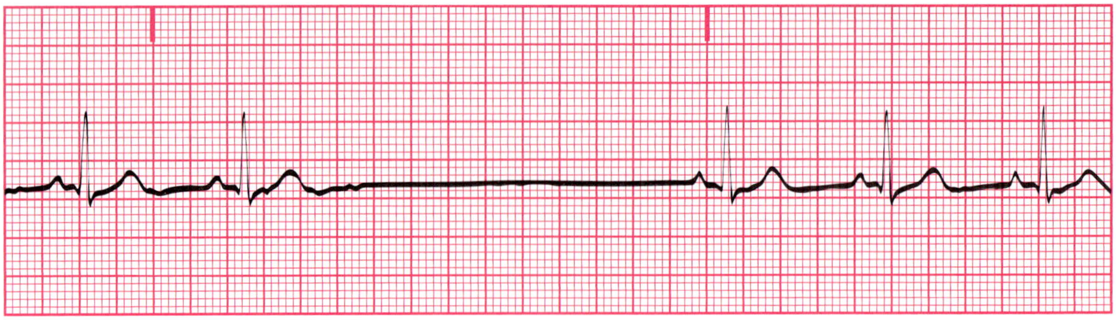

Rhythm (regular or irregular): ____________________ PR interval: ______________________________

Rate: ______________________________________ QRS: ______________________________

P wave: ______________________________________ Interpretation: ______________________________

32.

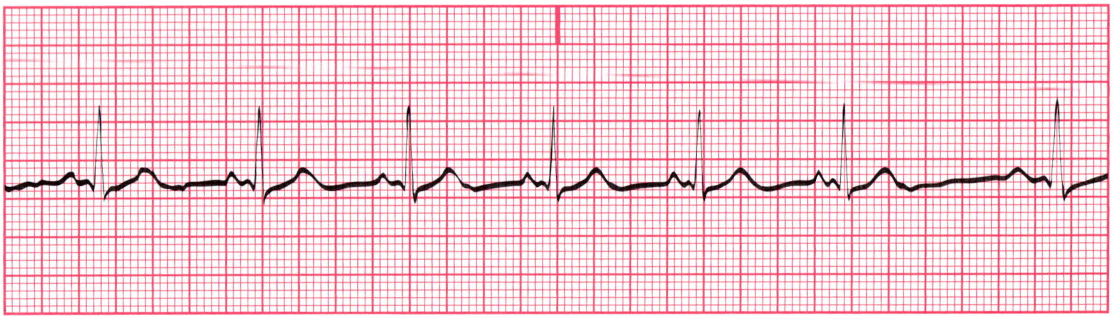

Rhythm (regular or irregular): ____________________ PR interval: ______________________________

Rate: ______________________________________ QRS: ______________________________

P wave: ______________________________________ Interpretation: ______________________________

Connect® Now that you have completed the material in the chapter text, go to Connect and complete any chapter activities you have not yet done.

Atrial Dysrhythmias

6

Learning Outcomes

6.1 Summarize the similarities and differences among atrial dysrhythmias.

6.2 Identify premature atrial complexes using the criteria for classification, and explain how the rhythm may affect the patient, including basic patient care and treatment.

6.3 Identify wandering atrial pacemaker using the criteria for classification, and explain how the rhythm may affect the patient, including basic patient care and treatment.

6.4 Identify multifocal atrial tachycardia using the criteria for classification, and explain how the rhythm may affect the patient, including basic patient care and treatment.

6.5 Identify atrial flutter using the criteria for classification, and explain how the rhythm may affect the patient, including basic patient care and treatment.

6.6 Identify atrial fibrillation using the criteria for classification, and explain how the rhythm may affect the patient, including basic patient care and treatment.

Key Terms

atrial kick
automaticity
biphasic
cerebrovascular accident (CVA)
ectopic impulse
focus (plural: foci)
myocardial infarction (MI; heart attack)
neurological
pulmonary embolism
renal infarction
thrombus
trigeminy

6.1 Introduction to Atrial Dysrhythmias

ectopic impulse An electrical impulse that comes from outside the normal pacemaker site or electrical conduction pathway.

Atrial dysrhythmias are caused by an **ectopic impulse** in either the right or the left atrium. The atrial origin is outside the SA node, which interrupts the inherent rate of the SA node. The heart works on the principle that the fastest impulse will control the heart rate. If the atrial ectopic beat is generating electrical impulses faster than the sinoatrial node, the ectopic beat overrides the sinoatrial node impulse and causes the atria and ventricles to depolarize. Dysrhythmias that are caused by the atrial ectopic site include premature atrial complexes, atrial tachycardia, atrial flutter, and atrial fibrillation. Because the P wave occurs as a result of atrial depolarization, rhythms in this category primarily affect the P wave.

neurological Pertaining to the nervous system, its diseases, and its functions.

Atrial dysrhythmias occur from conditions that cause pressure on the atria, such as damage to the atria from myocardial infarction, valvular problems, or **neurological** influences (pertaining to the nervous system). When the area is stressed or damaged, the cells become unstable and the electrical state may cause depolarization to occur more easily.

Checkpoint Question (LO 6.1)

1. Which wave is affected by the change in electrical activity within the atria?

____

____

6.2 Premature Atrial Complexes

Premature atrial complexes (PACs) are early electrical impulses that originate in the atria, interrupting the inherent regular rhythm (Figure 6-1).

Criteria for Classification

- ***Rhythm:*** The regularity between the P-P interval and R-R interval is constant with the exception of the early complexes.
- ***Rate:*** The rates of the atria and ventricles are usually within normal limits of 60 to 100, depending on the frequency of the PACs.
- ***P wave morphology:*** The P waves associated with the normal complexes have the same morphology and shape. The P waves associated with the early complex have a different shape than the rest of the P waves on the strip. The abnormal P waves may be flattened, notched, **biphasic** or equiphasic (have two phases), or otherwise unusual. They may even be hidden within the T wave of the preceding complex. Evidence that the P wave is hidden within the T wave includes a notch in the T wave, a pointed shape, or being taller than the other T waves.

biphasic A waveform that has positive (upward) and negative (downward) deflections (phases) on the ECG tracing.

- ***PR interval:*** The PR interval measures within normal limits of 0.12 to 0.20 second. The early beat will probably have a different PR measurement than the normal complexes but will be within normal limits.
- ***QRS duration and morphology:*** The QRS duration will be within normal limits of 0.06 to 0.10 second.

Figure 6-1 Premature atrial complex.

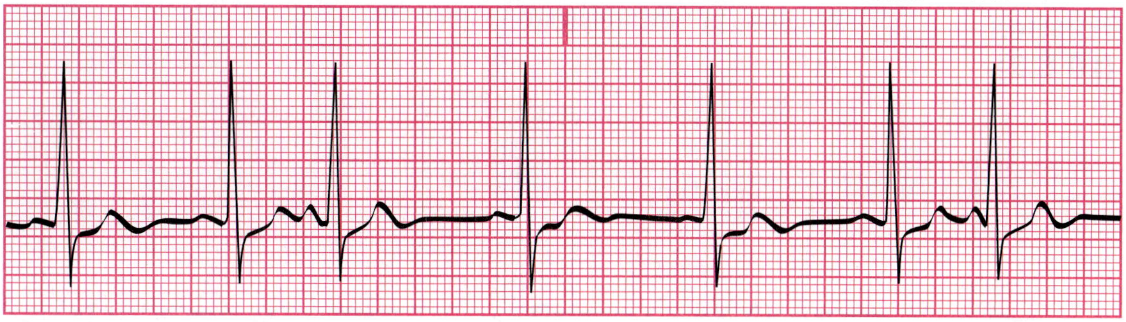

Interpret-TIP

Premature Atrial Complexes

A PAC is a cardiac complex that occurs too soon. It has a positively deflected P wave. Other than being "early," this complex does not possess any abnormal features.

trigeminy Pattern in which every third complex is a premature beat.

Determine the underlying rhythm of sinus rhythm, sinus bradycardia, sinus tachycardia, or sinus dysrhythmia when identifying PACs. The rhythm strip must be labeled with this underlying rhythm and the type of PAC. An example of this terminology is "sinus rhythm with trigeminal PACs" (**trigeminy** refers to a pattern in which every third complex is a premature beat). Refer to the chapter *Ventricular Dysrhythmias* for more information about types and patterns of premature complexes.

How the Patient Is Affected and What You Should Know

With each PAC, the atria do not have time to fill completely prior to contraction. This causes less volume in the ventricles prior to ventricular contraction and may cause a decrease in cardiac output. Therefore, in the patient who has prior cardiac disease, frequent PACs can cause the patient to experience signs and symptoms of low cardiac output.

When caring for a patient with PACs, observe the patient for signs and symptoms of low cardiac output. Monitoring the number or frequency of PACs is essential. The patient may complain of palpitations from the early beats. The severity of the patient's complaints is related to the frequency of the PACs. In addition, frequent PACs may indicate that a more serious atrial dysrhythmia may follow. The more frequent occurrence indicates that the ectopic **focus** (cardiac cell that produces an ectopic beat) may continue and take control of the heart rate. Any observation of low cardiac output should be communicated to a licensed practitioner for appropriate treatment.

focus (plural: foci) A cardiac cell or group of cells that produces an ectopic beat.

Checkpoint Question (LO 6.2)

Using the criteria for classification, select the rhythm that most closely resembles premature atrial complex (PAC).

A.

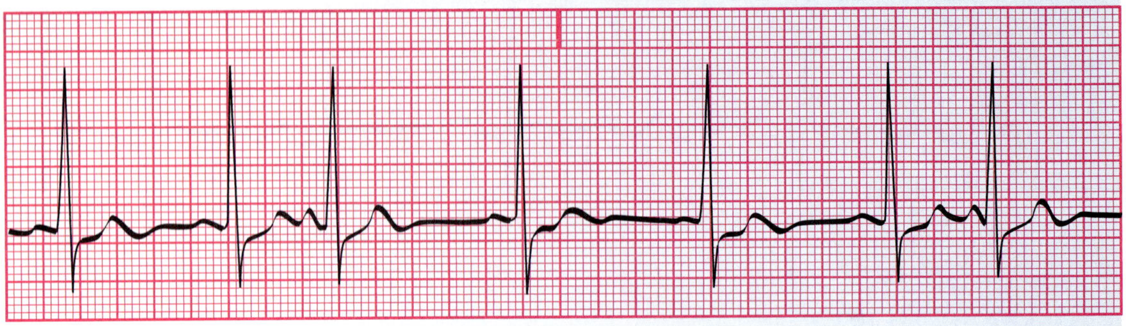

B.

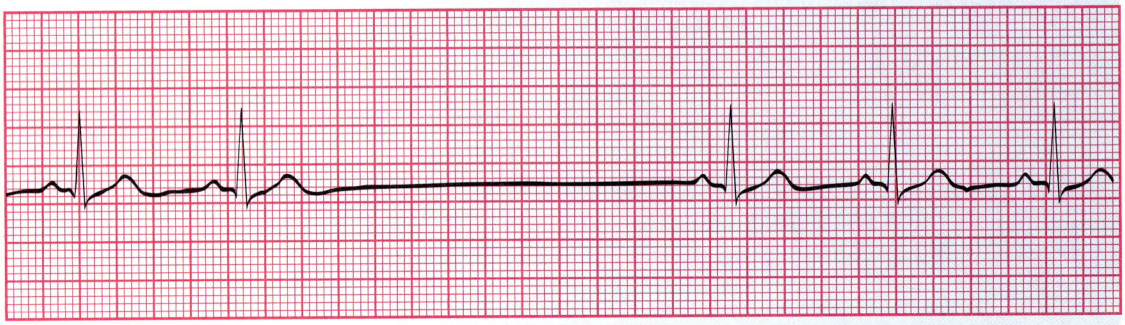

1. Which distinguishing feature(s) led you to make the selection?

____

____

____

6.3 Wandering Atrial Pacemaker

Wandering atrial pacemaker (WAP) is a rhythm in which the pacemaker site shifts between the SA node, other sites in the atria, and/or the AV junction. The P wave morphology changes in appearance during the pacemaker shift. At least three different P wave morphologies in the same lead indicate a wandering atrial pacemaker (Figure 6-2).

Criteria for Classification

- ***Rhythm:*** Slightly irregular
- ***Rate:*** Should be within normal limits of 60 to 100 beats per minute
- ***P wave morphology:*** Continuous change in appearance
- ***PR interval:*** Varies
- ***QRS duration and morphology:*** Usually within normal limits

How the Patient Is Affected and What You Should Know

WAP is a normal finding in children, older adults, and well-conditioned athletes and does not usually cause clinical signs and symptoms. However, it may also be related to some types of organic heart disease and drug toxicity.

Figure 6-2 Wandering atrial pacemaker.

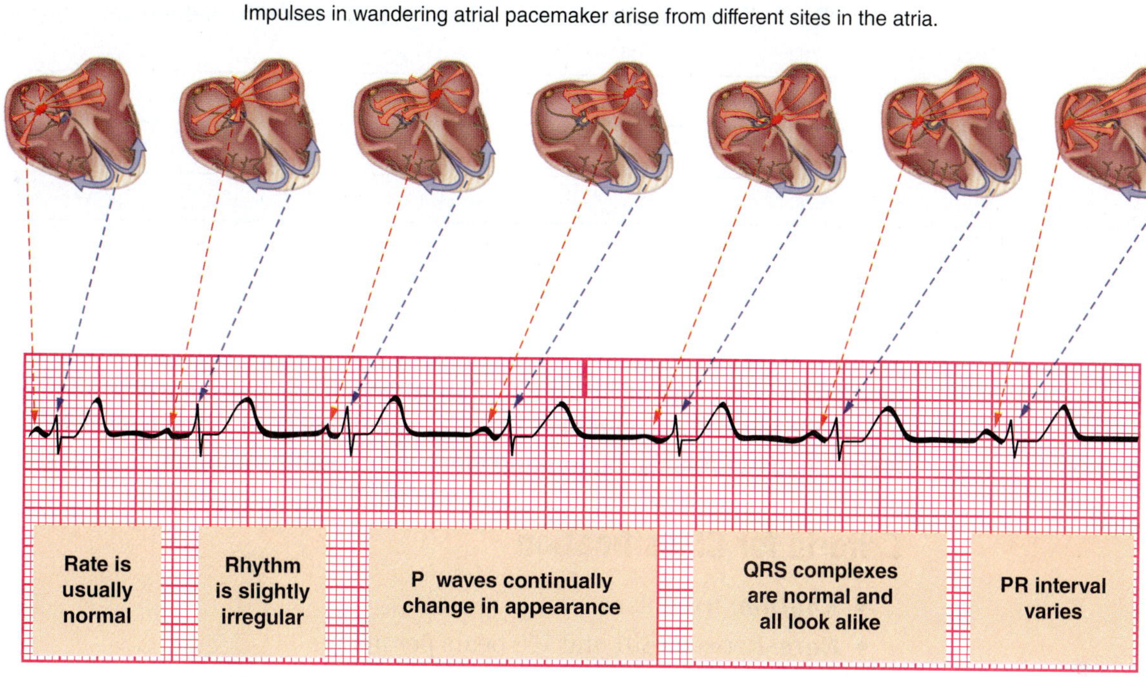

Interpret-TIP

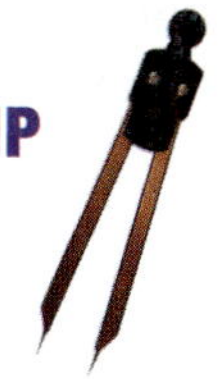

Wandering Atrial Pacemaker Rhythm

WAP has a changing P wave morphology with at least three variations in one lead. The rhythm may be irregular.

Checkpoint Question (LO 6.3)

Using the criteria for classification, select the rhythm that most closely resembles the wandering atrial pacemaker (WAP) rhythm.

A.

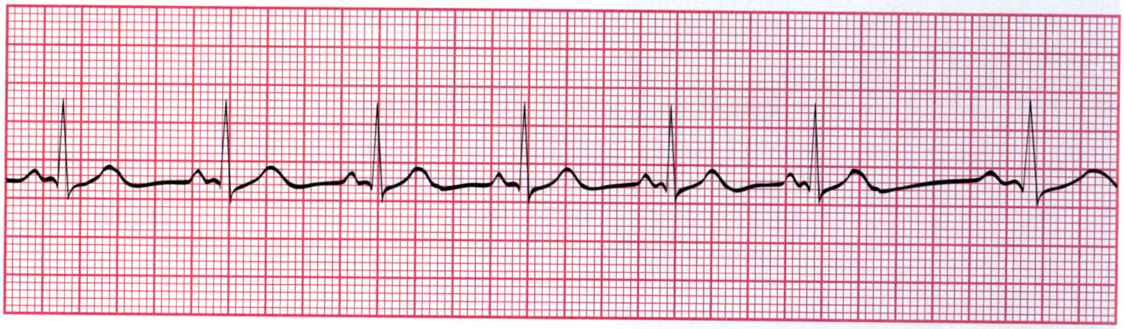

B.

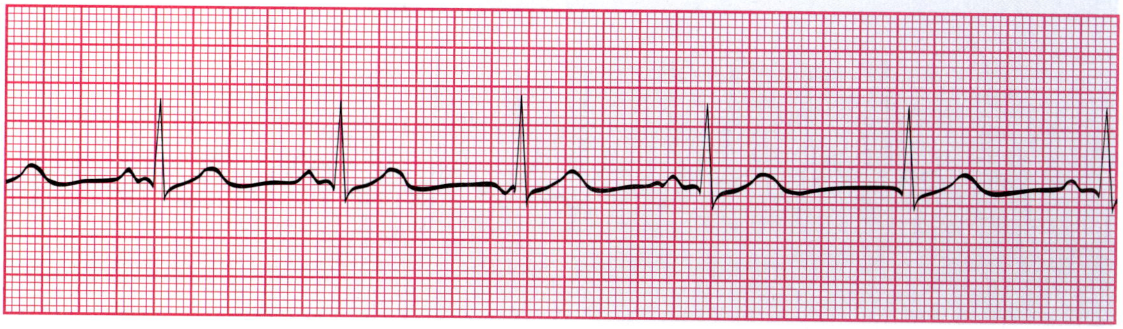

(Continued)

1. Which distinguishing feature(s) led you to make the selection?

____

____

____

6.4 Multifocal Atrial Tachycardia

Multifocal atrial tachycardia (MAT) has a P wave that changes from beat to beat and a heart rate of 101 to 150 (Figure 6-3). It has the same characteristics as wandering atrial pacemaker (WAP), except that the rate is in excess of 100. It can be distinguished by looking closely for visibly changing P waves.

Criteria for Classification

- ***Rhythm:*** Irregular
- ***Rate:*** Between 101 and 150 beats per minute
- ***P wave morphology:*** P waves change in appearance from beat to beat. They may be upright, rounded, notched, inverted, biphasic, or buried in the QRS complex.
- ***PR interval:*** Varies due to the changing origin of the electrical activity
- ***QRS duration and morphology:*** Normal in duration and all complexes look alike

Interpret-TIP

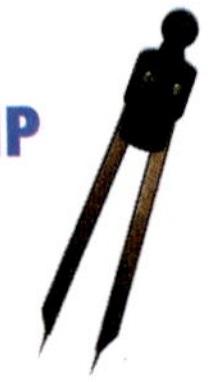

Multifocal Atrial Tachycardia

MAT has a clearly changing P wave and a heart rate of 101 to 150 beats per minute.

How the Patient Is Affected and What You Should Know

MAT is usually triggered by an acute exacerbation of emphysema, congestive heart failure (CHF), or acute mitral valve regurgitation. This rhythm should be reported to the licensed practitioner, and the patient's vital signs and condition should be monitored.

Figure 6-3 Multifocal atrial tachycardia.

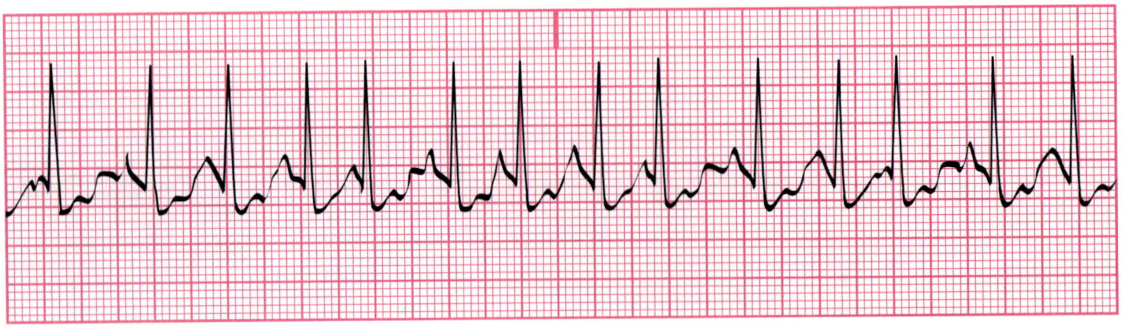

Checkpoint Question (LO 6.4)

Using the criteria for classification, select the rhythm that most closely resembles multifocal atrial tachycardia (MAT).

A.

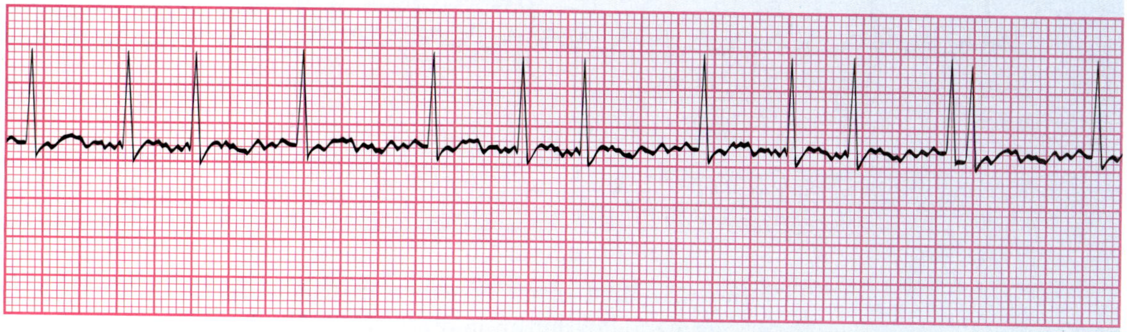

B.

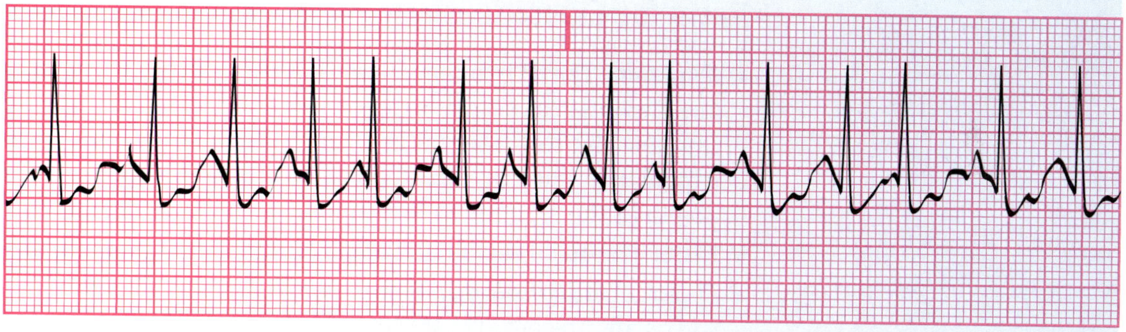

1. Which distinguishing feature(s) led you to make the selection?

____

____

____

6.5 Atrial Flutter

automaticity The ability of the heart to initiate an electrical impulse without being stimulated by an independent source.

Atrial flutter (A-flutter) occurs when a rapid impulse originates in the atrial tissue. The ectopic focus may be originating from ischemic areas of the heart with enhanced **automaticity** (ability to initiate an electrical current) or from a reentry pathway. A reentry pathway is an extra pathway that has developed in which a group of cells are generating an impulse faster than the SA node. This impulse then follows a route that allows the impulse to reach the AV node quicker than the normal conduction pathway. The reentry pathway is similar to finding a shortcut to work or school to bypass the normal traffic route to get you to your destination faster. The electrical current or rhythm has a characteristic sawtooth pattern (Figure 6-4). This atrial activity is called flutter (F) waves. As shown in Figure 6-4, F waves are often seen in a ratio of 2, 3, 4, and even 5 F waves to each QRS complex. This means that the atria (represented by the F waves) are depolarizing and contracting at a rate equal to the ratio of F waves to QRS complexes. When interpreting this rhythm, the ratio of F waves to QRS complexes is usually included; for example, atrial

Figure 6-4 Atrial flutter.

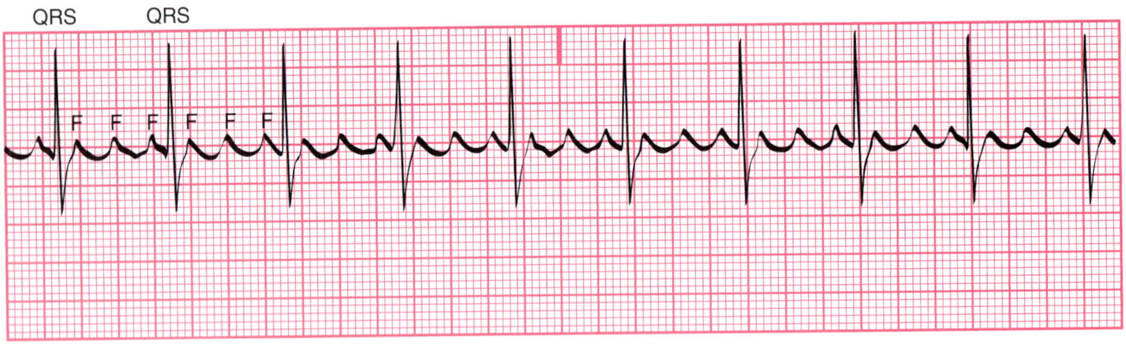

flutter 3:1. Most often this is a transient dysrhythmia that leads to more serious atrial dysrhythmia if not treated.

Criteria for Classification

- ***Rhythm:*** The P-P interval or flutter-to-flutter wave interval is regular. The interval set with the calipers will stay constant throughout the rhythm. The R-R interval is usually regular, but occasionally it may be irregular in pattern. The regularity of the R-R interval depends on the ability of the AV node to limit impulses to the ventricles.
- ***Rate:*** The atrial rate is between 250 and 350 beats per minute.
- ***P wave morphology:*** P waves are not seen, and only flutter (or F) waves are present. These flutter waves resemble a "sawtooth" or "picket fence." They are most easily seen in leads II, III, and aVF. The correlation between P waves and QRS complexes no longer exists. There are more flutter waves than QRS complexes.
- ***PR interval:*** No identifiable P wave exists, so the PR interval cannot be measured.
- ***QRS duration and morphology:*** The QRS duration is within normal limits of 0.06 to 0.10 second.

Interpret-TIP

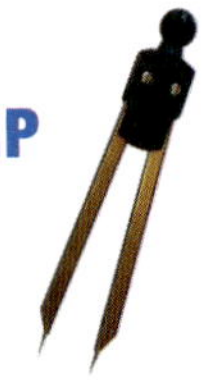

Atrial Flutter

Atrial flutter has a "sawtooth" atrial pattern between the QRS complexes.

How the Patient Is Affected and What You Should Know

atrial kick The extra blood that can be ejected into the ventricles by the atria as a result of the electrical impulse slowing as it enters the AV node.

The **atrial kick,** which occurs when blood is ejected into the ventricles by the atria immediately prior to ventricular systole, is no longer present because the atria do not contract completely, followed by a delay in the ventricular contraction. This loss of atrial kick contributes to a 10% to 30% decrease in cardiac output. Some patients may tolerate this if the heart rate is within normal limits of 60 to 100 beats per minute. But once the heart rate increases significantly and loss of the atrial kick occurs, the patient will demonstrate signs and symptoms of low cardiac output.

When atrial flutter occurs, notify the licensed practitioner to implement a treatment plan, which usually includes oxygen therapy to ensure adequate supply to the vital organs. The patient is monitored continuously to determine if the rhythm converts to a sinus rhythm or progresses to atrial fibrillation. A continuous rhythm strip is needed to document whether any changes occurred as a result of the medical intervention. Always indicate on the rhythm strip the type of intervention that is being implemented. The ECG strips are kept in the patient's medical record or chart. In some cases the rhythm strip is printed, mounted, and saved.

Checkpoint Question (LO 6.5)

Using the criteria for classification, select the rhythm that most closely resembles atrial flutter rhythm.

A.

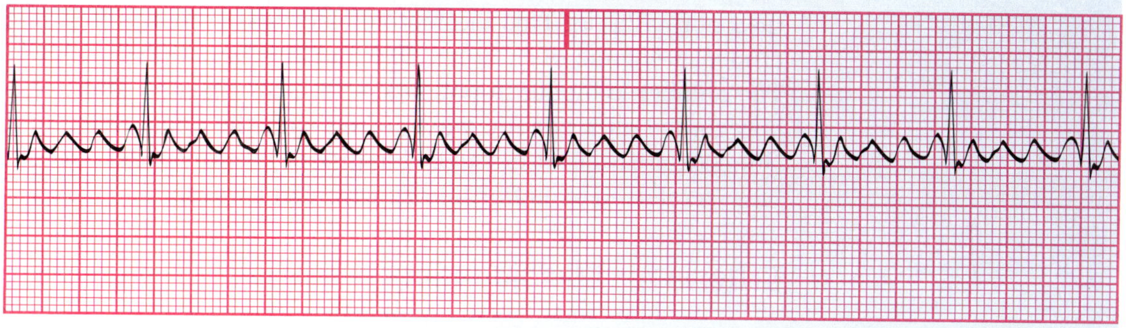

B.

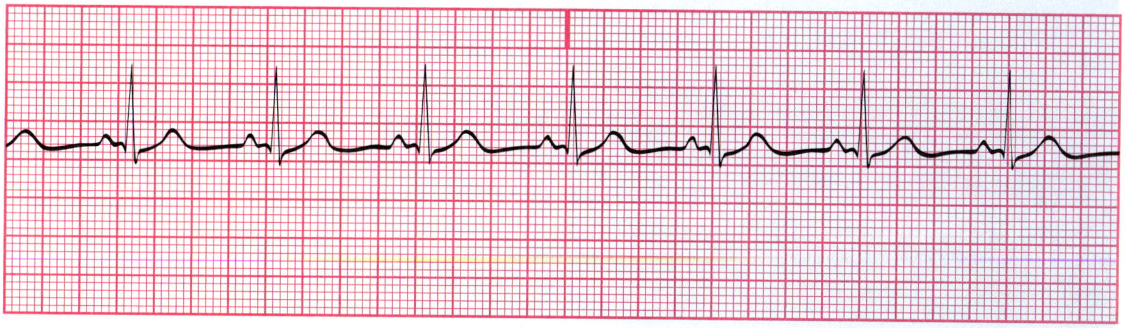

1. Which distinguishing feature(s) led you to make the selection?

____

____

____

6.6 Atrial Fibrillation

Atrial fibrillation (A-fib) occurs when electrical impulses come from areas of reentry pathways or multiple ectopic foci. Each electrical impulse results in depolarization of only a small group of atrial cells rather than the whole atrium. This results in the atrium not contracting as a whole. Instead, it quivers, similar to a bowl of Jell-O® when shaken. The result of

Figure 6-5 Atrial fibrillation.

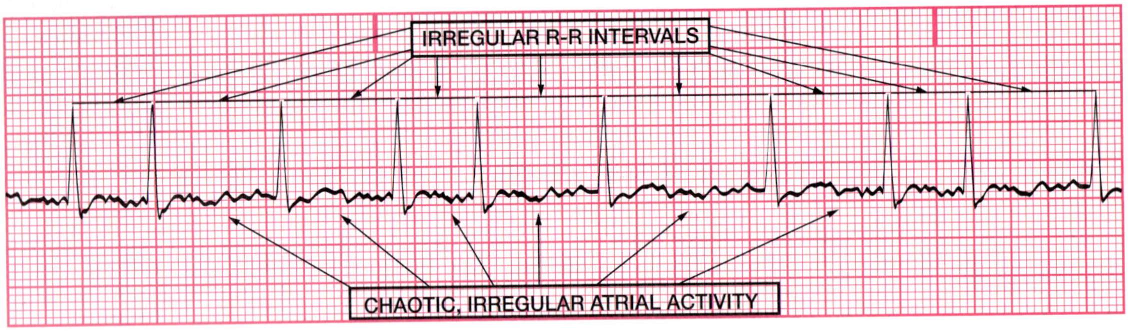

this disorganized electrical activity is that the atria do not pump blood as they normally do. This ineffective electrical activity often results in a loss of stroke volume of between 20% and 30% in patients with a normal heart. The number is higher in patients with heart disease. Multiple atrial activity is recorded as a chaotic wave, often with the appearance of fine scribbles (Figure 6-5). No P wave can be identified. The waveform of the chaotic "scribbles" is referred to as fibrillatory waves or f waves.

Criteria for Classification

- ***Rhythm:*** The P-P interval cannot be determined because of the fibrillatory waves or "f" waves. The R-R interval is irregular.
- ***Rate:*** The atrial rate cannot be determined due to the chaotic nature of the waveforms. The atria are not contracting and pumping blood due to this activity. The numbers referred to are electrical impulse activity, not contractions. Electrical impulse activity often is in the range of 375–700.
- ***P wave morphology:*** The P waves cannot be identified. There is chaotic electrical activity, or f waves may be seen.
- ***PR interval:*** The PR interval cannot be measured because the P wave is not identifiable.
- ***QRS duration and morphology:*** The QRS duration is within normal limits of 0.06 to 0.10 second and irregular.

Interpret-TIP

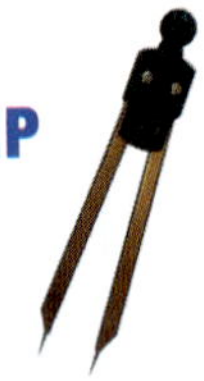

Atrial Fibrillation

Atrial fibrillation shows chaotic atrial electrical activity with irregular R-R intervals.

thrombus A blood clot attached to a diseased area of the wall of the endocardium or the wall of an injured blood vessel.

cerebrovascular accident (CVA) A stroke caused by a hemorrhage in the brain or more often by a clot lodged in a cerebral artery.

How the Patient Is Affected and What You Should Know

The patient exhibits signs and symptoms of decreased cardiac output. The patient usually has limited cardiac function because of preexisting cardiac conditions, so with the loss of atrial kick, the patient's cardiac output decreases significantly. When patients first present with atrial fibrillation, the ventricular response is often over 100 beats per minute. This is referred to as "uncontrolled" A-fib. Patients with "new onset" A-fib often complain of dizziness, nausea, and other signs of low cardiac output. The initial goal in the treatment of uncontrolled A-fib is to stabilize the patient by slowing the ventricular response via the use of medications first, then cardioversion if

myocardial infarction (MI; heart attack) Damage to the heart muscle caused by lack of oxygen due to a blockage of one or more of the coronary arteries.

pulmonary embolism A blocked artery in the lungs, usually caused by a blood clot.

renal infarction A lack of oxygen to kidney tissue due to a blocked blood vessel.

necessary. Once the heart rate is controlled within the range of 60 to 100 beats per minute, the patient may be able to tolerate the loss of the atrial kick.

During A-fib, blood begins to collect in the atria because they are not contracting completely, allowing the opportunity for a clot or **thrombus** to form. Therefore, the patient has an increased risk of developing and sending an embolism (traveling blood clot) out into the body's pulmonary or systemic circulation, which can then migrate to other vital organs, such as the lungs or brain. The patient may develop a **cerebrovascular accident (CVA), myocardial infarction (MI; heart attack), pulmonary embolism, renal infarction,** or an embolism in any place that the arterial blood is transported. Essentially there is no way to predict where the embolism will travel in the body to cause serious damage or even sudden death.

Patients who exhibit atrial fibrillation must be observed for low cardiac output. The rhythm needs to be monitored closely as the medication or electrical cardioversion is attempted. Report any complications or vital sign changes to the licensed practitioner immediately.

Checkpoint Question (LO 6.6)

Using the criteria for classification, select the rhythm that most closely resembles atrial fibrillation rhythm.

A.

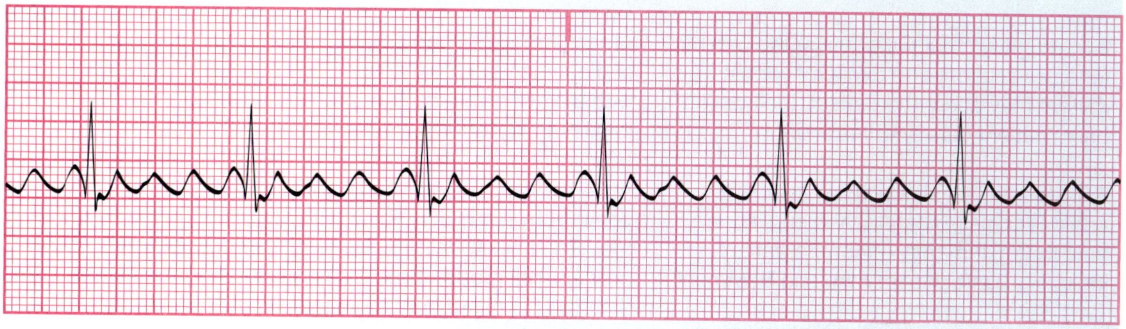

B.

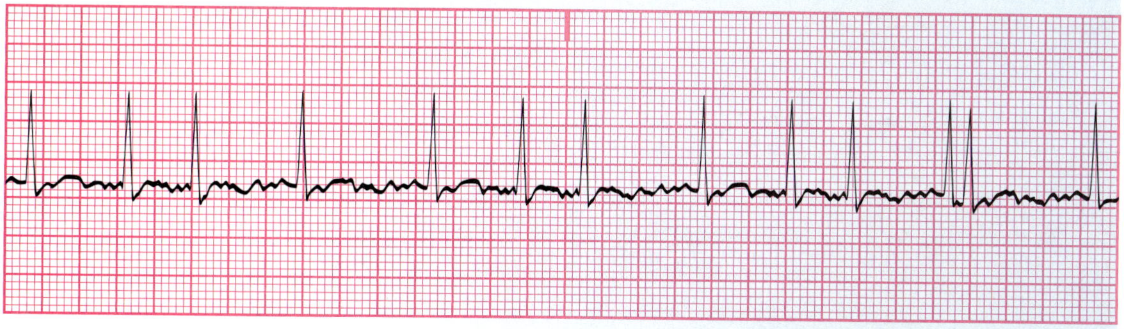

1. Which distinguishing feature(s) led you to make the selection?

____

____

____

Chapter Summary

Learning Outcomes	Summary	Pages
6.1 Summarize the similarities and differences among atrial dysrhythmias.	Atrial dysrhythmias are caused by an ectopic impulse in either of the atria.	147–148
6.2 Identify premature atrial complexes using the criteria for classification, and explain how the rhythm may affect the patient, including basic patient care and treatment.	Premature atrial complexes (PACs) are electrical impulses that originate in the atria and initiate an early impulse that interrupts the inherent regular rhythm.	148–150
6.3 Identify wandering atrial pacemaker using the criteria for classification, and explain how the rhythm may affect the patient, including basic patient care and treatment.	A wandering atrial pacemaker (WAP) is a rhythm in which the pacemaker site shifts between the SA node, other sites in the atria, and/or the AV junction. The P wave morphology changes in appearance during the pacemaker shift.	150–152
6.4 Identify multifocal atrial tachycardia using the criteria for classification, and explain how the rhythm may affect the patient, including basic patient care and treatment.	Multifocal atrial tachycardia (MAT) has a P wave that changes from beat to beat and a heart rate of 101 to 150 beats per minute.	152–153
6.5 Identify atrial flutter using the criteria for classification, and explain how the rhythm may affect the patient, including basic patient care and treatment.	Atrial flutter (A-flutter) occurs when a rapid impulse originates in the atrial tissue. This dysrhythmia presents with a classic sawtooth or picket fence appearance known as flutter or F waves.	153–155
6.6 Identify atrial fibrillation using the criteria for classification, and explain how the rhythm may affect the patient, including basic patient care and treatment.	Atrial fibrillation (A-fib) occurs when electrical impulses come from areas of reentry pathways or multiple ectopic foci. Each electrical impulse results in depolarization of only a small group of atrial cells rather than the whole atrium. This dysrhythmia presents with classic chaotic ("f" or fibrillatory) waves between the irregular R-R intervals.	155–157

Chapter Review

Matching

Match the terms on the left with their definitions on the right.

_______ **1.** ectopic (LO 6.1)
_______ **2.** trigeminy (LO 6.2)
_______ **3.** focus (LO 6.2)
_______ **4.** neurological (LO 6.1)
_______ **5.** automaticity (LO 6.5)
_______ **6.** atrial kick (LO 6.5)
_______ **7.** thrombus (LO 6.6)
_______ **8.** biphasic (LO 6.2)
_______ **9.** cerebrovascular accident (LO 6.6)
_______ **10.** renal (LO 6.6)
_______ **11.** pulmonary embolism (LO 6.6)
_______ **12.** myocardial (LO 6.6)

a. pertaining to the heart
b. pertaining to the kidneys
c. outside the normal pacemaker site
d. blood is ejected completely by the atria prior to ventricular systole
e. cell produces an ectopic impulse
f. every third complex is premature
g. pertaining to the nervous system
h. cardiac cell initiates an electrical impulse
i. stroke
j. traveling blood clot in the lungs
k. blood clot
l. having two equal but opposite deflections

Multiple Choice

Circle the correct answer.

13. What is the rate of wandering atrial pacemaker rhythm? (LO 6.3)
  a. 60 to 100 beats per minute
  b. 50 to 90 beats per minute
  c. 101 to 150 beats per minute
  d. 60 to 80 beats per minute

14. Which dysrhythmia is similar to wandering atrial pacemaker, except that the rate exceeds 100 beats per minute? (LO 6.4)
  a. Sinus tachycardia
  b. Multfocal atrial tachycardia
  c. Atrial flutter
  d. Atrial fibrillation

15. What is the major health risk for patients who have atrial fibrillation? (LO 6.6)
   a. Hypertension
   b. Thrombus formation and embolization
   c. Bundle branch block
   d. Bleeding problems

16. Which atrial dysrhythmia has capital “F” waves and a classic sawtooth or picket fence appearance? (LO 6.5)
   a. PACs
   b. Multifocal atrial tachycardia
   c. Atrial fibrillation
   d. Atrial flutter

17. Which atrial dysrhythmia has lowercase “f” waves, chaotic atrial electrical activity, and irregular R-R intervals? (LO 6.6)
   a. PACs
   b. Multifocal atrial tachycardia
   c. Atrial fibrillation
   d. Atrial flutter

18. Wandering atrial pacemaker rhythm must have ______________ or more differently shaped P waves. (LO 6.3)
   a. two
   b. three
   c. four
   d. none of the answers are correct

19. When premature complexes occur in a rhythm, they interrupt the underlying rhythm, causing it to be _____ when analyzing it. (LO 6.2)
   a. regular
   b. irregular
   c. a wider QRS complex
   d. bradycardic

20. Which of the following is a common sign of low cardiac output? (LO 6.1)
   a. High blood pressure
   b. Alert and oriented
   c. Increased perfusion of vital organs
   d. Low blood pressure

Fill in the Blank

21. Multifocal atrial tachycardia may occasionally be confused with ______________________. (LO 6.4)

22. When analyzing atrial flutter, you note that there are four F waves for each QRS complex. How will you represent this pattern in your interpretation? ______________________. (LO 6.5)

Short Answer

23. The patient has coronary artery disease. How would you expect PACs to affect this patient? (LO 6.1)

____

____

24. What treatment is usually indicated for patients with atrial flutter? (LO 6.5)

____

____

25. What is the best way to describe the rhythm pattern for atrial fibrillation? (LO 6.6)

____

____

26. Which rhythm is considered more serious, MAT or WAP, and why? (LO 6.3, 6.4)

____

____

Critical Thinking Application *Rhythm Identification*

Review the dysrhythmias pictured here and, using the criteria for classification provided in the chapter as clues, identify each rhythm and provide what information you used to make your decision. *Note:* Be certain to include the ratio for atrial flutter rhythms. (LO 6.2–6.6)

27.

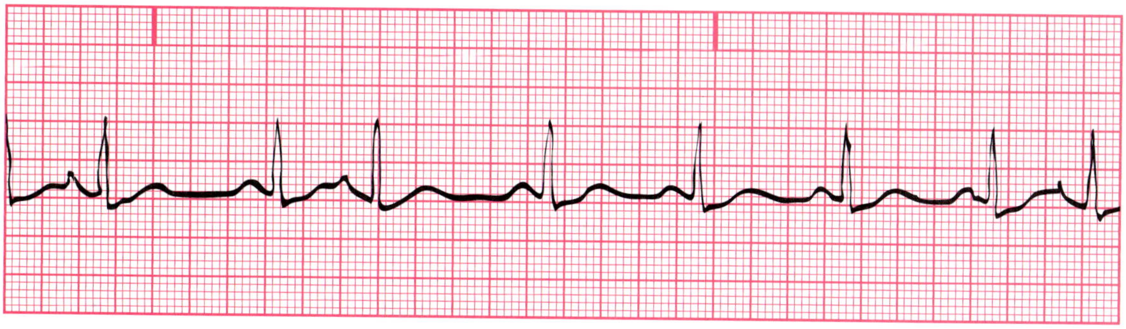

Rhythm (regular or irregular): ____________ PR interval: ____________

Rate: ____________ QRS: ____________

P wave: ____________ Interpretation: ____________

28.

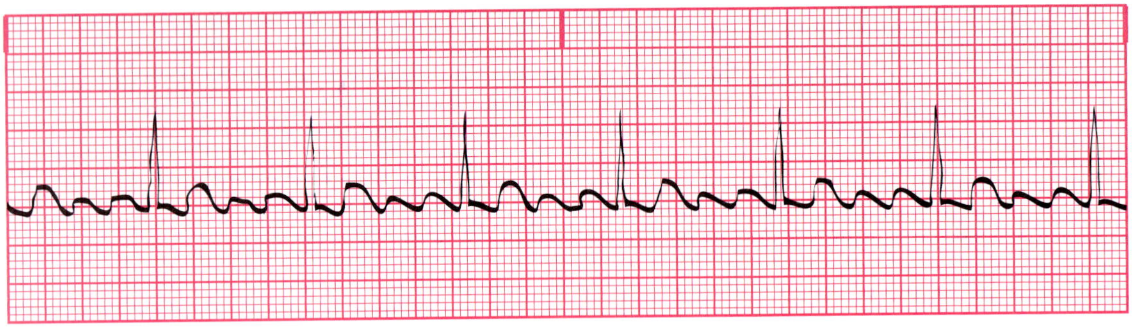

Rhythm (regular or irregular): ______________________ PR interval: ______________________

Rate: ______________________ QRS: ______________________

P wave: ______________________ Interpretation: ______________________

29.

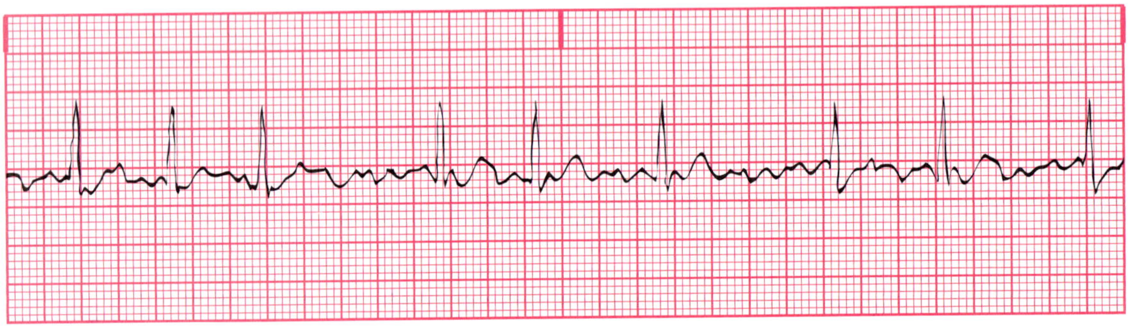

Rhythm (regular or irregular): ______________________ PR interval: ______________________

Rate: ______________________ QRS: ______________________

P wave: ______________________ Interpretation: ______________________

30.

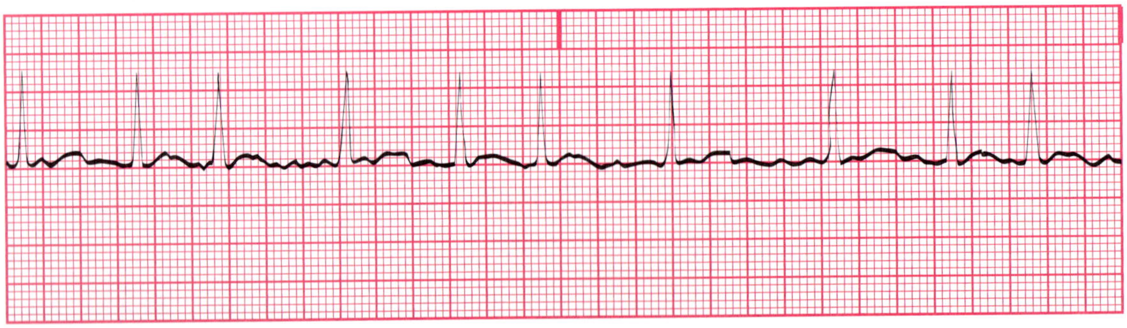

Rhythm (regular or irregular): ______________________ PR interval: ______________________

Rate: ______________________ QRS: ______________________

P wave: ______________________ Interpretation: ______________________

31.

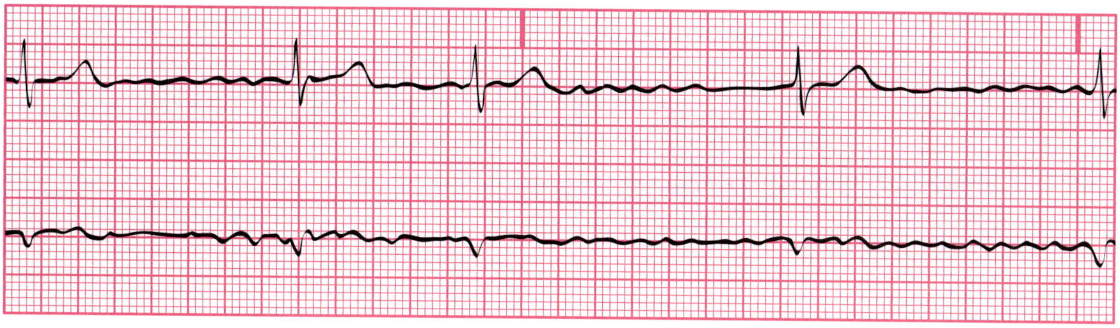

Rhythm (regular or irregular): ________________ PR interval: ________________

Rate: ________________ QRS: ________________

P wave: ________________ Interpretation: ________________

32.

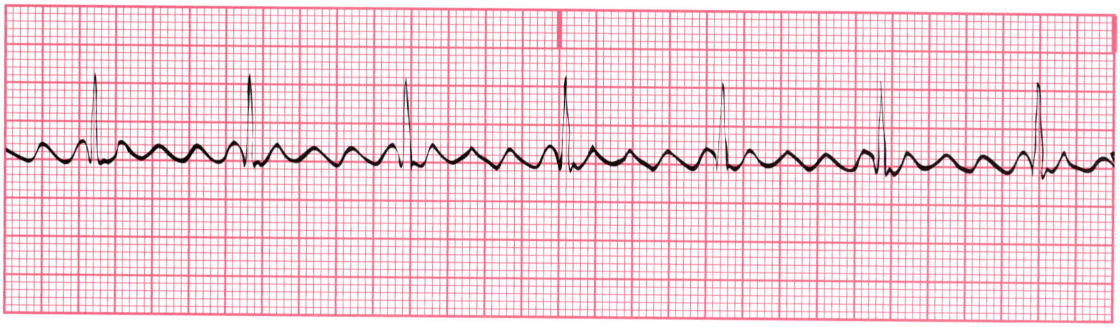

Rhythm (regular or irregular): ________________ PR interval: ________________

Rate: ________________ QRS: ________________

P wave: ________________ Interpretation: ________________

33.

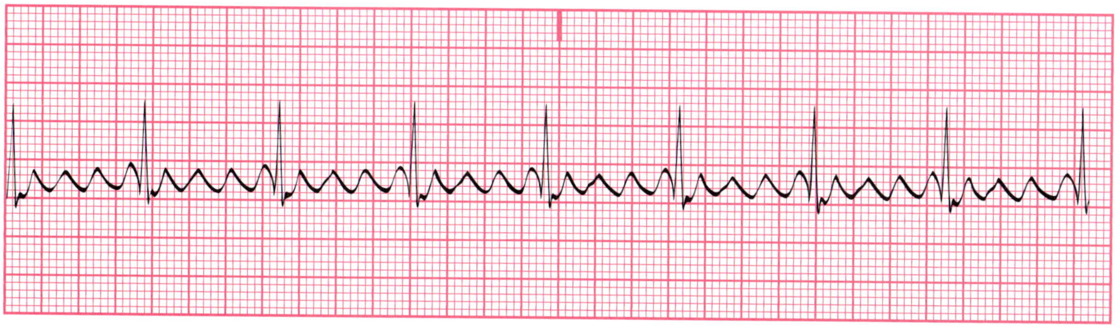

Rhythm (regular or irregular): ________________ PR interval: ________________

Rate: ________________ QRS: ________________

P wave: ________________ Interpretation: ________________

34.

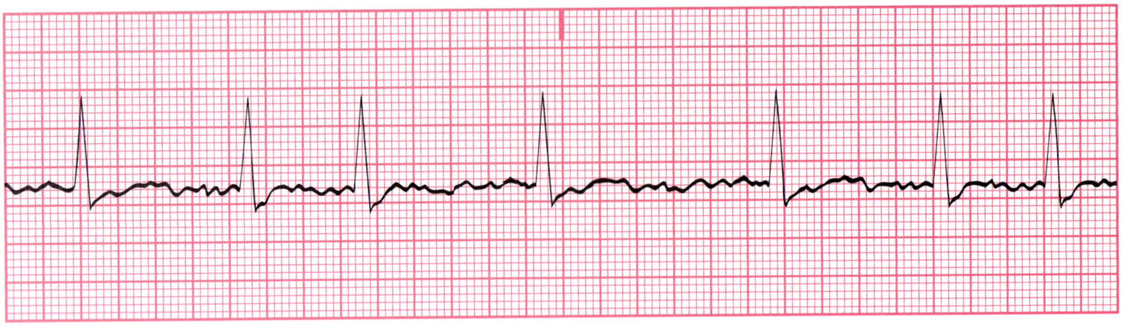

Rhythm (regular or irregular): ______ PR interval: ______

Rate: ______ QRS: ______

P wave: ______ Interpretation: ______

35.

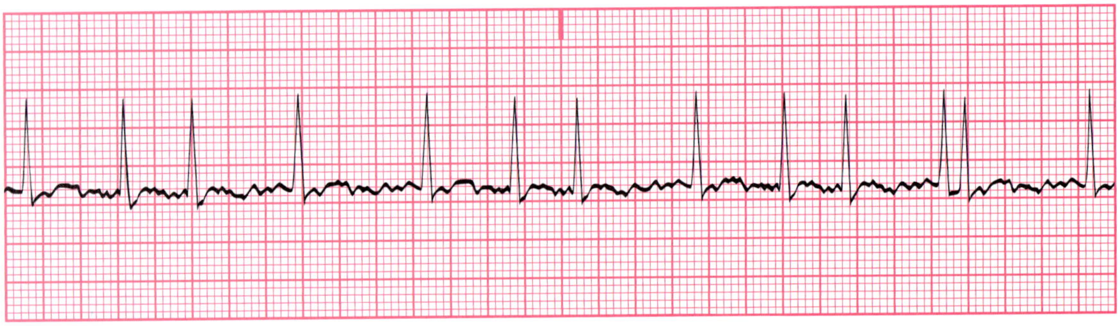

Rhythm (regular or irregular): ______ PR interval: ______

Rate: ______ QRS: ______

P wave: ______ Interpretation: ______

36.

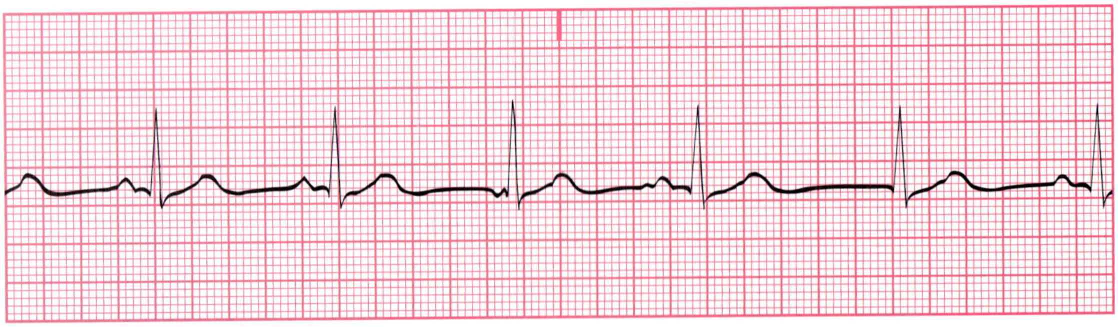

Rhythm (regular or irregular): ______ PR interval: ______

Rate: ______ QRS: ______

P wave: ______ Interpretation: ______

37.

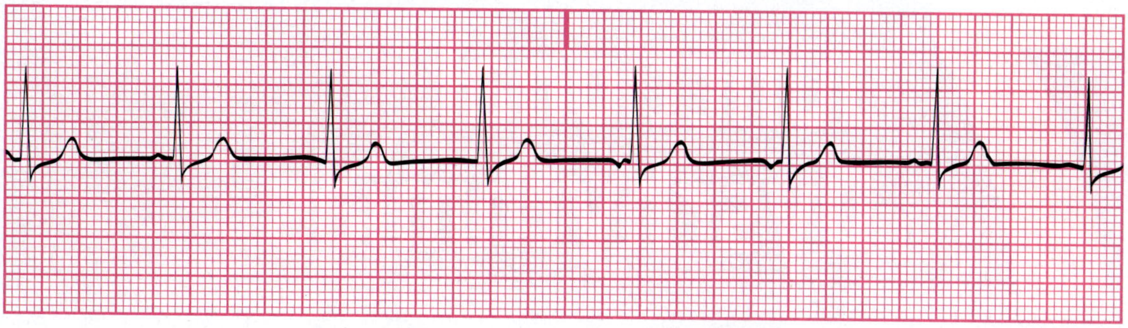

Rhythm (regular or irregular): ______________________ PR interval: ______________________

Rate: ______________________ QRS: ______________________

P wave: ______________________ Interpretation: ______________________

connect® Now that you have completed the material in the chapter text, go to Connect and complete any chapter activities you have not yet done.

7 Junctional Dysrhythmias

Learning Outcomes

7.1 Describe the various junctional dysrhythmias.

7.2 Identify premature junctional complexes using the criteria for classification, and explain how the rhythm may affect the patient, including basic patient care and treatment.

7.3 Identify junctional escape rhythm using the criteria for classification, and explain how the rhythm may affect the patient, including basic patient care and treatment.

7.4 Identify accelerated junctional rhythm using the criteria for classification, and explain how the rhythm may affect the patient, including basic patient care and treatment.

7.5 Identify junctional tachycardia using the criteria for classification, and explain how the rhythm may affect the patient, including basic patient care and treatment.

7.6 Identify supraventricular tachycardia using the criteria for classification, and explain how the rhythm may affect the patient, including basic patient care and treatment.

Key Terms

AV junction
delta wave
hypotension
junctional escape rhythm
retrograde
supraventricular
underlying rhythm
Wolfe-Parkinson-White syndrome

7.1 Introduction to Junctional Dysrhythmias

AV junction The AV node and surrounding tissue, including the bundle of His.

The atrioventricular (AV) node and the surrounding area, including the bundle of His, are collectively known as the **AV junction.** Cells in the AV junction have automaticity and can function as a pacemaker, although the AV junction is not the heart's normal pacemaker. Junctional rhythms are the result of electrical impulses coming from the AV junction rather than the SA node. The inherent rate of the AV junction is between 40 and 60 beats per minute.

retrograde Moving backward.

With junctional rhythms, it is important to understand that the electrical current is initiated *from* the AV junction. As a result, the electrical impulses that cause depolarization of the atria flow **retrograde,** or backward. This reverse flow of electrical activity causes the inverted P wave morphology seen in junctional dysrhythmias.

Another feature of junctional complexes and rhythms is the orientation of the P wave in relation to the QRS complex. The P wave can occur before, during (hidden or buried), or after the QRS complex. This is due to the region of tissue from which the impulse originates. When the impulse leaves the AV junction, it travels backward to the atria, but it also travels forward into the ventricles. Therefore, location, distance, and speed of the impulse play a role in junctional complexes.

If the impulse is initiated high up in the AV junction (higher in the atrium, near the AV node), atrial depolarization occurs before ventricular depolarization, so the P wave occurs before the QRS complex. If the impulse comes from the midpoint of the AV junction, atrial and ventricular depolarization occur at the same time. As a result, the P wave is buried by the QRS complex. Remember that the cardiac monitor or ECG machine records only electrical activity in the form of voltage, and it can record only what it "sees." If the P wave and QRS complex occur at the same time, whichever has the larger voltage is reflected on the tracing. Finally, if the electrical impulse comes from the lowest aspect of the AV junction, the ventricles depolarize before the atria, and the P wave occurs after the QRS complex. See Figure 7-1.

Think of it as a kiddie pool in your backyard. If you drop a stone in the middle of the pool, the little waves will reach all sides of the pool at the same time. If you drop another stone closer to one side of the pool, the waves reach one side before the other.

Figure 7-1 For junctional rhythms the electrical impulses are retrograde and the P wave location on the ECG tracing depends on where the ectopic impulse occurs. (A) The P wave precedes the QRS complex; (B) the P wave is buried in the QRS complex; (C) the P wave follows the QRS complex.

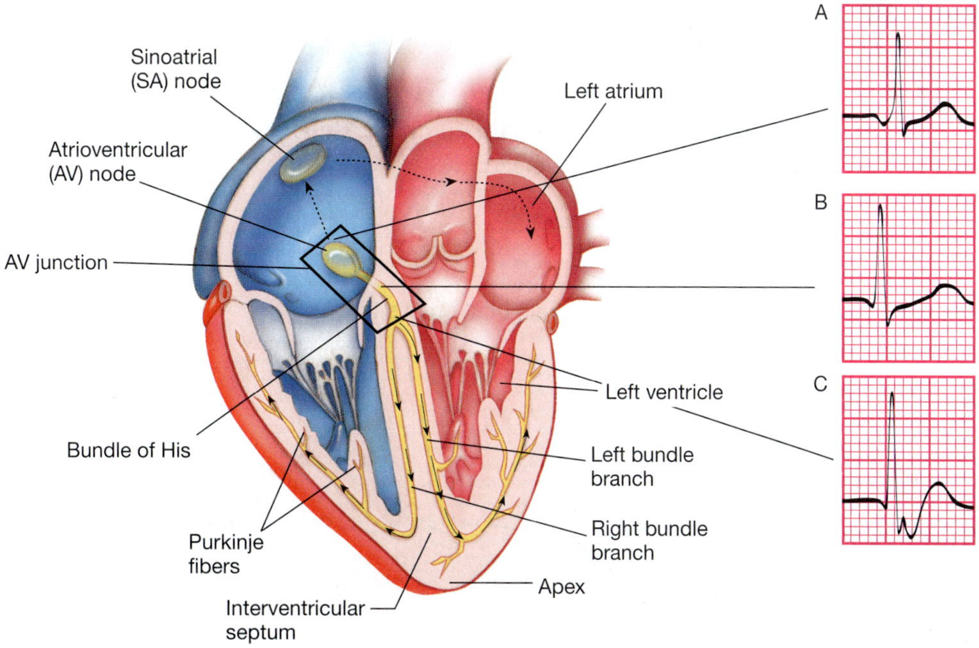

Checkpoint Question (LO 7.1)

1. Explain what causes the inverted P wave morphology found with junctional rhythms.

____

____

7.2 Premature Junctional Complex (PJC)

A premature junctional complex (PJC) is a single early electrical impulse that originates in the atrioventricular junction. It occurs before the next expected sinus impulse, causing an irregularity in the **underlying rhythm** (Figure 7-2).

underlying rhythm The heart rhythm that would be present if the abnormal impulses were ignored or removed from the tracing.

Criteria for Classification

- ***Rhythm:*** May be occasionally irregular or frequently irregular, depending on the underlying rhythm and the number of PJCs present.
- ***Rate:*** Depends on the underlying rhythm.
- ***P wave morphology:*** The P wave is inverted and may immediately precede or follow the QRS complex, or it may be buried within the QRS complex.
- ***PR interval:*** May be shorter than normal if the P wave precedes the QRS complex, absent if the P wave is buried in the QRS, or not measurable if it occurs after the QRS complex. *Note:* Remember that the PR interval can be measured only if the P wave (regardless of shape) occurs prior to the QRS complex.
- ***QRS duration and morphology:*** The QRS duration is between the normal limits of 0.06 and 0.10 second.

Interpret-TIP

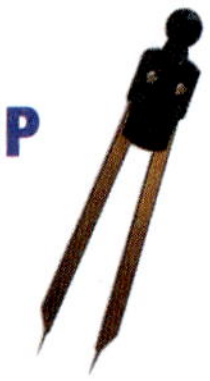

Premature Junctional Complexes

PJCs cause the rhythm to be irregular, and the P wave may appear before, during, or after the QRS complex. Regardless of location, if the P wave is seen, it will be inverted.

Figure 7-2 The premature junctional complex is the sixth beat on this tracing.

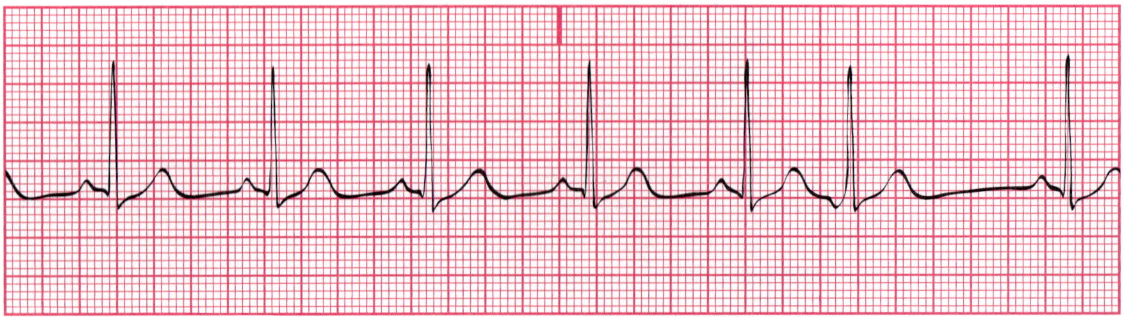

hypotension A lower than normal blood pressure that can cause reduction of blood flow to vital organs.

How the Patient Is Affected and What You Should Know

When the patient has a healthy heart, isolated PJCs cause no signs or symptoms. If more than four to six PJCs occur per minute, this warns of a more serious condition. An irregular pulse would be noted, and the patient may experience **hypotension** due to low cardiac output.

Checkpoint Question (LO 7.2)

Using the criteria for classification, select the rhythm that most closely resembles premature junctional complex.

A.

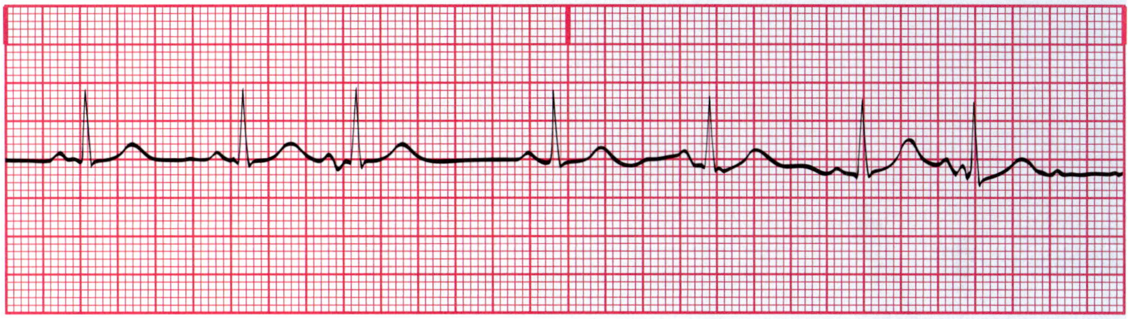

B.

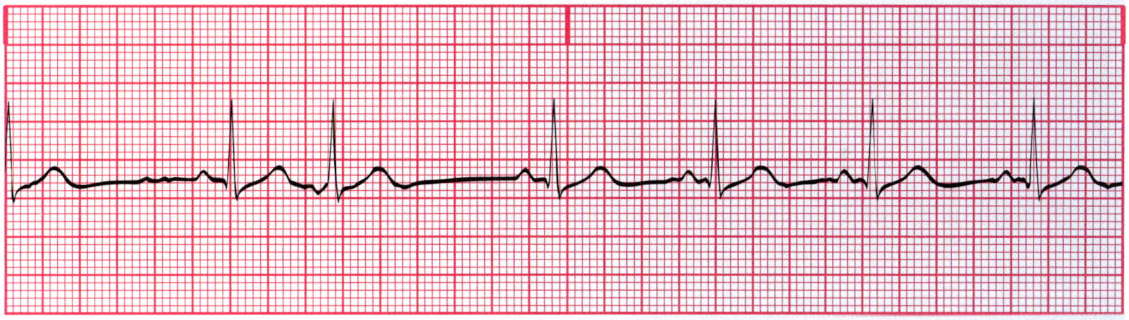

1. Which distinguishing feature(s) led you to make the selection?

____

____

____

junctional escape rhythm A rhythm that occurs when the SA node fails to initiate the electrical activity and one of the backup pacemaker sites takes over.

7.3 Junctional Escape Rhythm

Junctional rhythm, also known as **junctional escape rhythm,** originates at the AV junction, producing retrograde (backward) depolarization of atrial tissue and, at the same time, stimulating the depolarization of ventricles (Figure 7-3). Escape rhythms occur when the SA node fails to initiate the electrical activity. When this happens, one of the backup pacemaker sites takes over.

Criteria for Classification

- ***Rhythm:*** The P-P and R-R intervals are regular and occur at similar intervals. The P-P interval may be difficult to measure due to the location of the P wave.
- ***Rate:*** The ventricular rate is 40 to 60 beats per minute. The atrial rate is 40 to 60 beats per minute, but this may not be measurable if the P waves are not identifiable.
- ***P wave morphology:*** The P wave is usually inverted and may precede, follow, or fall within the QRS complex. It may not be visible at all on the rhythm strip.
- ***PR interval:*** If the P wave is before the QRS complex, the PR interval measures less than 0.12 second and is constant. If the P wave is not before the QRS complex, the PR interval cannot be determined because this P wave is not associated with the next QRS complex.
- ***QRS duration and morphology:*** The QRS duration is within normal limits of 0.06 to 0.10 second.

Interpret-TIP

Junctional Escape Rhythm

The P wave may occur before, during (buried in), or after the QRS. If the P wave is seen, it will be inverted. The heart rate is between 40 and 60 beats per minute.

How the Patient Is Affected and What You Should Know

The patient with junctional escape rhythm has a slower heart rate than normal and loses the atrial kick due to the shortening of the interval between the atrial depolarization and ventricular depolarization. These conditions often cause the patient to exhibit signs and symptoms of low cardiac output. Common signs and symptoms of low cardiac output displayed include hypotension (low blood pressure) and altered mental status, such as confusion or disorientation. Observe for symptoms and monitor the ECG tracing in case a more serious dysrhythmia occurs. Report the presence of junctional rhythm and your observations of the patient to a licensed practitioner for appropriate medical treatment.

Figure 7-3 Junctional escape rhythm.

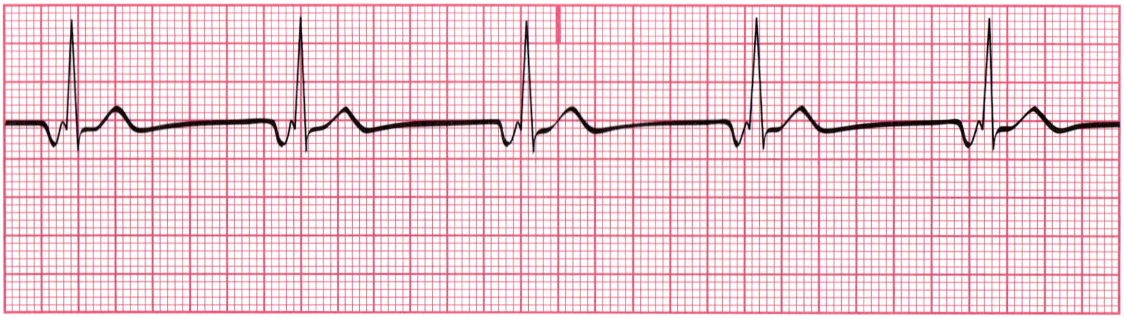

Checkpoint Questions (LO 7.3)

Using the criteria for classification, select the rhythm that most closely resembles junctional escape rhythm.

A.

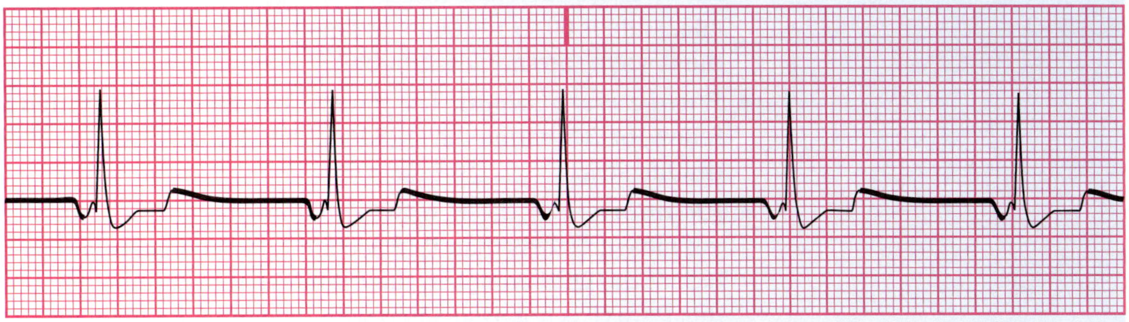

B.

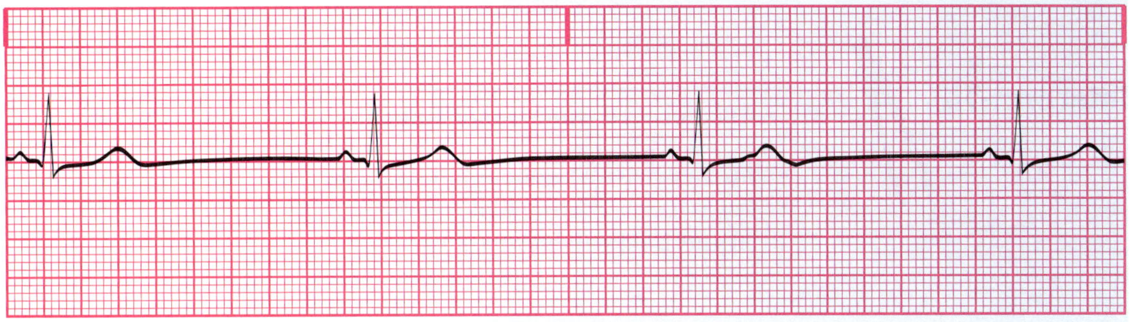

1. Which distinguishing feature(s) led you to make the selection?

2. What are the differences between a rhythm with a PJC in it and a junctional escape rhythm?

7.4 Accelerated Junctional Rhythm

The morphology of accelerated junctional rhythm is similar to that of junctional escape rhythm; the distinguishing factor is the heart rate. This rhythm originates at the AV junction, producing retrograde depolarization of atrial tissue, and, at the same time, stimulates the depolarization of ventricles (Figure 7-4).

Criteria for Classification

- ***Rhythm:*** The P-P and R-R intervals are regular and occur at similar intervals. The P-P interval may be difficult to measure due to the location of the P wave.
- ***Rate:*** The ventricular rate is between 60 and 100 beats per minute. The atrial rate is 60 to 100 beats per minute, but this may not be measurable if the P waves are not identifiable.
- ***P wave morphology:*** The P wave is usually inverted and may precede, follow, or fall within the QRS complex. It may not be visible at all on the rhythm strip.
- ***PR interval:*** If the P wave is before the QRS complex, the PR interval measures less than 0.12 second and is constant. If the P wave is not before the QRS complex, the PR interval cannot be determined because this P wave is not associated with the next QRS complex.
- ***QRS duration and morphology:*** The QRS duration is within normal limits of 0.06 to 0.10 second.

Interpret-TIP

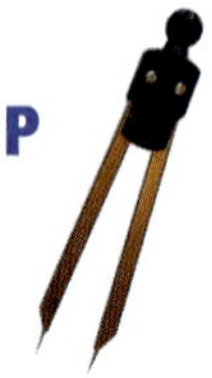

Accelerated Junctional Rhythm

An accelerated junctional rhythm may have an inverted or absent P wave or a P wave that follows the QRS complex. Heart rate is between 60 and 100 beats per minute.

How the Patient Is Affected and What You Should Know

It is unlikely that the patient will show signs and symptoms of low cardiac output because the rate is the same as normal sinus rhythm. It is still very important to observe your patient for symptoms and to monitor the ECG tracing in case a more serious dysrhythmia occurs. Report the presence of accelerated junctional rhythm and your observations of the patient to a licensed practitioner for appropriate medical treatment.

Figure 7-4 Accelerated junctional rhythm.

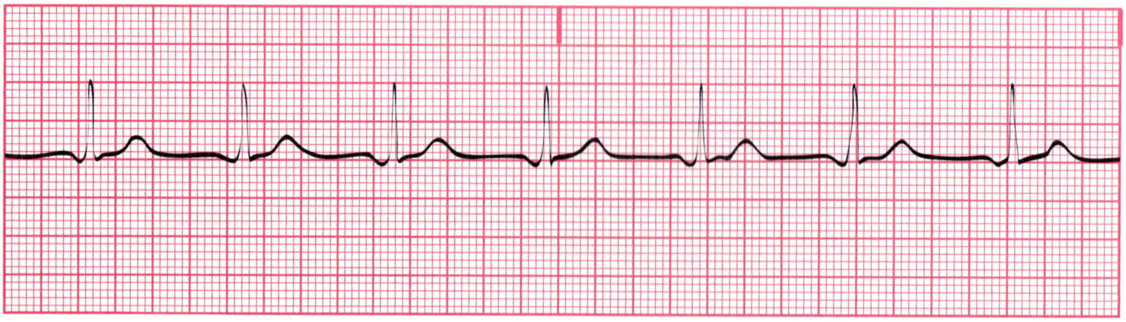

Checkpoint Question (LO 7.4)

Using the criteria for classification, select the rhythm that most closely resembles accelerated junctional rhythm.

A.

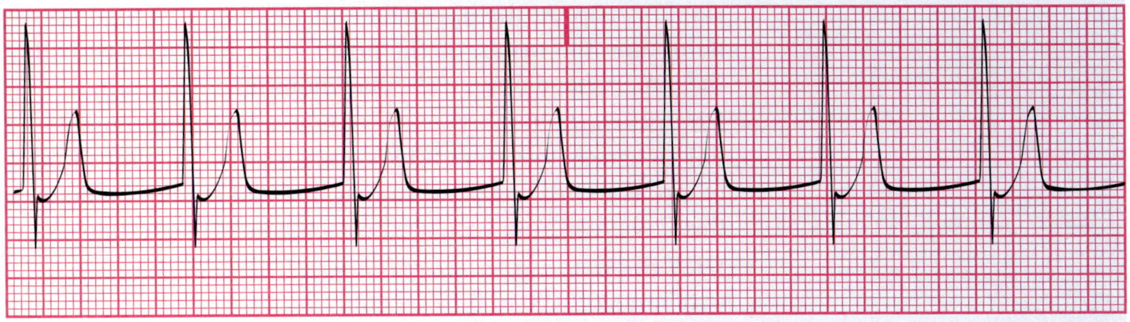

B.

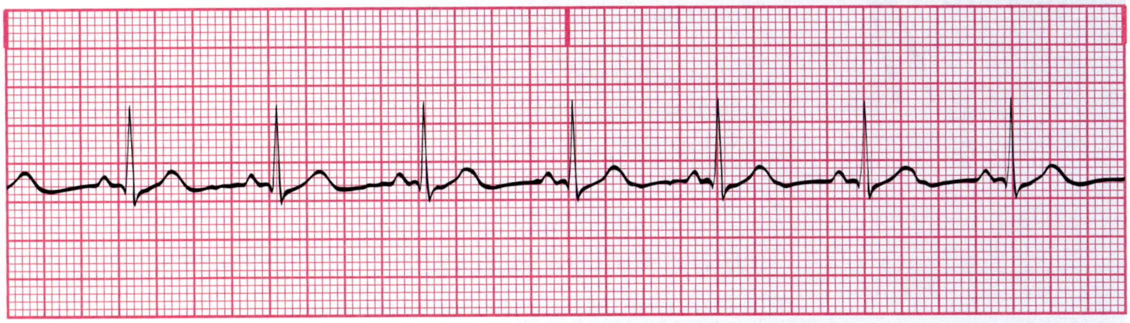

1. Which distinguishing feature(s) led you to make the selection?

____

____

____

7.5 Junctional Tachycardia

The morphology of junctional tachycardia rhythm is similar to that of junctional escape rhythm and accelerated junctional rhythm. The distinguishing factor is that the heart rate is faster in junctional tachycardia. The electrical activity originates at the AV junction from an irritable and ectopic focus (location) that overrides the SA node due to its rate, producing retrograde depolarization of atrial tissue, and at the same time stimulates the depolarization of ventricles (Figure 7-5).

Criteria for Classification

- ***Rhythm:*** The P-P and R-R intervals are regular and occur at similar intervals. The P-P interval may be even more difficult to measure because of the combination of location of the P wave and the increased rate of automaticity.

- ***Rate:*** The ventricular rate is between 100 and 180 beats per minute. The atrial rate is 100 to 180 beats per minute, but this may not be measurable if the P waves are not identifiable.
- ***P wave morphology:*** The P wave is usually inverted and may precede, follow, or fall within the QRS complex. It may not be visible at all on the rhythm strip. At the upper limit of this range, it may be very difficult to determine the origin of the atrial electrical activity without increasing the paper speed of your cardiac monitor.
- ***PR interval:*** If the P wave is before the QRS complex, the PR interval measures less than 0.12 second and is constant. If the P wave is not before the QRS complex, the PR interval cannot be determined because this P wave is not associated with the next QRS complex.
- ***QRS duration and morphology:*** The QRS duration is within the normal limits of 0.06 to 0.10 second.

Interpret-TIP

Junctional Tachycardia Rhythm

A junctional tachycardia rhythm may have an inverted or absent P wave or a P wave that follows the QRS complex. Heart rate is between 100 and 180 beats per minute.

How the Patient Is Affected and What You Should Know

The effect of this rhythm on the patient depends on the rate of junctional tachycardia. For example, if the patient's normal resting heart rate is 90 and now the patient is exhibiting a rate of 108 beats per minute after walking the hallway, tachycardia would be expected and is viewed as the patient's normal response to exercise. However, if the patient's normal heart rate is 60 and it is now 140, the patient is probably experiencing symptoms of low cardiac output. Often the patient will complain of palpitations or "heart fluttering" with faster rates. If the patient has had a recent myocardial infarction, junctional tachycardia or tachycardia of any type is considered to be more serious or even life threatening.

Observe the patient for symptoms, and monitor the ECG tracing in case a more serious dysrhythmia occurs. Report the presence of junctional tachycardia rhythm and your observations of the patient to a licensed practitioner for appropriate medical treatment. Medication may need to be administered to terminate this dysrhythmia.

Figure 7-5 Junctional tachycardia rhythm.

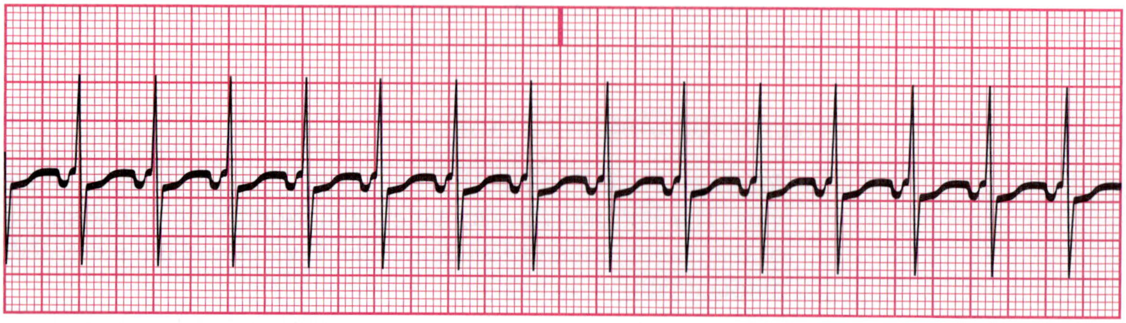

Checkpoint Question (LO 7.5)

Using the criteria for classification, select the rhythm that most closely resembles junctional tachycardia rhythm.

A.

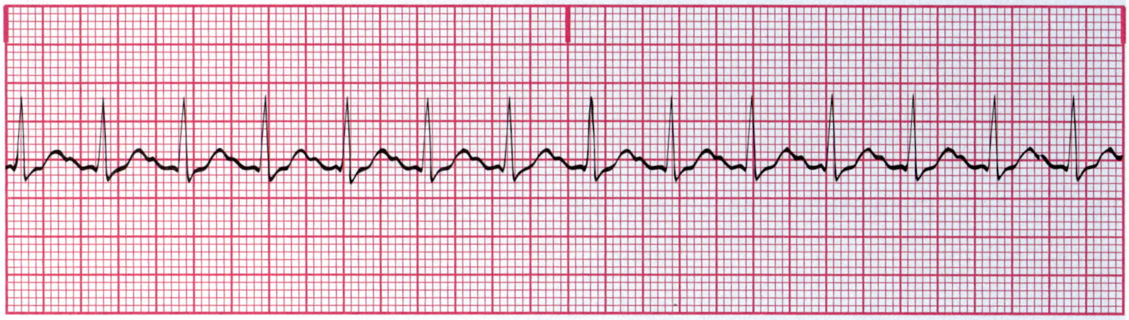

B.

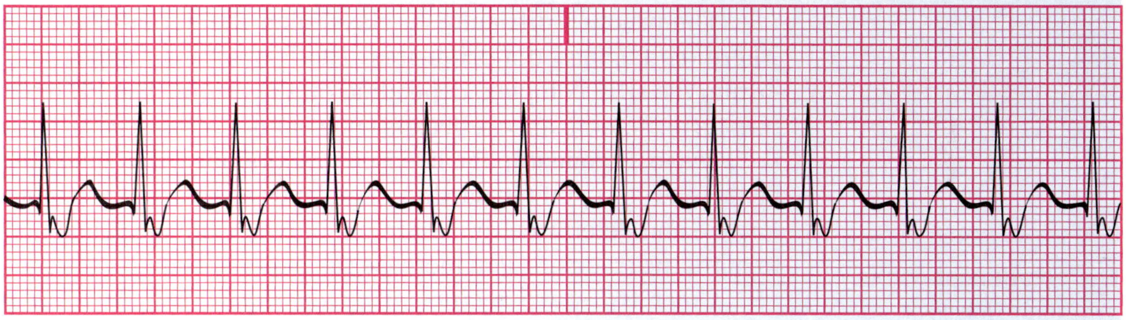

1. Which distinguishing feature(s) led you to make the selection?

____

____

____

7.6 Supraventricular Tachycardia (SVT)

supraventricular An ectopic focus originating above the ventricles in the atria or junctional region of the heart.

A supraventricular tachycardia (SVT) is a category of rapid rhythms in which the heartbeats faster than 100 beats per minute (Figure 7-6). *Supra* means "above," so the term **supraventricular** refers to an ectopic focus originating above the ventricles; in other words, in the atria or in the AV junction of the heart. Only those cases of SVT that originate in the AV junction are technically junctional dysrhythmias. However, the heart is beating so fast that it is difficult to determine whether the origin is from the SA node, the atria, or the AV junction.

Because the heart rate is so rapid, the atria contract as soon as the ventricles relax. This causes the P waves, which represent atrial contraction, to be difficult to identify because they occur at the same time as the QRS complexes or T waves (ventricular relaxation). Rhythms that fall into this category are identified in Table 7-1.

Some SVTs are *reentry dysrhythmias*. They occur when there is a blockage or short circuit in the normal electrical conduction pathway. This forces the electrical impulse to follow a different pathway, which often leads to a series of rapid depolarizations that in turn lead to tachydysrhythmias such as atrial fibrillation, atrial flutter, or junctional tachycardia.

Figure 7-6 Supraventricular tachycardia.

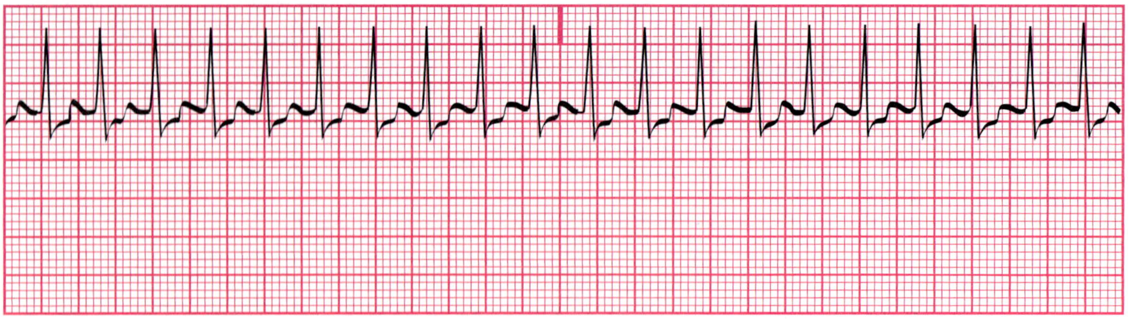

TABLE 7-1 Dysrhythmias Associated with Supraventricular Tachycardia

Sinus Node	Atrium	Junctional
Sinus tachycardia	Atrial flutter Atrial fibrillation	Junctional tachycardia Wolfe-Parkinson-White syndrome

Wolfe-Parkinson-White syndrome A type of supraventricular tachycardia in which an extra electrical pathway between an atrium and a ventricle short-circuits the normal pathway, resulting in tachycardia.

delta wave A widening at the beginning of the QRS complex due to ventricular pre-excitation.

The primary difficulty in classifying the actual rhythm is identifying where the tachycardia originates. The P wave may appear before, after, or during the QRS complex, depending on the origin. The PR interval measurement is difficult to assess because you cannot often see the initial upswing of the P wave. Frequently, the licensed practitioner will request the paper speed be increased to pull the cardiac complexes apart in an attempt to expose the P wave and determine the origin or source of the electrical activity. Be sure to mark the tracing if you increase the paper speed.

Other SVTs are *reciprocating dysrhythmias.* An example is **Wolfe-Parkinson-White syndrome,** which occurs as a result of an abnormal electrical conduction pathway between one of the atria and a ventricle. This abnormal pathway allows a portion of the electrical impulse causing atrial depolarization to enter the ventricle directly (prematurely), bypassing the AV node. The tracing presents with a P wave, but the P wave may not completely reach the isoelectric line before it starts into an early QRS complex. Whether the P wave is able to complete or not, the tracing will have a short PR interval due to ventricular *pre-excitation* (early start). Due to this pre-excitation, the QRS is abnormally wide (greater than 0.12 second). The pre-excitation period often looks like a slur, as shown in Figure 7-7. This portion of the cardiac complex is commonly referred to as the **delta wave.**

Criteria for Classification

- ***Rhythm:*** The ventricular (R-R) rhythm is usually regular or has minimal irregularity. The atrial rhythm may or may not be seen because other electrical activity is occurring at the same time. Remember, the

Figure 7-7 Delta waves due to Wolfe-Parkinson-White syndrome.

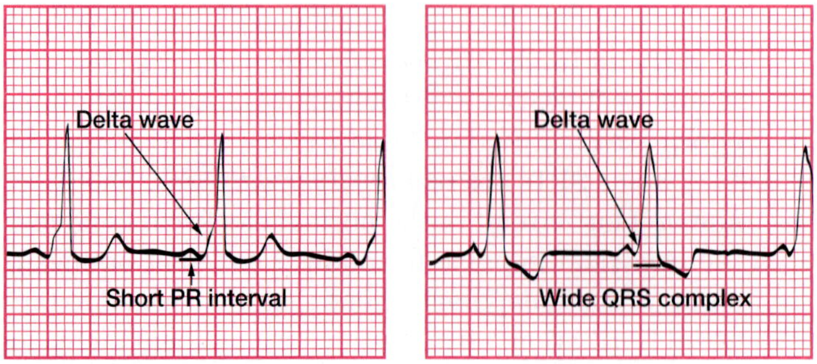

ECG records only the activity it "sees" in each lead. The atrial activity is small compared to ventricular activity; therefore, the ventricular activity is the largest amount of energy seen when the ECG tracing is recorded. Depending on whether the P waves are seen, you may not be able to determine regular P waves. If identifiable, they are usually regular.

- ***Rate:*** The ventricular rate is 150 to 250 beats per minute. The atrial rate is difficult to determine when P waves are unidentifiable.
- ***P wave morphology:*** The P waves are usually not identified when the heart rate is this rapid. Remember that when the heart rate increases, the time interval between atrial contraction and ventricular relaxation decreases. Therefore, if there is a P wave present, it may occur simultaneously with the T wave and may be buried within it. The P wave may occur before, during, or after the QRS complex.
- ***PR interval:*** Usually the PR interval cannot be determined because the beginning of the P wave cannot be clearly identified.
- ***QRS duration and morphology:*** The QRS measurement is considered within normal limits when measured at 0.06 to 0.10 second.

Interpret-TIP

Supraventricular Dysrhythmias

Supraventricular tachycardia describes a group of dysrhythmias that present with a normal-to-narrow QRS complex and a rate of greater than 150 beats per minute.

How the Patient Is Affected and What You Should Know

There are various supraventricular dysrhythmias, all of which may cause the patient to exhibit the same signs and symptoms. The patient may be in either a stable or an unstable condition. The stable patient (one without signs and symptoms of decreased cardiac output) may complain only of palpitations and state, "I'm just not feeling right" or "My heart is fluttering." When the patient's condition is *unstable*, he or she may experience any symptom of low cardiac output because the heart is not pumping effectively to other body systems. Many patients may present initially with a stable condition and then a few minutes later experience unstable symptoms.

Observe the patient for signs and symptoms of low cardiac output. Signs, symptoms, and rhythm changes need to be communicated quickly to a licensed practitioner for appropriate medical treatment. Because tachycardia significantly increases myocardial oxygen demand, treatment should begin as early as possible. It is difficult to predict how long a patient's heart can beat at a rapid rate before it begins to affect the other body systems.

Law & Ethics

Scope of Practice

Your role regarding evaluation of the rhythm strip and assessment of the patient will depend on your training and place of employment. Working outside your scope of practice is illegal, and you could be held liable for performing tasks that are not part of your role as a healthcare professional.

Checkpoint Questions (LO 7.6)

1. What are the rate and the origination point of a supraventricular tachycardia?

____

____

2. What might you be asked to do when a patient has a supraventricular dysrhythmia?

____

____

3. List common sensations described by patients experiencing SVT.

____

____

4. Using the criteria for classification, select the rhythm that most closely resembles a supraventricular tachycardia (SVT) rhythm and identify the specific rhythm.

A.

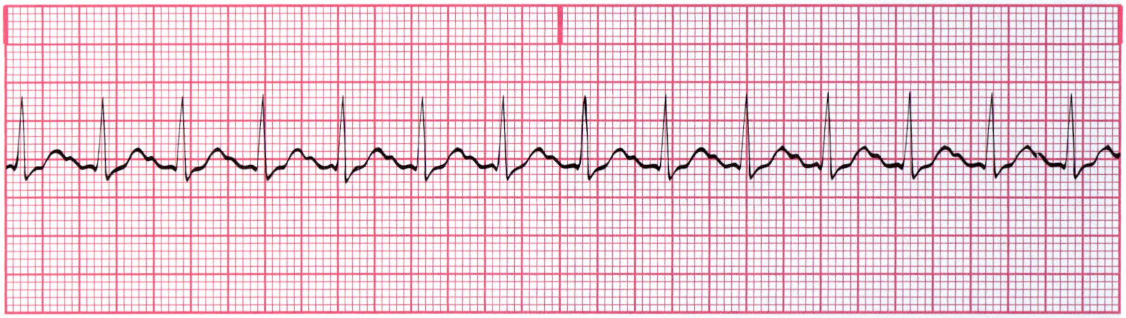

B.

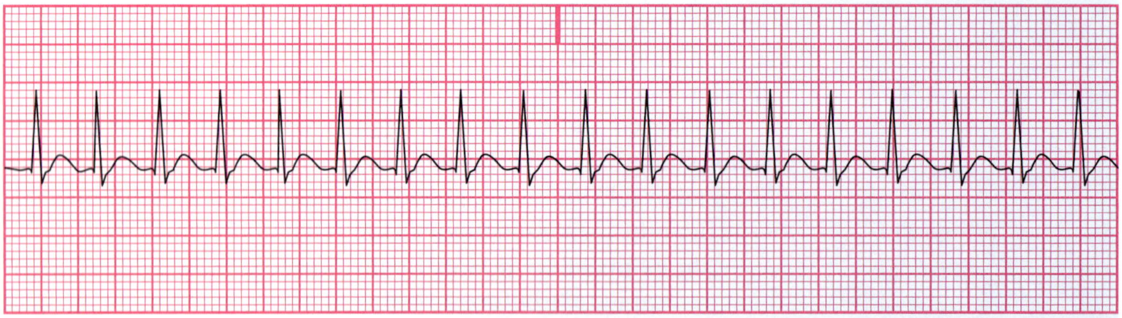

5. Which distinguishing feature(s) led you to make the selection?

____

____

Chapter Summary

Learning Outcomes	Summary	Pages
7.1 Describe the various junctional dysrhythmias.	Junctional rhythms occur as a result of electrical impulses coming from the AV junction rather than the SA node. As a result of this change in origination site, the electrical impulses causing depolarization of the atria flow retrograde (backward). This reverse flow of electrical activity causes the inverted P wave morphology seen in junctional dysrhythmias.	166–168
7.2 Identify premature junctional complex using the criteria for classification, and explain how the rhythm may affect the patient, including basic patient care and treatment.	A premature junctional complex (PJC) is a single early electrical impulse that originates in the AV junction. It occurs before the next expected sinus impulse, causing an irregularity in the rhythm.	168–169
7.3 Identify junctional escape rhythm using the criteria for classification, and explain how the rhythm may affect the patient, including basic patient care and treatment.	Junctional rhythm, also known as junctional escape rhythm, originates at AV junctional tissue, producing retrograde (backward) depolarization of atrial tissue and, at the same time, stimulates the depolarization of ventricles. This rhythm may be lifesaving and occurs when a higher pacemaker (the SA node) has failed to fire impulses to initiate depolarization. The inherent rate of the AV junction is 40 to 60 beats per minute.	169–171
7.4 Identify accelerated junctional rhythm using the criteria for classification, and explain how the rhythm may affect the patient, including basic patient care and treatment.	Accelerated junctional rhythm is similar to junctional escape rhythm, except that the heart rate is between 60 and 100 beats per minute for accelerated junctional rhythm.	171–173
7.5 Identify junctional tachycardia rhythm using the criteria for classification, and explain how the rhythm may affect the patient, including basic patient care and treatment.	Junctional tachycardia rhythm is similar to junctional escape rhythm in its morphology; however, while junctional escape rhythm is lifesaving and occurs in failure of a higher pacemaker (the SA node), junctional tachycardia occurs when the rate exceeds 100 beats per minute. It commonly arises from an irritable and ectopic focus and overrides the SA node due to its rate.	173–175
7.6 Identify supraventricular tachycardia rhythm using the criteria for classification, and explain how the rhythm may affect the patient, including basic patient care and treatment.	Although supraventricular tachycardia is not specifically a junctional dysrhythmia, the origin causing this rapid heart rhythm may come from any location "above the ventricles." Supraventricular tachycardia presents with a normal- to narrow-appearing QRS complex and a rate of greater than 150 beats per minute. Supraventricular tachycardia includes all forms of tachycardia that originate above the ventricles.	175–178

Chapter Review

Multiple Choice

Circle the correct answer.

1. What is the normal, inherent rate for the AV junction? (LO 7.1)
   a. 60–100 beats per minute
   b. 40–60 beats per minute
   c. 100–160 beats per minute
   d. 20–40 beats per minute
2. Which of the following dysrhythmias is *not* considered part of the supraventricular tachycardia classification? (LO 7.6)
   a. Atrial fibrillation
   b. Sinus tachycardia
   c. Ventricular tachycardia
   d. Junctional tachycardia
3. What sign or symptom might a patient complain about when experiencing a supraventricular tachycardia in an unstable condition? (LO 7.6)
   a. Back pain
   b. Palpitations
   c. Flank pain
   d. Chest pain and discomfort
4. The criterion needed to classify a dysrhythmia as a supraventricular tachycardia is (LO 7.6)
   a. a heart rate between 150 and 350 beats per minute.
   b. a wide QRS complex.
   c. a clear, easily identifiable P wave with the entire wave visualized.
   d. atrial and ventricular rates that are not the same.
5. What is the primary difficulty in determining a supraventricular rhythm? (LO 7.6)
   a. Determining the ventricular rate
   b. Determining the regularity
   c. Measuring the QRS interval
   d. Determining the origin of the tachycardia
6. When is the identification of the specific dysrhythmia important in terms of treatment of the patient? (LO 7.6)
   a. When the patient first complains of any signs or symptoms
   b. When the patient's heart rate has decreased to a rate of 100 beats per minute
   c. During the treatment of a fast tachycardia situation
   d. After the rhythm has been converted to a normal rhythm and/or the heart rate is between 60 and 100 beats per minute

7. What is the heart rate range for junctional escape rhythm? (LO 7.2)
   a. 20–40 beats per minute
   b. 100–150 beats per minute
   c. 40–60 beats per minute
   d. 60–100 beats per minute

8. What is the heart rate range for accelerated junctional rhythm? (LO 7.3)
   a. 20–40 beats per minute
   b. 100–150 beats per minute
   c. 40–60 beats per minute
   d. 60–100 beats per minute

9. What is the heart rate range for junctional tachycardia? (LO 7.4)
   a. 20–40 beats per minute
   b. 100–150 beats per minute
   c. 40–60 beats per minute
   d. 60–100 beats per minute

Short Answer

10. Describe why P waves are inverted or buried within the QRS complex with junctional dysrhythmias. (LO 7.1)

____

____

Critical Thinking Application *Rhythm Identification*

Review the dysrhythmias pictured here and, using the criteria for classification provided in the chapter as clues, identify each rhythm and provide the information you used to make your decision. (LO 7.2–7.6)

11.

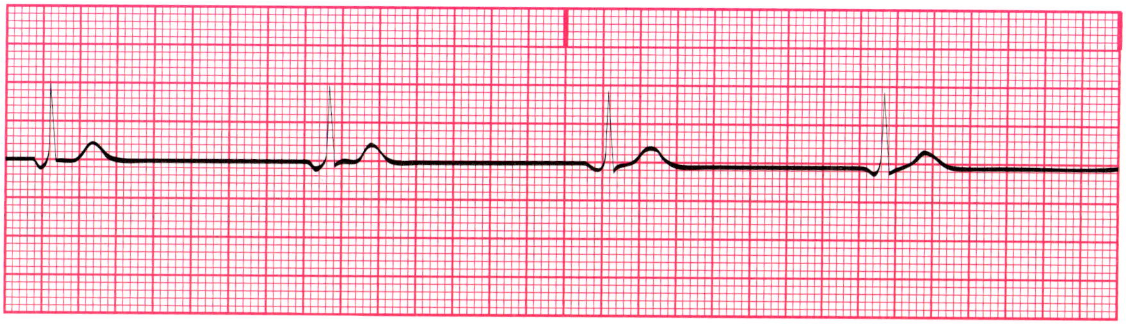

Rhythm (regular or irregular): ____________________ PR interval: ____________________

Rate: ____________________ QRS: ____________________

P wave: ____________________ Interpretation: ____________________

18.

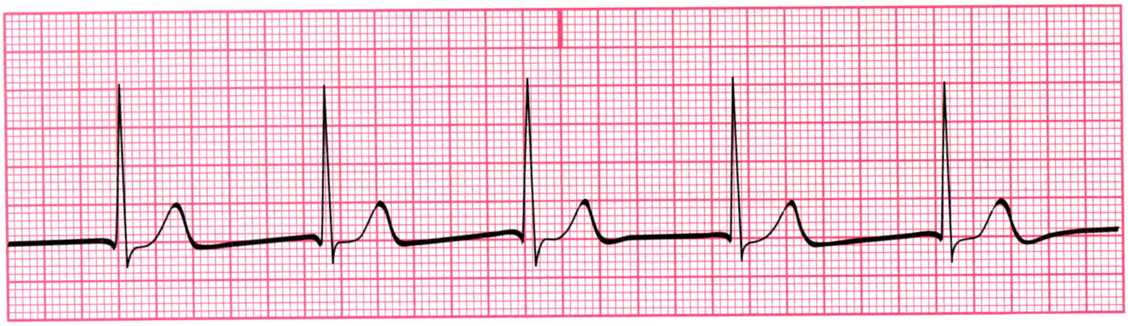

Rhythm (regular or irregular): ____________ PR interval: ____________

Rate: ____________ QRS: ____________

P wave: ____________ Interpretation: ____________

19.

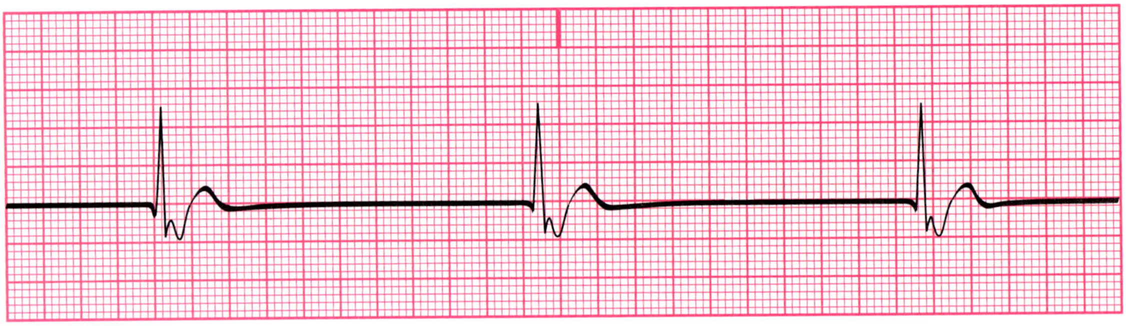

Rhythm (regular or irregular): ____________ PR interval: ____________

Rate: ____________ QRS: ____________

P wave: ____________ Interpretation: ____________

20.

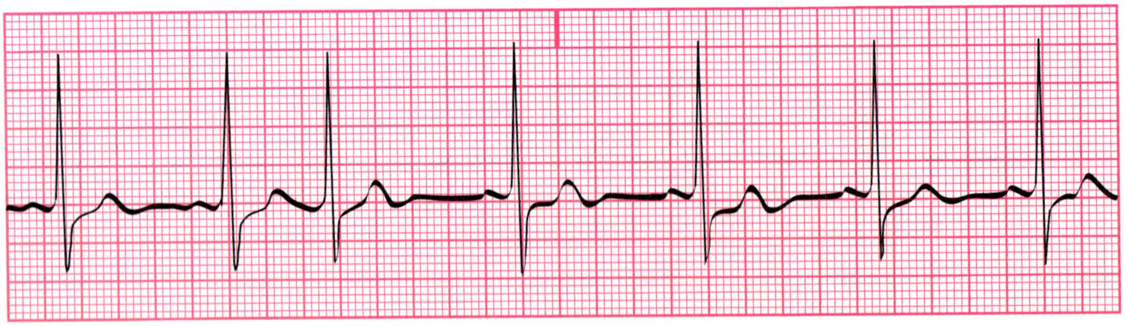

Rhythm (regular or irregular): ____________ PR interval: ____________

Rate: ____________ QRS: ____________

P wave: ____________ Interpretation: ____________

21.

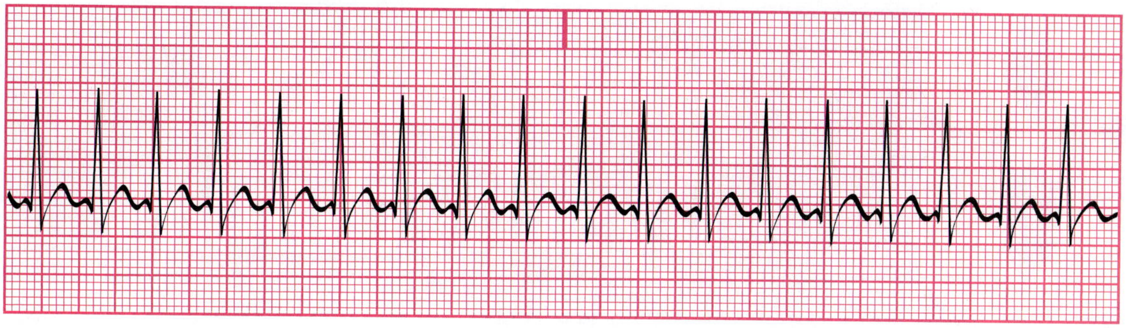

Rhythm (regular or irregular): ____________ PR interval: ____________

Rate: ____________ QRS: ____________

P wave: ____________ Interpretation: ____________

connect® Now that you have completed the material in the chapter text, go to Connect and complete any chapter activities you have not yet done.

8 Heart Block Dysrhythmias

Learning Outcomes

8.1 Describe the various heart block dysrhythmias.

8.2 Identify first degree atrioventricular (AV) block using the criteria for classification, and explain how the rhythm may affect the patient, including basic patient care and treatment.

8.3 Identify second degree atrioventricular (AV) block, Mobitz I, using the criteria for classification, and explain how the rhythm may affect the patient, including basic patient care and treatment.

8.4 Identify second degree atrioventricular (AV) block, Mobitz II, using the criteria for classification, and explain how the rhythm may affect the patient, including basic patient care and treatment.

8.5 Identify third degree atrioventricular (AV) block using the criteria for classification, and explain how the rhythm may affect the patient, including basic patient care and treatment.

Key Terms

blocked or nonconducted impulse
cardiac output parameters
dissociative

8.1 Introduction to Heart Block Dysrhythmias

In heart block rhythms, the electrical current has difficulty traveling along the normal conduction pathway, causing a delay in or absence of ventricular depolarization. The degree of blockage depends on the area affected and the cause of the delay or blockage. There are three levels of heart blocks.

Checkpoint Question (LO 8.1)

1. What is the cause of a heart block dysrhythmia?

____

____

8.2 First Degree Atrioventricular (AV) Block

First degree AV block is a *delay* in electrical conduction from the SA node to the AV node, usually around the AV node, which slows or delays an electrical impulse from traveling to the ventricular conduction system. This is reflected by a longer than normal PR interval as shown in Figure 8-1. The condition is similar to being in a traffic jam. You still arrive at your destination, but it takes you longer to get there. Electrical current from the SA node still stimulates ventricular depolarization, but the time the impulse takes to arrive in the ventricles is longer than normal.

Criteria for Classification

- ***Rhythm:*** The regularity between the P-P interval and the R-R interval is constant.
- ***Rate:*** The rate of the atria and ventricles is usually within normal limits of 60 to 100 beats per minute.
- ***P wave morphology:*** The P waves will have the same morphology and shape. Each QRS complex has a P wave before it. There is the same number of P waves as QRS complexes.
- ***PR interval:*** The PR interval is greater than 0.20 second.
- ***QRS duration and morphology:*** The QRS duration and morphology are within normal limits of 0.06 to 0.10 second.

Interpret-TIP

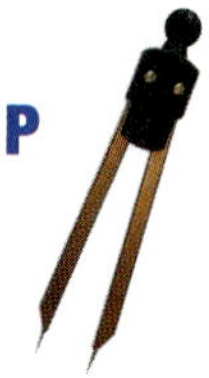

First Degree AV Block

With first degree atrioventricular block, the PR interval is constant and measures greater than 0.20 second.

How the Patient Is Affected and What You Should Know

cardiac output parameters Observation guidelines used to assess the blood supply to the vital organs of the body to maintain normal function.

The patient will be able to maintain normal cardiac output consistent with the underlying rhythm. No change in the patient should occur from this AV block alone as long as all other measuring parameters are within the normal range. Monitor and observe for further degeneration and development of other heart blocks and report if they occur. It is important to observe

Figure 8-1 First degree AV block.

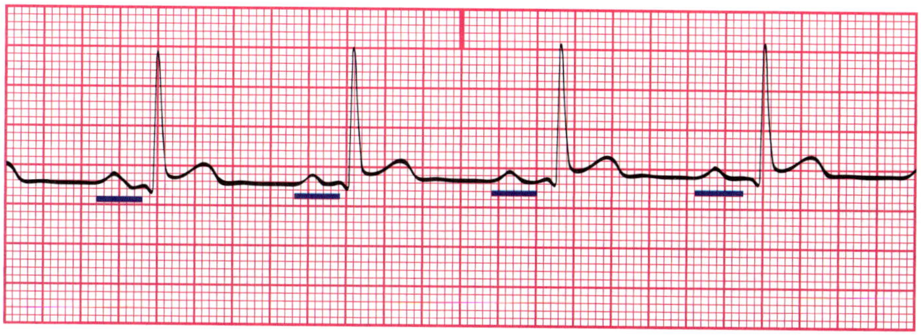

the **cardiac output parameters**—to assess the blood supply to the vital organs—and to determine how well the patient is tolerating the dysrhythmia.

Checkpoint Question (LO 8.2)

Using the criteria for classification, select the rhythm that most closely resembles first degree AV block.

A.

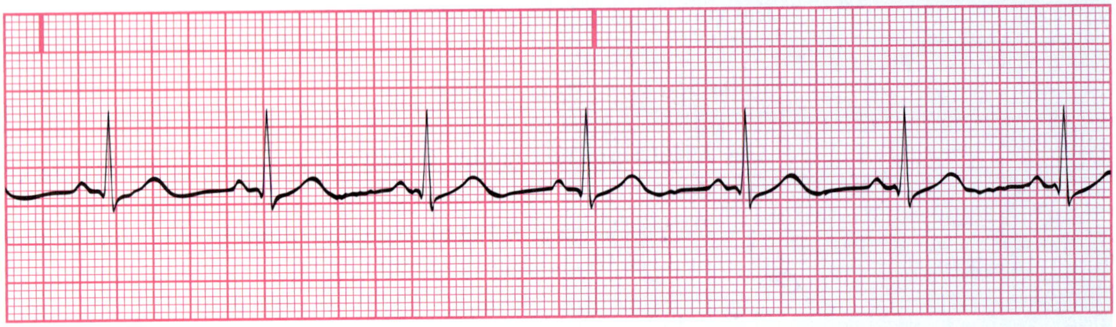

B.

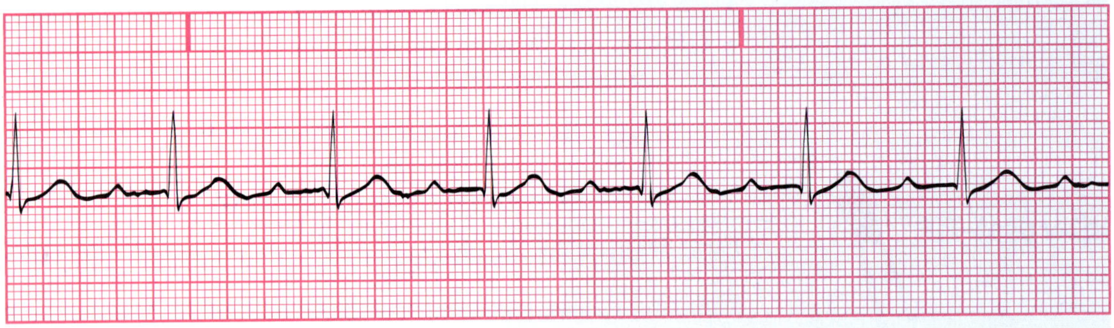

1. Which distinguishing feature(s) led you to make the selection?

____

____

____

8.3 Second Degree Atrioventricular (AV) Block, Type I (Mobitz or Wenckebach)

There are two types of second degree heart blocks: second degree type I and second degree type II. This category of heart block has some blocked or nonconducted electrical impulses from the SA node to the ventricles at the atrioventricular junction region. A **blocked or nonconducted impulse** occurs too soon after the preceding impulse, causing a period when no other impulses can occur in the ventricles. As a result, there are missing QRS complexes. The impulses from the atria are regular, but depending on which type of second degree block is present, the conduction through the AV node may be delayed and at some point blocked in a pattern, or the impulse may be blocked entirely, resulting in missing QRS complexes.

blocked or nonconducted impulse Impulse occurs too soon after the preceding impulse, causing a period when no other impulses can occur in the ventricles.

Note: Second degree heart blocks are the only blocks with an irregular ventricular response.

There are currently two known types of second degree heart blocks. The first was discovered by Dr. Woldemar Mobitz, a German internist, in the early 20th century. Dr. Karel Frederik Wenckebach further investigated the rhythm and was able to identify a similar blockage pattern, but it was different from the one Dr. Mobitz observed. The rhythm Dr. Wenckebach observed was specifically labeled second degree atrioventricular block, Mobitz I, but it is often referred to as a Wenckebach rhythm. It is caused when diseased or injured atrioventricular node tissue conducts the electrical impulse to the ventricular conduction pathway with increasing difficulty, causing a delay in time until one of the atrial impulses fails to be conducted or is blocked. After the dropped ventricular impulse, the atrioventricular node resets itself to be able to handle future impulses more quickly and then progressively gets more difficult until it drops or is blocked again. This pattern repeats itself. Notice in Figure 8-2 that the PR interval becomes longer and longer until a QRS complex is missed.

Criteria for Classification

- ***Rhythm:*** The P-P interval is regular. The R-R interval is irregular due to the blocked impulse(s).
- ***Rate:*** The atrial rate is within normal limits. The ventricular rate is slower than the atrial rate.
- ***P wave morphology:*** The P wave morphology is normal size with an upright P wave. There is a P wave for every QRS complex, but there are extra P waves.
- ***PR interval:*** The PR interval varies from one measurement to the next. The PR interval becomes progressively longer with each subsequent conducted P wave until the QRS wave is dropped. The next PR interval is short, and then the cycle begins again.
- ***QRS duration and morphology:*** The QRS duration and morphology should be within normal limits of 0.06 to 0.10 second.

Interpret-TIP

Second Degree AV Block, Mobitz I (Wenckebach)

A Mobitz I rhythm has a cyclical prolonging PR interval until the QRS is dropped. Then the cycle resets and begins again (irregular ventricular response).

Figure 8-2 Second degree AV block, Mobitz I (Wenckebach).

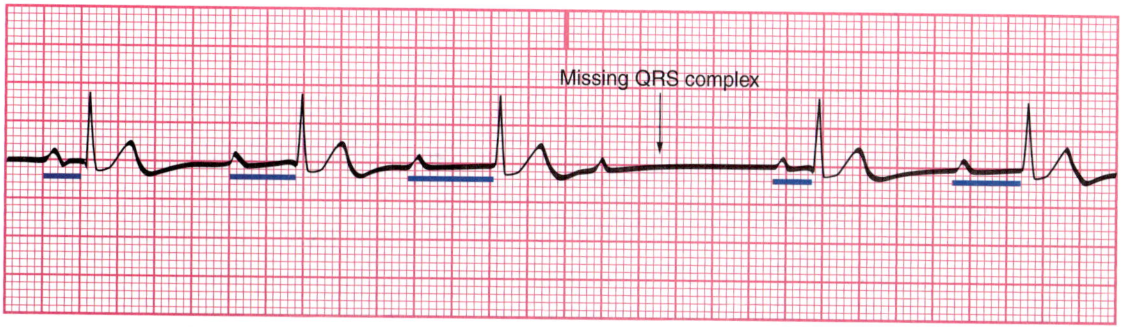

How the Patient Is Affected and What You Should Know

The patient may or may not exhibit symptoms of decreased cardiac output, depending on the rate of ventricular contraction. As this rate decreases and reaches levels of 40 beats per minute or lower, the patient will show signs and symptoms of low cardiac output. This rhythm is usually due to inflammation around the atrioventricular node, and it is often a temporary condition that will resolve itself and return to a normal heart rhythm.

Because treatment is based on how the patient is tolerating the rhythm, the patient is observed for signs and symptoms of low cardiac output. If the patient is experiencing difficulties, a licensed practitioner administers medication; if not, the patient is monitored for further progression to third degree heart block.

Checkpoint Question (LO 8.3)

Using the criteria for classification, select the rhythm that most closely resembles second degree AV block, type I.

A.

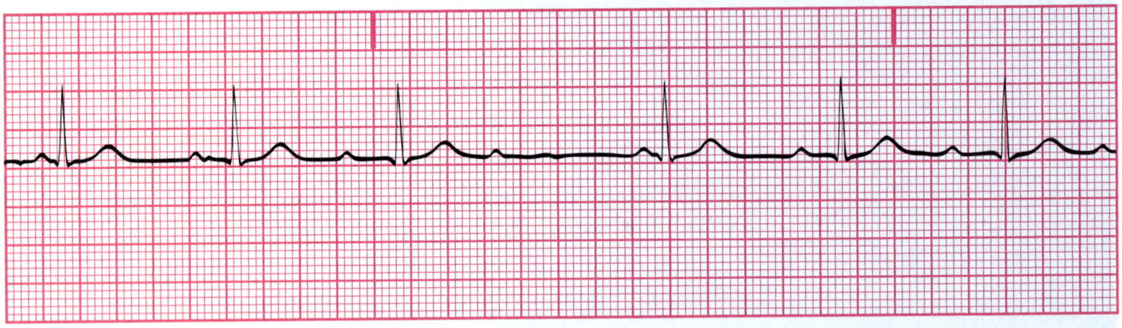

B.

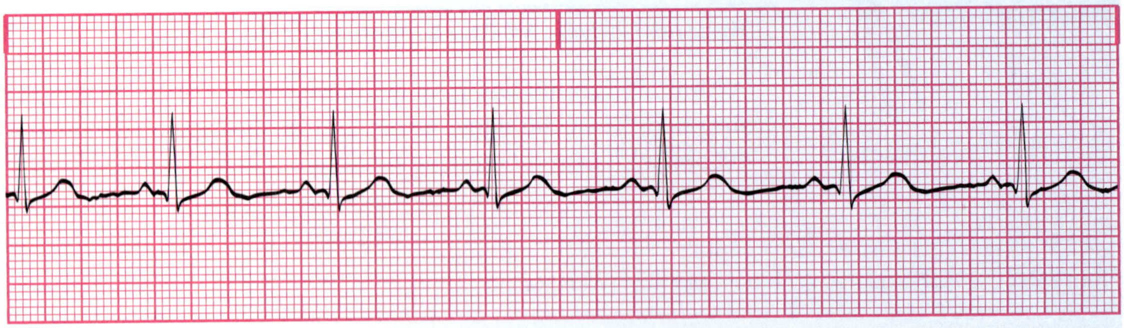

1. Which distinguishing feature(s) led you to make the selection?

____

____

____

Figure 8-3 Second degree AV block, type II (Mobitz II).

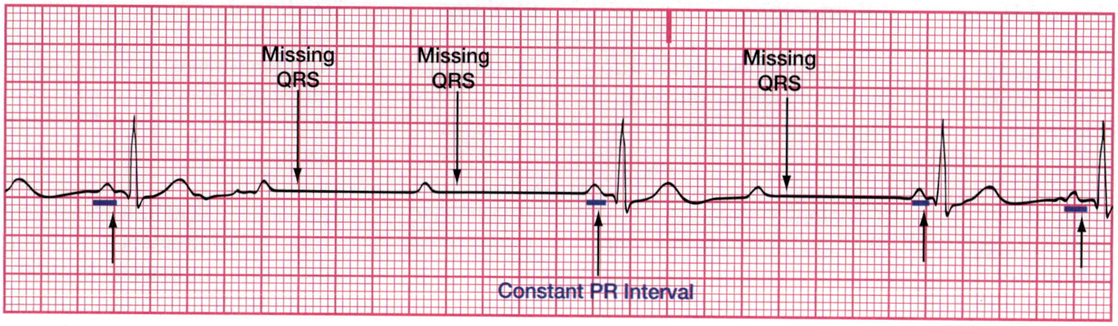

8.4 Second Degree Atrioventricular (AV) Block, Type II (Mobitz II)

Second degree atrioventricular block, Mobitz II, is often referred to as the classical heart block because it was the first rhythm observed to have an occasional dropped complex (Figure 8-3). The atrioventricular node selects which electrical impulses it will block. Occasionally, the blocked QRS complexes will occur in a pattern. It might be seen as two, three, or four P waves between each QRS complex. When second degree type II occurs in this fashion, it is often referred to by the ratio of P waves to each QRS (e.g., second degree type II 3:1). When in doubt, refer to the Interpret-TIP for this dysrhythmia. There is usually no pattern or reason for the dropping of the QRS complex. This dysrhythmia frequently progresses to third degree atrioventricular block.

Criteria for Classification

- ***Rhythm:*** The P-P interval is regular. The R-R interval may or may not be irregular due to the unpredictable nature of the blocked impulse(s). R-R intervals are occasionally in a pattern.
- ***Rate:*** The atrial rate is within normal limits. The ventricular rate is slower than the atrial rate. The atrial and ventricular rates are not the same.
- ***P wave morphology:*** The P wave morphology will be normal, with a normal size and upright wave. There is at least one P wave for every QRS complex, and there are more P waves than QRS complexes.
- ***PR interval:*** The PR interval is constant and remains constant even after the QRS drop occurs.
- ***QRS duration and morphology:*** The QRS duration and morphology should be within normal limits of 0.06 to 0.10 second.

Interpret-TIP

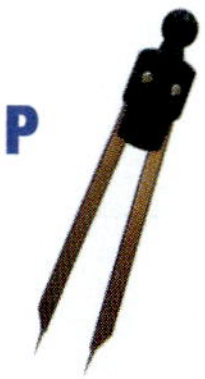

Second Degree AV Block, Mobitz Type II

QRS complexes are missing, but, wherever a P is with the QRS complex, the PR interval always measures the same.

TABLE 8-1 Differences Between Second Degree Heart Blocks

Type of Heart Block	PR Interval	Etiology	Treatment
Second degree AV block, Type I (Mobitz I or Wenckebach)	Varies from one complex to another; resets itself after the dropped complex	Temporary	May resolve itself; observe cardiac output and wait until the PR intervals vary and the dropped QRS complexes occur
Second degree AV block, Type II (Mobitz II or classical block)	Constant PR interval throughout the rhythm strip	Chronic and more critical	Can quickly lead to a complete heart block, a life-threatening situation that needs immediate attention: call 911 or Code Blue. Transcutaneous pacing may be placed on stand-by. The use of this device may be directly related to the speed of ventricular depolarization or the frequency of dropped QRS complexes. Either of these circumstances may dramatically affect cardiac output.

How the Patient Is Affected and What You Should Know

Observe the patient for signs and symptoms of low cardiac output, because this rhythm frequently progresses very quickly to a third degree atrioventricular block, or complete heart block (CHB), usually within seconds. Recognition of the classical block pattern versus the Wenckebach pattern is essential. See Table 8-1 for differences between second degree heart blocks. The classical (Mobitz II) block is more critical and can quickly lead to a complete heart block and a life-threatening situation. When your patient is experiencing second degree heart block, Mobitz II, you should immediately report it to a licensed practitioner; and, if trained, you should prepare for a Code Blue and application of a temporary external pacemaker.

Troubleshooting

Mobitz I versus Mobitz II

To quickly determine the difference between a second degree, Mobitz I (type I, or Wenckebach) and a second degree, Mobitz II (classical) AV block, first look for missing QRS complexes. Once this is determined, analyze the PR interval of the rhythm. If the PR interval is in a progressively pronging pattern, followed by a missing QRS, then you have second degree type I (Wenckebach). If the PR interval remains the same, then you have second degree type II.

Remember the mnemonic "Lengthen, Lengthen, drop equals Wenckebach."

Both rhythms should be reported; however, second degree type II is a highly unstable dysrhythmia and is a critical condition. Second degree type I is typically a much more stable rhythm; it is usually transient with a low degree of conversion to complete heart block.

What does the mnemonic "Lengthen, Lengthen, drop equals Wenckebach" mean?

____

____

Checkpoint Question (LO 8.4)

Using the criteria for classification, select the rhythm that most closely resembles second degree AV block type II.

A.

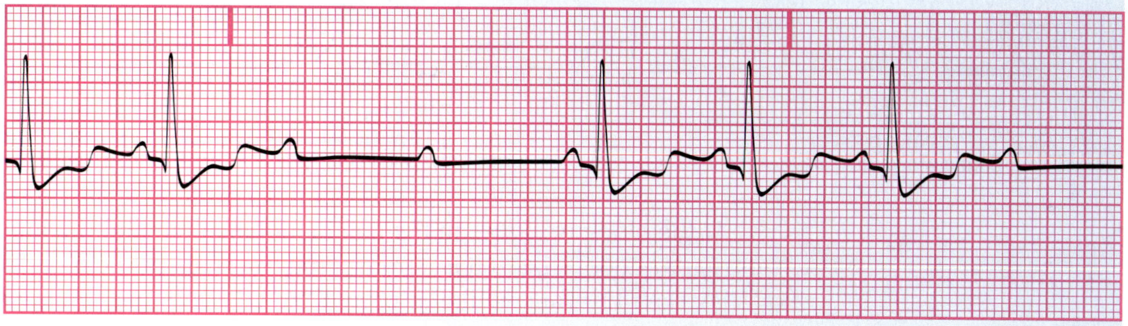

B.

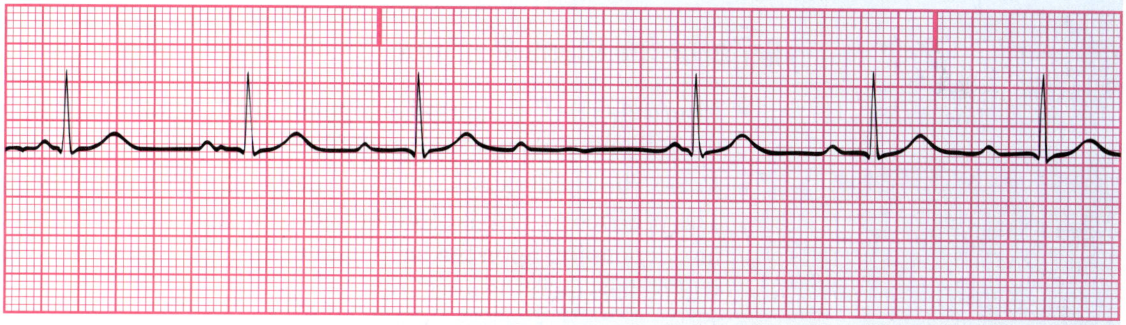

1. Which distinguishing feature(s) led you to make the selection?

____

____

____

8.5 Third Degree Atrioventricular (AV) Block (Complete)

Third degree atrioventricular block is also known as *third degree heart block* or *complete heart block* (CHB). All electrical impulses originating above the ventricles are blocked and prevented from reaching the ventricles. There is no correlation between atrial and ventricular depolarization. As a result, the P-P and R-R intervals are noticeably and suspiciously **dissociative.** Although the intervals are regular when measured, the atria and ventricles fire at completely different rates, resulting in a variable PR interval. This is due to the block. The ventricular rate is slower than the atrial rate (Figure 8-4).

dissociative Not related at all; the atria and the ventricles beat entirely independently of each other.

The rate of the ventricular response and the morphology of the QRS complex depend on the level of the block. If the block is low in the bundle of His, the pacemaker comes from the slow (20 to 40 beats per minute) Purkinje network. The QRS complex in this instance would measure 0.12 second or greater.

Figure 8-4 Third degree AV block (complete heart block).

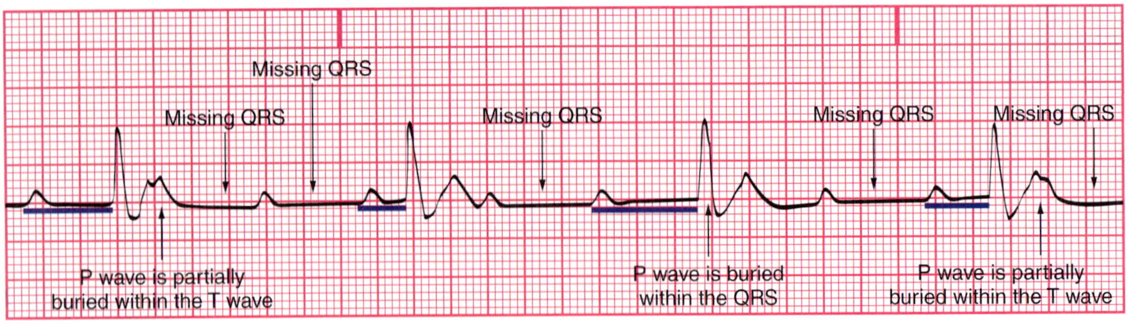

If the block is higher in the conduction system and the impulse causing ventricular depolarization is coming from the area of the AV junction (bundle of His), then the rate is likely to be 40 to 60 beats per minute and the QRS complex will present with a normal to narrow appearance measuring 0.06 to 0.10 second. The ventricular rate and QRS morphology are keys indicating the level of the heart block.

Criteria for Classification

- ***Rhythm:*** The P-P interval is regular. The R-R interval is also regular, but the P-P and R-R intervals are different.
- ***Rate:*** The atrial rate is within normal limits of 60 to 100 beats per minute. The ventricular rate is slow, between 20 and 40 or 40 to 60 beats per minute, depending upon the pacemaker site. (Either way, the ventricular rate will be less than the atrial rate.)
- ***P wave morphology:*** P waves are of normal size and morphology, but the location may be buried within the QRS, either before or after the QRS complex. There is no correlation between the P waves and the QRS complex. More P waves will be noted than QRS complexes, and not every P wave will have a QRS complex following it.
- ***PR interval:*** PR intervals are variable due to the atrial and ventricular tissue depolarizing at different rates.
- ***QRS duration and morphology:*** The QRS duration and morphology are the same, but the measurements may be either within normal limits or wide, depending on the area of the blockage.

Interpret-TIP

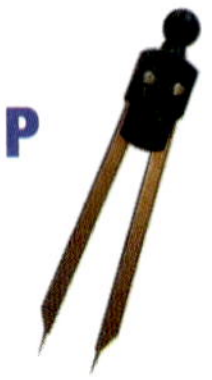

Third Degree (Complete) Heart Block

In third degree atrioventricular block, the P-P and R-R intervals are regular (constant), but the atria and ventricles are firing at different rates. This is the only heart block where the P waves can be buried inside a QRS complex or T wave.

How the Patient Is Affected and What You Should Know

With complete heart block, the atria and the ventricles are electrically separated from one another. This is often referred to as *AV dissociation.* As a result of this condition, the atria and ventricles are firing at different rates because different pacemaker sites are initiating depolarization of those areas of the heart. This condition results in a loss of atrial kick. Along with the loss of atrial kick and reduced ventricular rate, the patient often exhibits signs and symptoms of low cardiac output. The slower ventricular rate increases the likelihood that the patient will be unconscious and require immediate medical intervention.

When the patient is in third degree AV block, your first responsibility is to observe the patient for signs and symptoms of low cardiac output. If the patient displays any signs and symptoms, notify a licensed practitioner immediately.

It may be necessary to initiate a cardiac arrest, rapid response, or Code Blue alarm. A temporary pacemaker should be available and ready for application as deemed necessary by the licensed practitioner. All rhythm strips should be mounted and identified in the patient's medical record as documentation of the dysrhythmia.

Comparing Heart Blocks

Understanding the differences between the different heart block dysrhythmias is essential. Figure 8-5 shows a comparison so you can identify the distinguishing characteristics of each.

Checkpoint Question (LO 8.5)

Using the criteria for classification, select the rhythm that most closely resembles third degree AV block (complete heart block).

A.

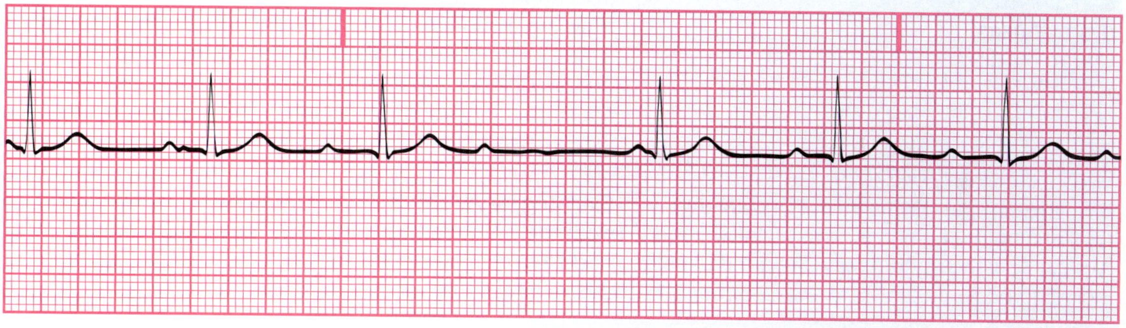

B.

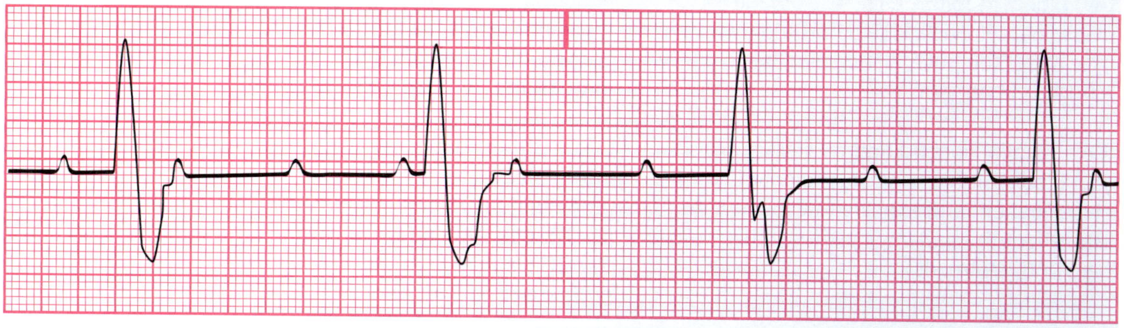

1. Which distinguishing feature(s) led you to make the selection?

____

____

____

Figure 8-5 Distinguishing features of heart block types.

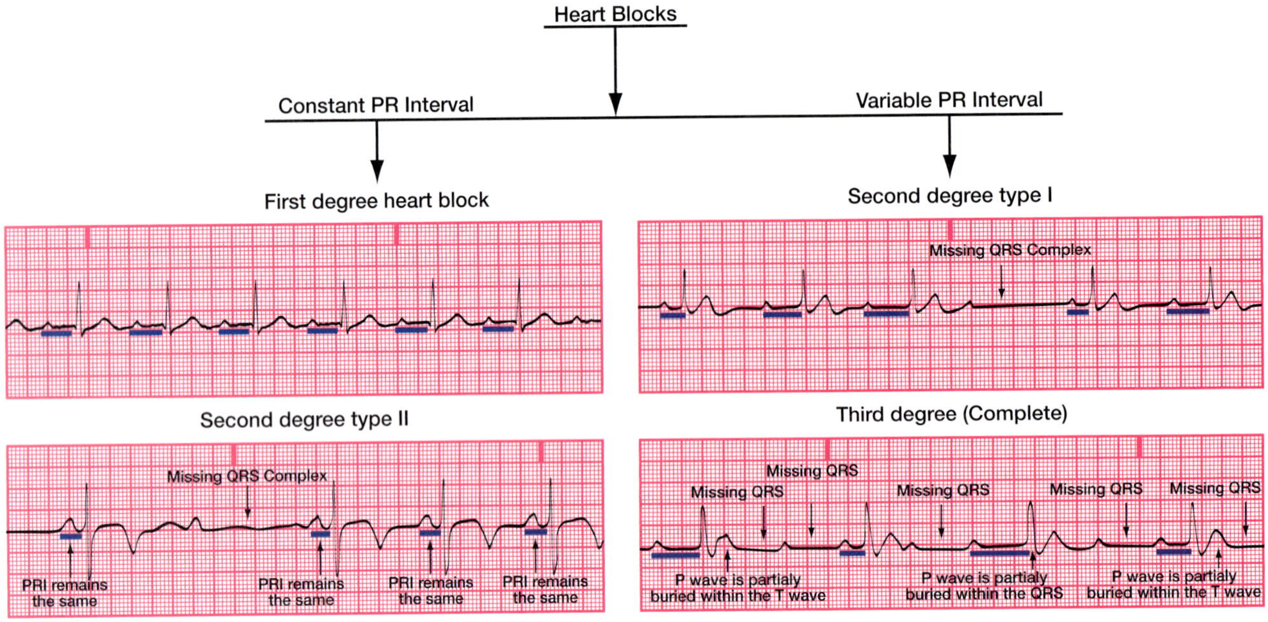

Chapter Summary

Learning Outcomes	Summary	Pages
8.1 Describe the various heart block dysrhythmias.	In heart block rhythms, the electrical current has difficulty traveling along the normal conduction pathway, causing a delay in or absence of ventricular depolarization. The degree of blockage depends on the area affected and the cause of the delay or blockage. The P-P interval is regular with all heart blocks. There are three levels of heart blocks.	186
8.2 Identify first degree atrioventricular (AV) block using the criteria for classification, and explain how the rhythm may affect the patient, including basic patient care and treatment.	First degree AV block is a delay in electrical conduction from the SA node to the AV node, usually around the AV node, which slows the electrical impulses as they travel to the ventricular conduction system.	187–188
8.3 Identify second degree atrioventricular (AV) block, Mobitz I, using the criteria for classification, and explain how the rhythm may affect the patient, including basic patient care and treatment.	Second degree heart block type I has some blocked or nonconducted electrical impulses from the SA node to the ventricles at the atrioventricular junction. The impulses coming from the atria are regular, but the conduction through the AV node gets delayed.	188–190
8.4 Identify second degree atrioventricular (AV) block, Mobitz II, using the criteria for classification, and explain how the rhythm may affect the patient, including basic patient care and treatment.	Second degree atrioventricular block, Mobitz II, is often referred to as the "classical" heart block. The atrioventricular node selects which electrical impulses it will block. No pattern or reason for the dropping of the QRS complex exists. Frequently this dysrhythmia progresses to third degree atrioventricular block.	191–193
8.5 Identify third degree atrioventricular (AV) block using the criteria for classification, and explain how the rhythm may affect the patient, including basic patient care and treatment.	Third degree atrioventricular block is also known as *third degree heart block* or *complete heart block (CHB).* All electrical impulses originating above the ventricles are blocked and prevented from reaching the ventricles. There is no correlation between atrial and ventricular depolarization. In third degree atrioventricular block, the P-P and R-R intervals are regular (constant) but firing at different rates.	193–196

Chapter Review

Multiple Choice

Circle the correct answer.

1. Which heart block rhythm is the one with the distinguishing feature of a PR interval that measures greater than 0.20 second and measures the same duration each time? (LO 8.2)
   - **a.** First degree heart block
   - **b.** Second degree type I
   - **c.** Second degree type II
   - **d.** Third degree heart block
2. Which of the following heart block dysrhythmias is identified by a repetitious prolonging PR interval pattern after each blocked QRS complex? (LO 8.3)
   - **a.** First degree heart block
   - **b.** Second degree type I
   - **c.** Second degree type II
   - **d.** Third degree heart block
3. Which of the following heart block dysrhythmias is identified by missing QRS complexes and a consistent PR interval measurement? (LO 8.4)
   - **a.** First degree heart block
   - **b.** Second degree type I
   - **c.** Second degree type II
   - **d.** Third degree heart block
4. Which of the following heart block dysrhythmias is identified by regular P-P and R-R intervals that are firing at two distinctly different rates? (LO 8.5)
   - **a.** First degree heart block
   - **b.** Second degree type I
   - **c.** Second degree type II
   - **d.** Third degree heart block
5. P-P intervals are ________________________ with all heart block dysrhythmias. (LO 8.2–8.5)
   - **a.** irregular
   - **b.** absent
   - **c.** regular
   - **d.** progressively prolonged
6. QRS complexes that measure 0.12 second or greater with a rate between 20 and 40 beats per minute indicate that the impulses causing ventricular depolarization are coming from the ________________________. (LO 8.5)
   - **a.** SA node
   - **b.** interatrial pathways
   - **c.** AV node
   - **d.** Purkinje fibers (ventricles)

7. What is the typical heart rate range for first degree heart block? (LO 8.2)
   a. 20–40 beats per minute
   b. 40–60 beats per minute
   c. 60–100 beats per minute
   d. 100–150 beats per minute
8. Frequent nonconducted QRS complexes are likely to cause signs of ______________________. (LO 8.3, 8.4, 8.5)
   a. high cardiac output
   b. low cardiac output
   c. kidney failure
   d. congestive heart failure
9. Which heart block dysrhythmia has regular P-P and R-R intervals with both having the same rate? (LO 8.2)
   a. First degree heart block
   b. Second degree type I
   c. Second degree type II
   d. Third degree heart block
10. Which heart block dysrhythmia is known as the "classical" heart block? (LO 8.4)
   a. First degree heart block
   b. Second degree type I
   c. Second degree type II
   d. Third degree heart block

Short Answer

11. Name the heart block rhythms described in this chapter. Which one is most serious? (LO 8.2–8.5)

    ____

    ____

12. How can you tell the difference between a Mobitz I and Mobitz II heart block? (LO 8.3, 8.4)

    ____

    ____

13. What should you do if the patient has a third degree heart block? (LO 8.5)

    ____

    ____

Critical Thinking Application *Rhythm Identification*

Review the dysrhythmias pictured here and, using the criteria for classification provided in the chapter as clues, identify each rhythm and provide what information you used to make your decision. (LO 8.2–8.5)

14.

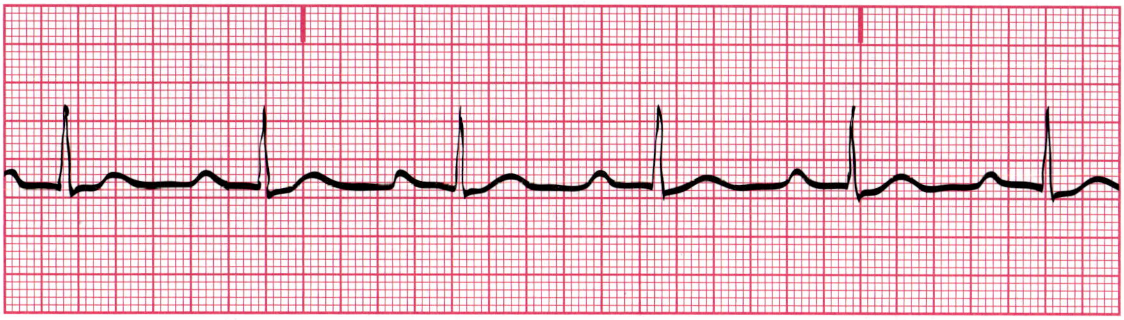

Rhythm (regular or irregular): ______________ PR interval: ______________

Rate: ______________ QRS: ______________

P wave: ______________ Interpretation: ______________

15.

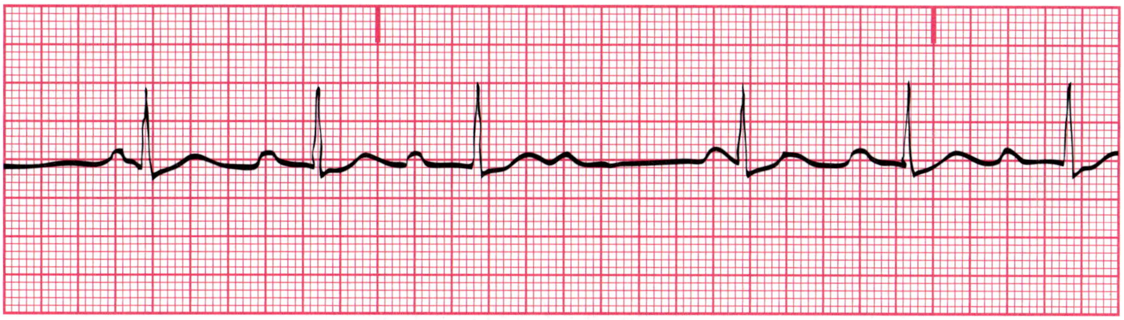

Rhythm (regular or irregular): ______________ PR interval: ______________

Rate: ______________ QRS: ______________

P wave: ______________ Interpretation: ______________

16.

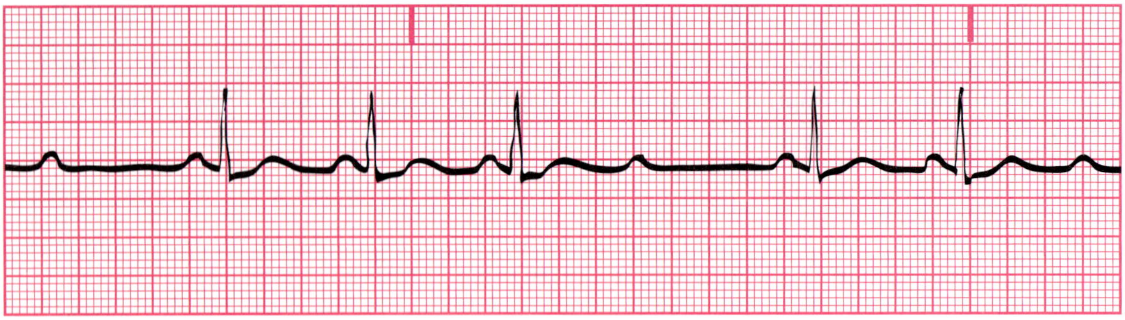

Rhythm (regular or irregular): ________________ PR interval: ________________

Rate: ________________ QRS: ________________

P wave: ________________ Interpretation: ________________

17.

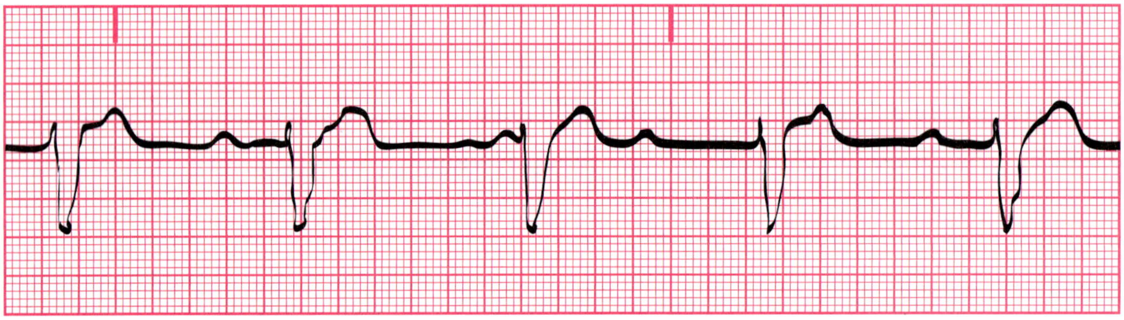

Rhythm (regular or irregular): ________________ PR interval: ________________

Rate: ________________ QRS: ________________

P wave: ________________ Interpretation: ________________

18.

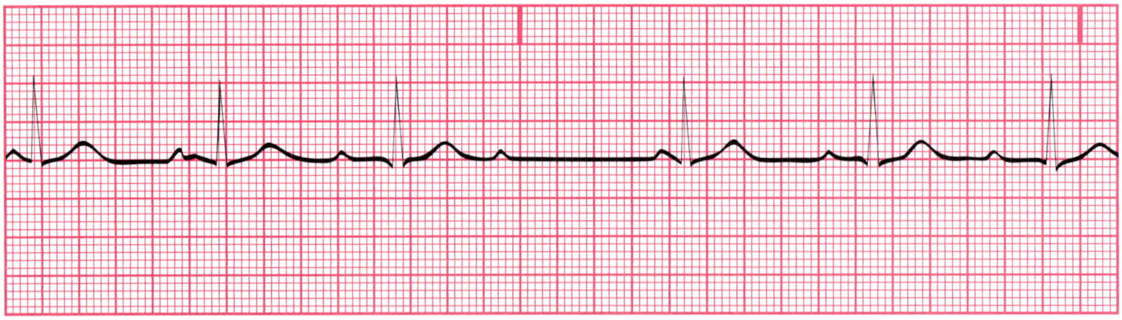

Rhythm (regular or irregular): ________________ PR interval: ________________

Rate: ________________ QRS: ________________

P wave: ________________ Interpretation: ________________

19.

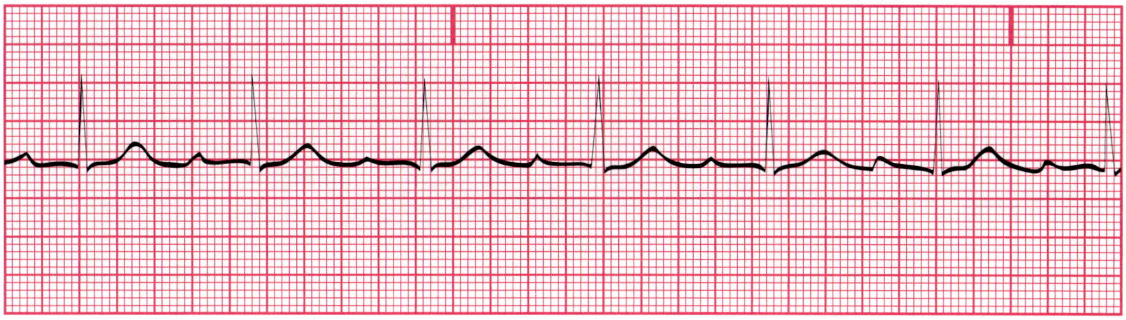

Rhythm (regular or irregular): ______________ PR interval: ______________

Rate: ______________ QRS: ______________

P wave: ______________ Interpretation: ______________

20.

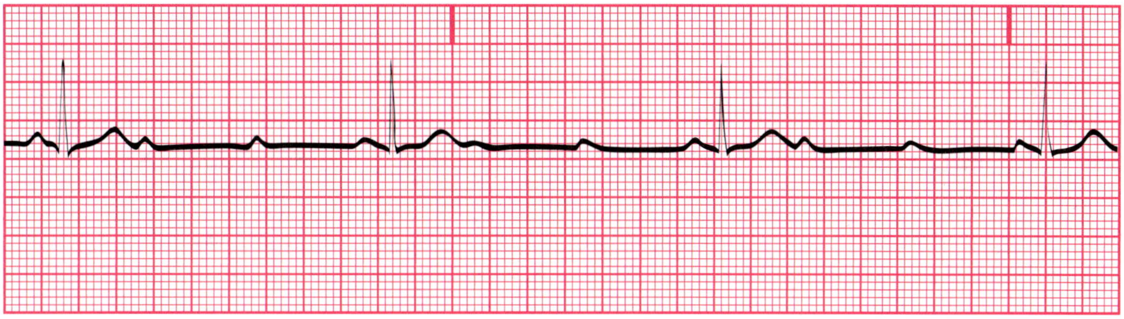

Rhythm (regular or irregular): ______________ PR interval: ______________

Rate: ______________ QRS: ______________

P wave: ______________ Interpretation: ______________

21.

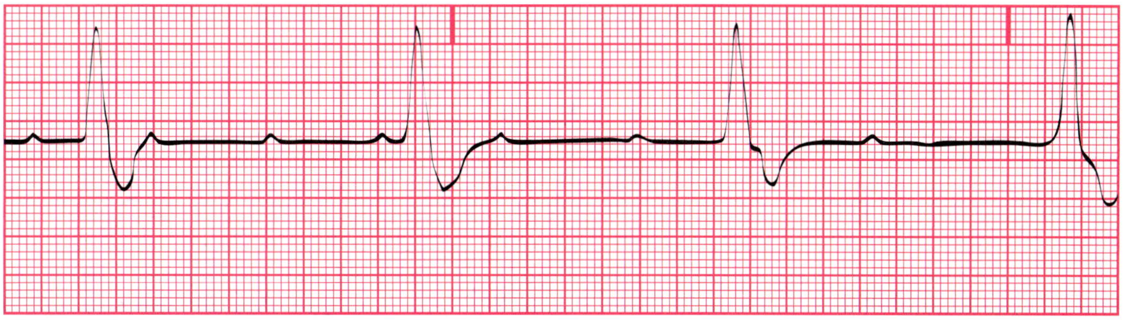

Rhythm (regular or irregular): ______________ PR interval: ______________

Rate: ______________ QRS: ______________

P wave: ______________ Interpretation: ______________

22.

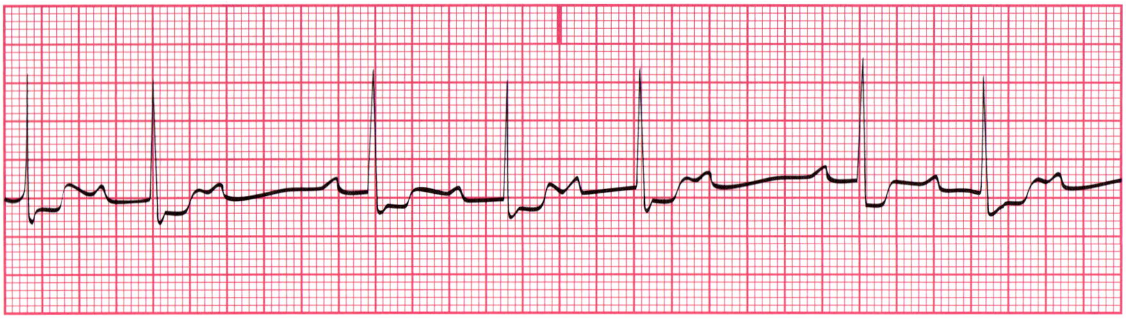

Rhythm (regular or irregular): ____________ PR interval: ____________

Rate: ____________ QRS: ____________

P wave: ____________ Interpretation: ____________

23.

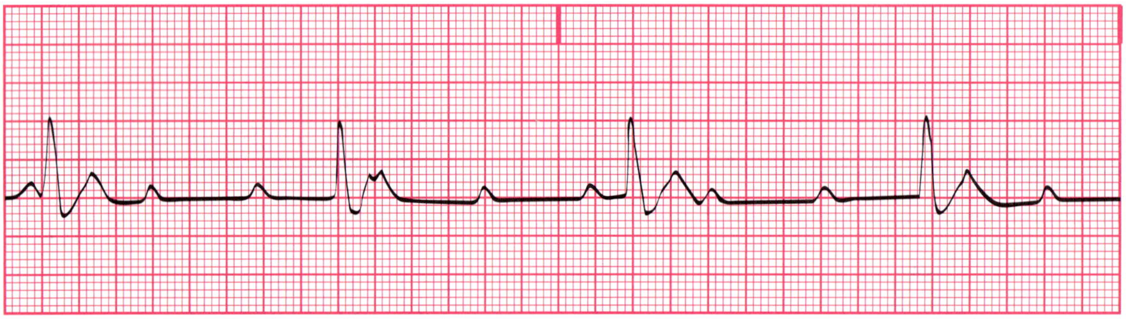

Rhythm (regular or irregular): ____________ PR interval: ____________

Rate: ____________ QRS: ____________

P wave: ____________ Interpretation: ____________

24.

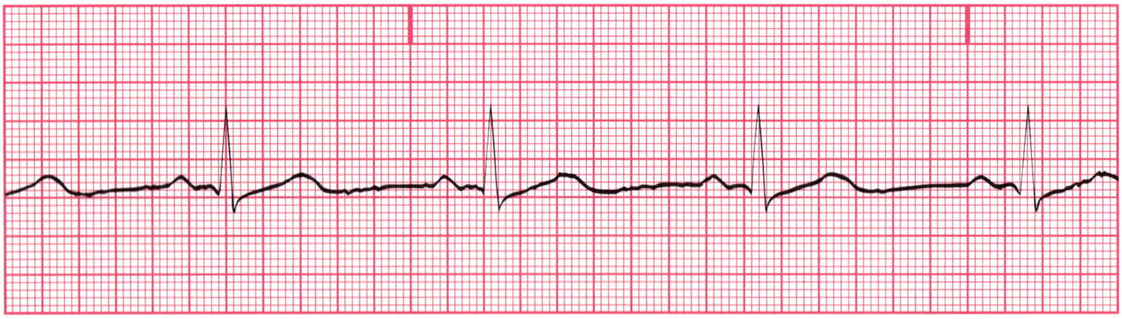

Rhythm (regular or irregular): ____________ PR interval: ____________

Rate: ____________ QRS: ____________

P wave: ____________ Interpretation: ____________

25.

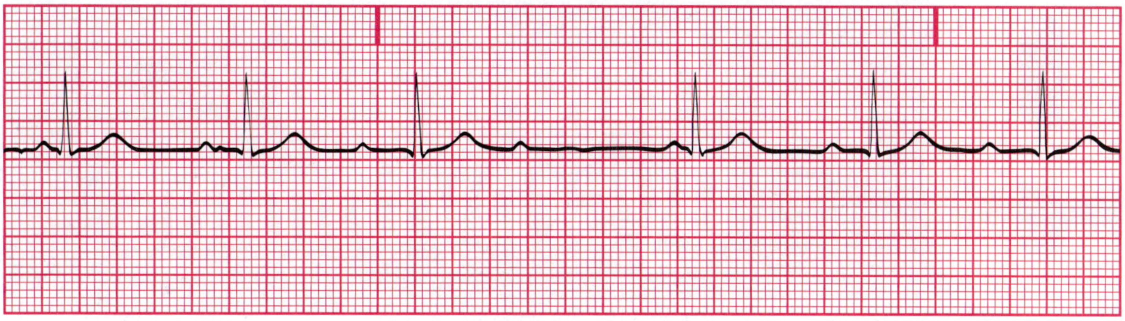

Rhythm (regular or irregular): ____________ PR interval: ____________

Rate: ____________ QRS: ____________

P wave: ____________ Interpretation: ____________

26.

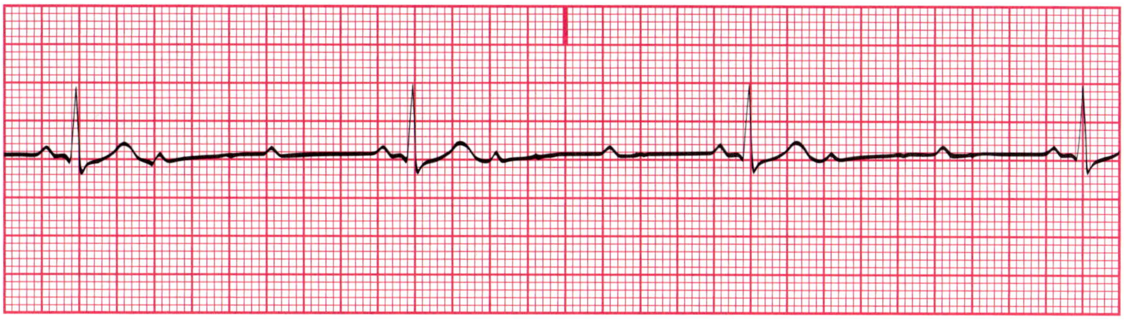

Rhythm (regular or irregular): ____________ PR interval: ____________

Rate: ____________ QRS: ____________

P wave: ____________ Interpretation: ____________

connect® Now that you have completed the material in the chapter text, go to Connect and complete any chapter activities you have not yet done.

9 Ventricular Dysrhythmias

Learning Outcomes

9.1 Describe the various ventricular dysrhythmias.

9.2 Identify premature ventricular complexes (PVCs) using the criteria for classification, and explain how the rhythm may affect the patient, including basic patient care and treatment.

9.3 Identify agonal rhythm using the criteria for classification, and explain how the rhythm may affect the patient, including basic patient care and treatment.

9.4 Identify idioventricular rhythm using the criteria for classification, and explain how the rhythm may affect the patient, including basic patient care and treatment.

9.5 Identify accelerated idioventricular rhythm using the criteria for classification, and explain how the rhythm may affect the patient, including basic patient care and treatment.

9.6 Identify ventricular tachycardia using the criteria for classification, and explain how the rhythm may affect the patient, including basic patient care and treatment.

9.7 Identify ventricular fibrillation using the criteria for classification, and explain how the rhythm may affect the patient, including basic patient care and treatment.

9.8 Identify asystole using the criteria for classification, and explain how the rhythm may affect the patient, including basic patient care and treatment.

Key Terms

advanced cardiac life support (ACLS)
apnea
bigeminy
coupling
crash cart
frequent PVC
interpolated PVC
multifocal PVC
occasional PVC
paroxysmal event
premature ventricular complex (PVC)
quadgeminy
R-on-T PVC
run of ventricular tachycardia
salvo
Torsades de Pointes
trigeminy
triplet PVCs
unifocal PVC

9.1 Introduction to Ventricular Dysrhythmias

The ventricular pacemaker cells are found at the Purkinje fibers. This pacemaker is the last of the group of inherent pacemaker cells within the heart. The rate of automaticity is between 20 and 40 beats per minute. Current is initiated within the Purkinje fibers and spreads the electrical stimulation from one ventricular cell to the next. Because current is not traveling down the normal ventricular conduction pathway to activate both the right and left ventricles simultaneously, it will take longer than normal to depolarize the ventricles. A QRS duration measurement of 0.12 second or greater suggests that this cell-by-cell stimulation of electrical current is occurring to depolarize the ventricles. Ventricular rhythms occurring within the range of the Purkinje network (20 to 40 beats per minute) are occasionally referred to as *ventricular escape rhythms.* Ventricular rhythms occur for one of these reasons:

1. The higher pacemaker sites within the heart fail.
2. The rate of automaticity from this portion of the heart is faster, so it takes over as the primary pacemaker within the heart.
3. In third degree block, the higher pacemaker is still functioning, but all supraventricular impulses are prevented from entering the ventricular conduction system due to the block. This results in the AV junction or Purkinje network having to fire in order to maintain ventricular depolarization.

Remember, the fastest electrical activity in the heart controls the heart rate.

Interpret-TIP

Ventricular Complexes and Rhythms

Ventricular complexes and rhythms share a conspicuous morphologic similarity—missing P waves and "wide and bizarre" QRS complexes that measure 0.12 or greater.

Checkpoint Question (LO 9.1)

1. Why does it take longer than normal to depolarize the ventricles during a ventricular dysrhythmia?

____

____

9.2 Premature Ventricular Complexes (PVCs)

premature ventricular complex (PVC) An ectopic impulse originating in either ventricle that occurs too early in the cycle.

A **premature ventricular complex (PVC)** is caused by an ectopic impulse that occurs early in the cycle and originates from the ventricles (Figure 9-1). These ectopic events are often caused by an ischemic region within the ventricles. Ischemia increases excitability (irritability) of the ventricular myocardium. Table 9-1 shows the various types of premature ventricular complexes.

Figure 9-1 Premature ventricular complexes.

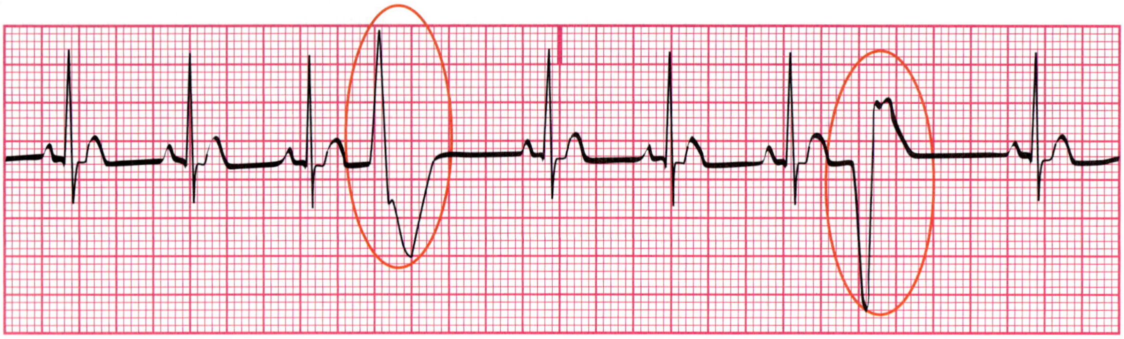

Criteria for Classification

- ***Rhythm:*** The P-P and R-R intervals are regular with early QRS complexes. Every early complex has a full compensatory pause, meaning that two R-R interval periods are required before another electrical impulse can be conducted. A compensatory pause measures longer than the underlying R-R and a noncompensatory pause measures less than the underlying R-R.
- ***Rate:*** Heart rate is influenced by the number of ectopic complexes (PVCs) present. This rhythm is irregular, so the six-second method must be used to determine the rate. Count all complexes, including PVCs, and multiply by 10 to determine the rate.
- ***P wave morphology:*** The P wave assumes the shape of the underlying rhythm. P waves are not identified on the early ventricular complex.
- ***PR interval:*** The PR interval measurement follows the underlying rhythm, but in the early complex no P wave is present.
- ***QRS duration and morphology:*** The QRS morphology and duration must be analyzed for both the underlying rhythm and the premature complexes. Typically, the QRS complexes of the underlying rhythm measure within the normal range (0.06–0.10). The QRS morphology of the premature complexes may be of different shapes but share the descriptive characteristic wide and bizarre, measuring 0.12 second or greater. The T wave will be in the opposite direction of the ventricular depolarization.

Interpret-TIP

Premature Ventricular Complexes

A PVC is an early QRS complex that measures 0.12 second or greater and has a wide and bizarre appearance. There is no P wave.

How the Patient Is Affected and What You Should Know

The clinical significance of the PVCs depends on their frequency and the amount of decrease in cardiac output that occurs with each PVC. Because PVCs can occur in normal hearts, patients may tolerate PVCs without a noticeable change in their cardiac output and have no obvious symptoms. In fact, they may be unaware they are having PVCs. Other patients may complain of the "thump or skipping" sensation with each PVC. They may also experience dizziness and other symptoms of low cardiac output. More complex PVCs, such as frequent PVCs, multifocal PVCs, R-on-T PVCs, and coupling, indicate an increased risk of developing a more serious ventricular dysrhythmia (see Table 9-1).

TABLE 9-1 Types and Patterns of Premature Complexes

Unifocal PVC	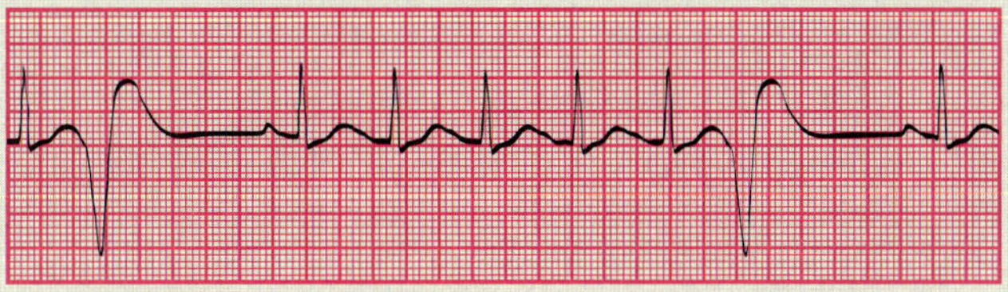	Early complex (has similar shape, suggesting only one irritable focus present)
Multifocal PVC	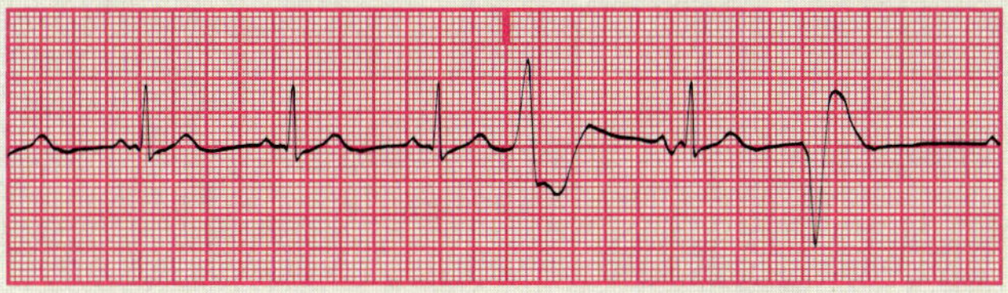	Varied shapes and forms of the PVCs, suggesting more than one irritable focus
Interpolated PVC	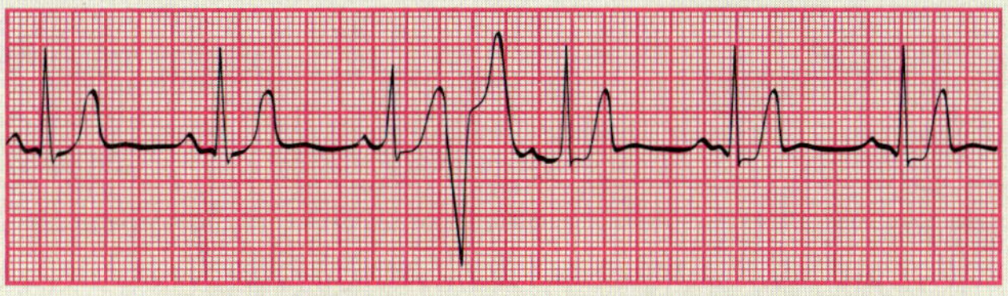	PVC occurs during the normal R-R interval without interrupting the underlying rhythm
Occasional PVC	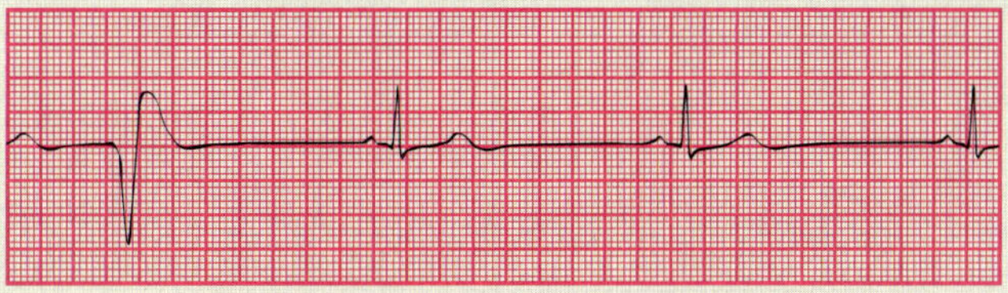	Less than six per minute
Frequent PVC	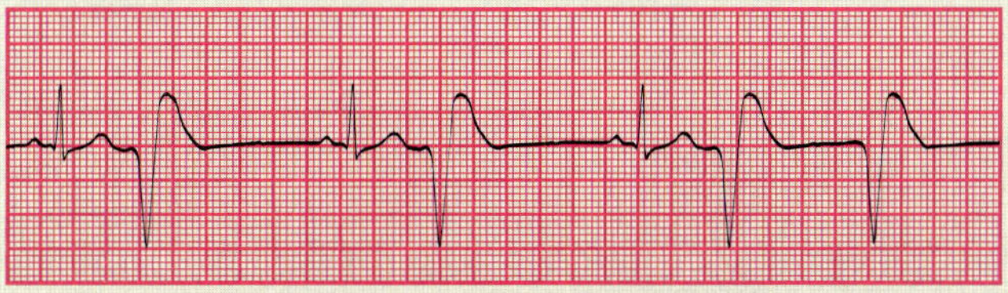	Six or more PVCs per minute
Bigeminy	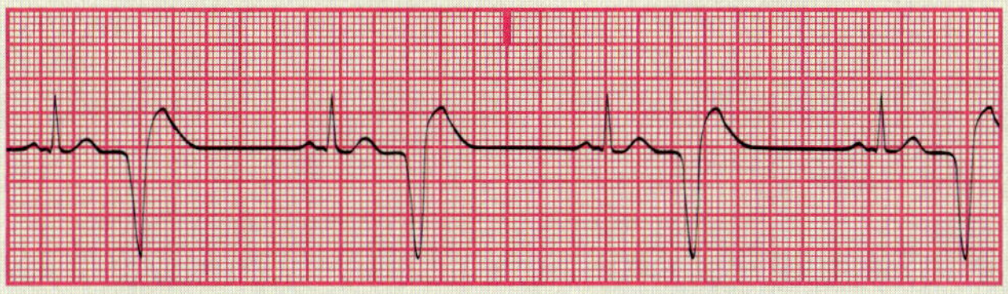	Every other complex is a PVC

(Continued)

(*Continued*)

Trigeminy	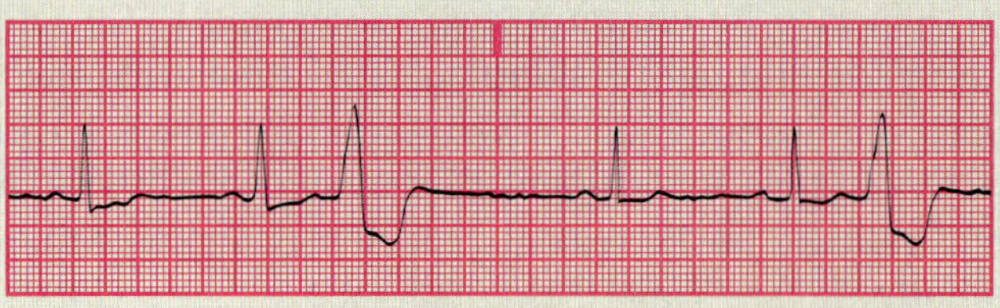	Every third complex is a PVC
Quadgeminy	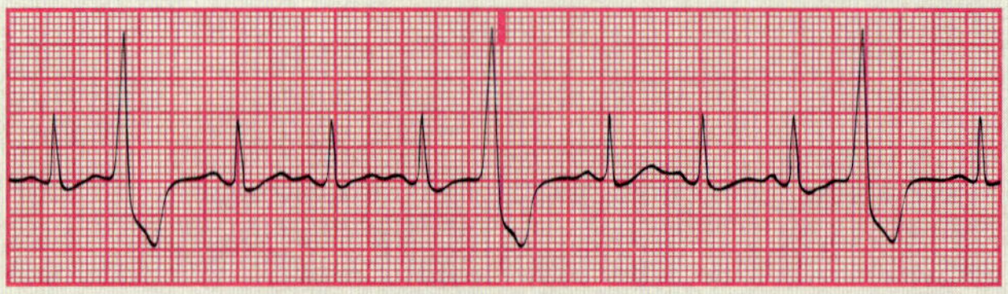	Every fourth complex is a PVC
R-on-T PVC	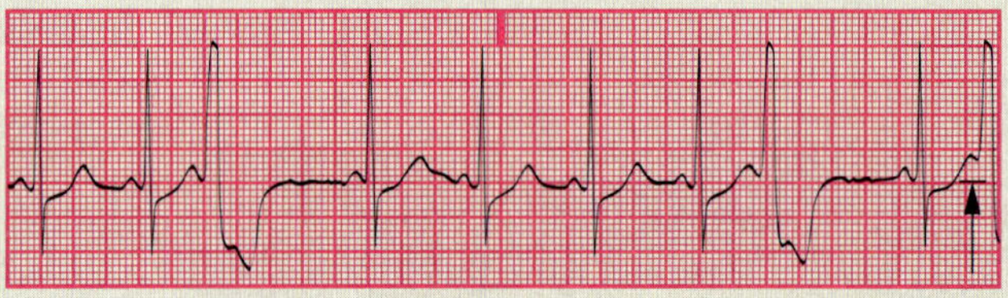	PVC occurs on the downslope of the T wave or the vulnerable period of the relative ventricular refractory period
Coupling	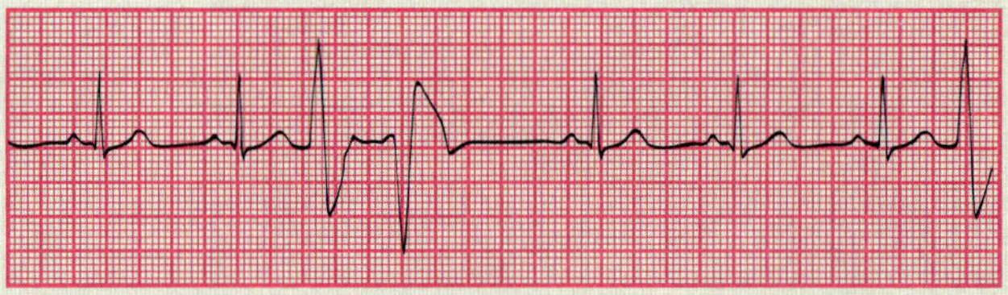	Two PVCs that occur back to back (multifocal couplet pictured)
Run of ventricular tachycardia	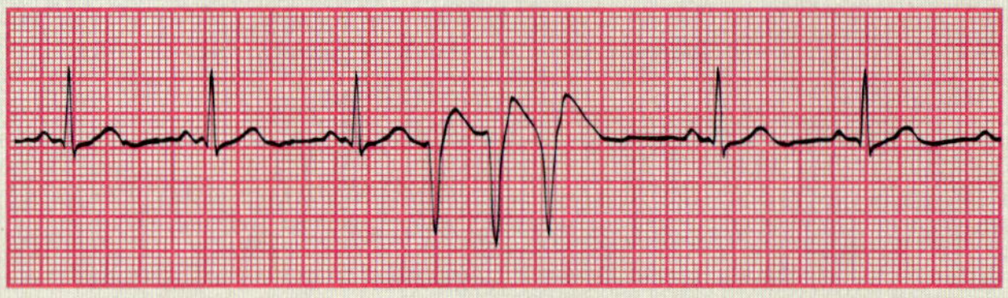	Three or more PVCs in a row at a rate greater than 100 bpm. Also known as **triplet PVCs** or **salvo**
Paroxysmal event	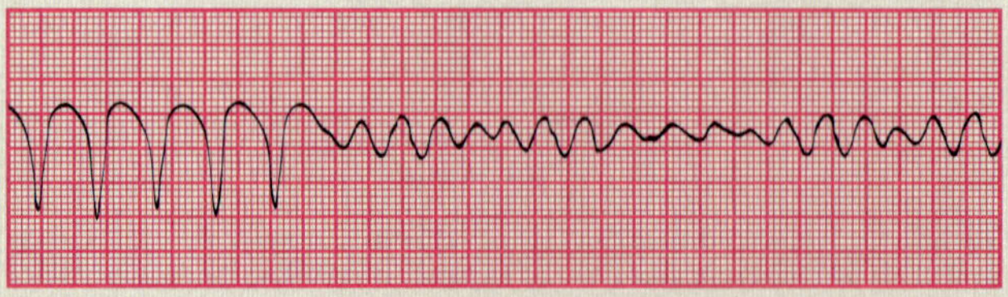	Witnessed change in any cardiac rhythm, including starting, stopping, or both. For example, sinus rhythm to SVT or ventricular tachycardia to ventricular fibrillation

Observe the patient for symptoms of low cardiac output. If symptoms exist, a licensed practitioner should be notified to begin appropriate treatment. Patients are provided oxygen because PVCs often occur due to hypoxic states (suffering from lack of oxygen). Blood samples are drawn to evaluate the hypoxic state as well as electrolyte values, specifically potassium and calcium levels.

Checkpoint Question (LO 9.2)

Using the criteria for classification, select the rhythm that most closely resembles a rhythm containing a premature ventricular complex (PVC).

A.

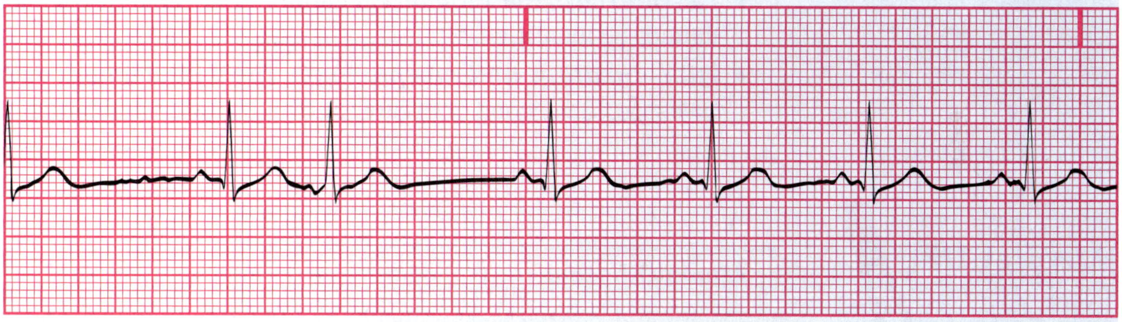

B.

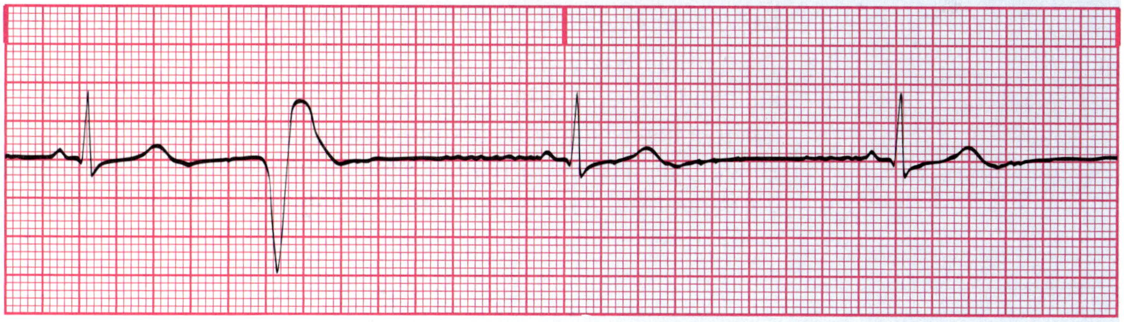

1. Which distinguishing feature(s) led you to make the selection?

____

____

____

9.3 Agonal Rhythm

Agonal rhythms occur when essentially all of the pacemakers in the heart have failed. This is the last semblance of ordered electrical activity in the heart. The heart is dying. The impulses showing on the monitor are ventricular but firing at a rate of less than 20 beats per minute. This dysrhythmia presents with wide and bizarre QRS complexes (0.12 second or greater) and an absence of P waves (Figure 9-2).

Criteria for Classification

- ***Rhythm:*** P-P interval cannot be determined. R-R interval may or may not be regular.
- ***Rate:*** Atrial rate cannot be determined due to the absence of atrial depolarization. The ventricular rate is less than 20 beats per minute.
- ***P wave morphology:*** The P wave is absent; therefore, no analysis of the P wave can be done.
- ***PR interval:*** The PR interval cannot be measured because the P wave cannot be identified.
- ***QRS duration and morphology:*** The QRS duration and morphology measure 0.12 second or greater and have a wide and bizarre appearance.

Interpret-TIP

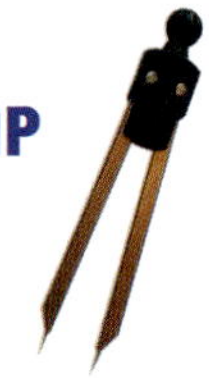

Agonal Rhythm

The agonal rhythm has an absence of P waves, a ventricular rate of less than 20 beats per minute, and wide and bizarre QRS complexes.

How the Patient Is Affected and What You Should Know

The patient has a profound loss of cardiac output due to the loss of atrial kick and the slow ventricular rate. The patient will be unconscious. You must notify a licensed healthcare practitioner immediately. This is a medical emergency that will likely require both basic life support and advanced cardiac life support interventions. ECG strips must be saved and added to the patient's medical record.

Figure 9-2 Agonal rhythm.

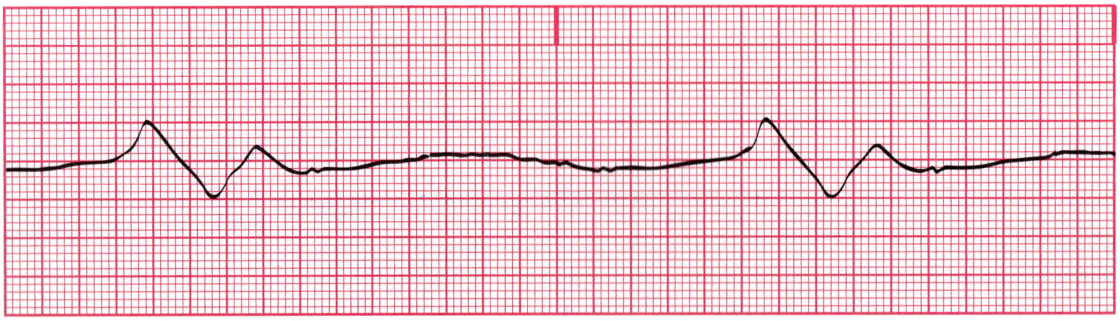

Checkpoint Question (LO 9.3)

Using the criteria for classification, select the rhythm that most closely resembles agonal rhythm.

A.

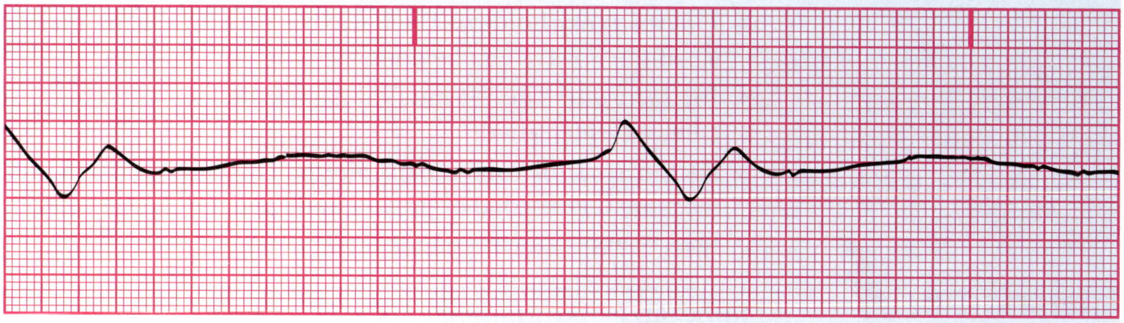

B.

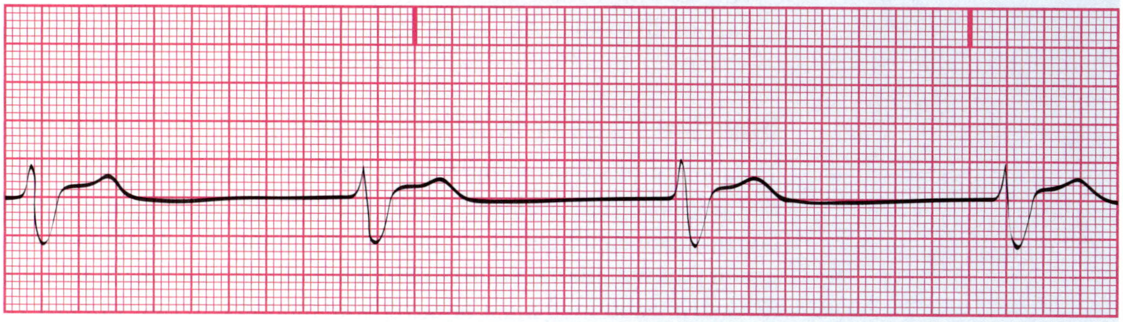

1. Which distinguishing feature(s) led you to make the selection?

____

____

9.4 Idioventricular Rhythm

Idioventricular rhythms occur when the sinoatrial and junctional pacemakers fail to initiate an impulse and all that remains is the slow ventricular pacemaker (20 to 40 beats per minute). Note that the prefix *idio-* means "distinct, separate, or by itself." This dysrhythmia presents with the classic "wide" QRS (0.12 second or greater), a slow ventricular rate (20 to 40), and an absence of P waves (Figure 9-3).

Figure 9-3 Idioventricular rhythm.

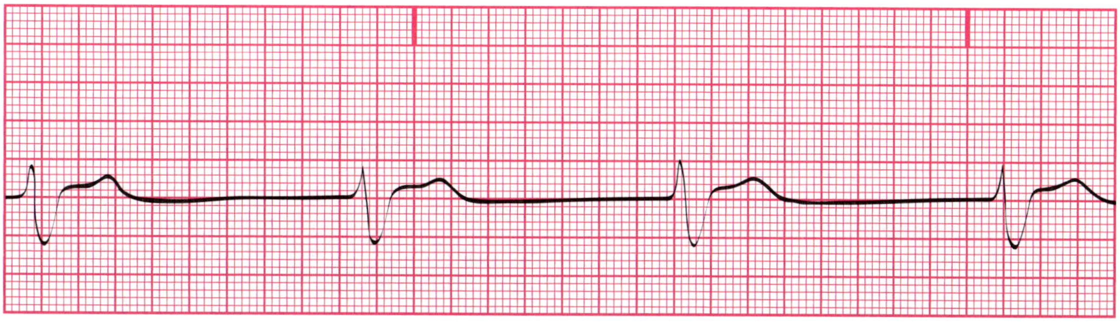

Criteria for Classification

- ***Rhythm:*** P-P interval cannot be determined; the R-R interval is regular.
- ***Rate:*** Atrial rate cannot be determined due to the absence of atrial depolarization. The ventricular rate is 20 to 40 beats per minute.
- ***P wave morphology:*** The P wave is usually absent; therefore, no analysis of the P wave can be done.
- ***PR interval:*** The PR interval cannot be measured because the P wave cannot be identified.
- ***QRS duration and morphology:*** The QRS duration and morphology measure 0.12 second or greater and have the classic ventricular wide and bizarre appearance.

Interpret-TIP

Idioventricular Rhythm

An idioventricular rhythm has an absence of P waves, a slow ventricular rate of 20 to 40 beats per minute, and wide and bizarre QRS complexes.

How the Patient Is Affected and What You Should Know

The patient has a profound loss of cardiac output due to the loss of atrial kick and the slow ventricular rate. The patient will likely be unconscious. You must notify a licensed healthcare practitioner immediately. This is a medical emergency that will likely require treatment with cardiac medications and/or pacing. ECG strips obtained must be saved and mounted in the patient's medical record.

Checkpoint Question (LO 9.4)

Using the criteria for classification, select the rhythm that most closely resembles idioventricular rhythm.

A.

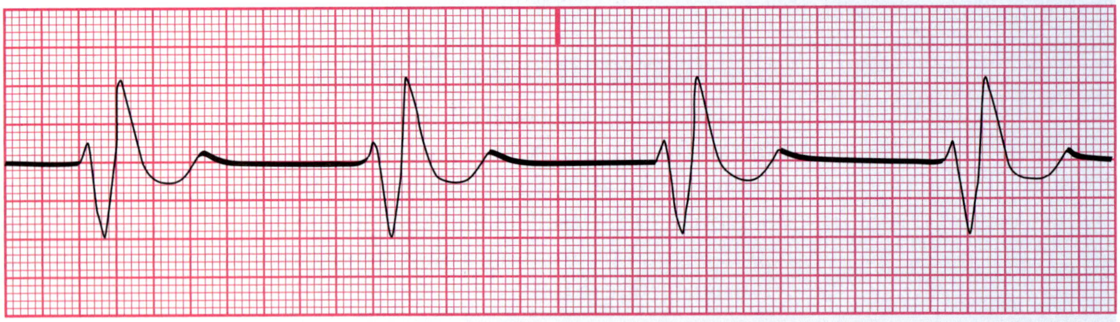

B.

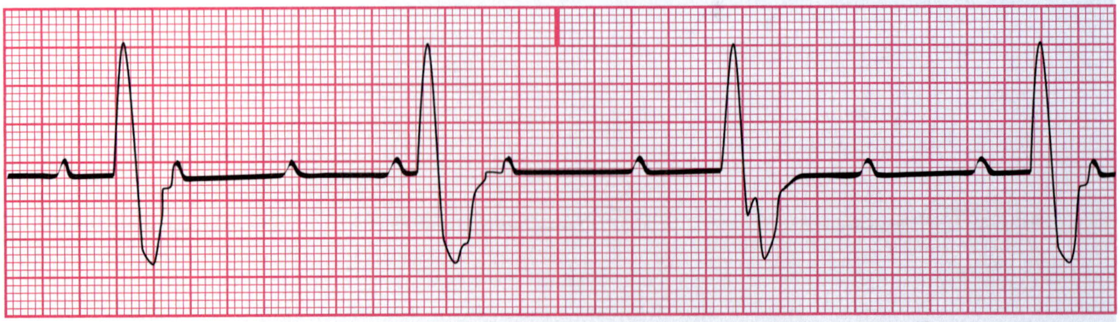

1. Which distinguishing feature(s) led you to make the selection?

____

____

____

9.5 Accelerated Idioventricular Rhythm

Accelerated idioventricular rhythms occur when the sinoatrial and junctional pacemakers fail to initiate an impulse and all that is remaining is the slow ventricular pacemaker. The primary difference between accelerated idioventricular and idioventricular dysrhythmias is the heart rate. This dysrhythmia still presents with the classic "wide" QRS complex (0.12 second or greater) and an absence of P waves. The impulse rate for this dysrhythmia is 40 to 100 beats per minute. It is simply a faster idioventricular rhythm (Figure 9-4).

Criteria for Classification

- ***Rhythm:*** P-P interval cannot be determined; the R-R interval is regular.
- ***Rate:*** Atrial rate cannot be determined due to the absence of atrial depolarization. The ventricular rate is 40 to 100 beats per minute.
- ***P wave morphology:*** The P wave is usually absent; therefore, no analysis of the P wave can be done.
- ***PR interval:*** The PR interval cannot be measured because the P wave cannot be identified.
- ***QRS duration and morphology:*** The QRS duration and morphology measure 0.12 second or greater and have the classic ventricular wide and bizarre appearance.

Interpret-TIP

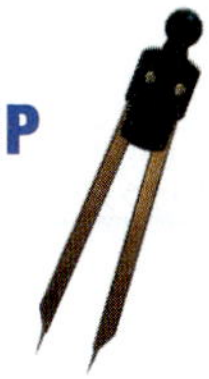

Accelerated Idioventricular Rhythm

The accelerated idioventricular rhythm has an absence of P waves, a ventricular rate of 40 to 100 beats per minute, and wide and bizarre QRS complexes.

Figure 9-4 Accelerated idioventricular rhythm.

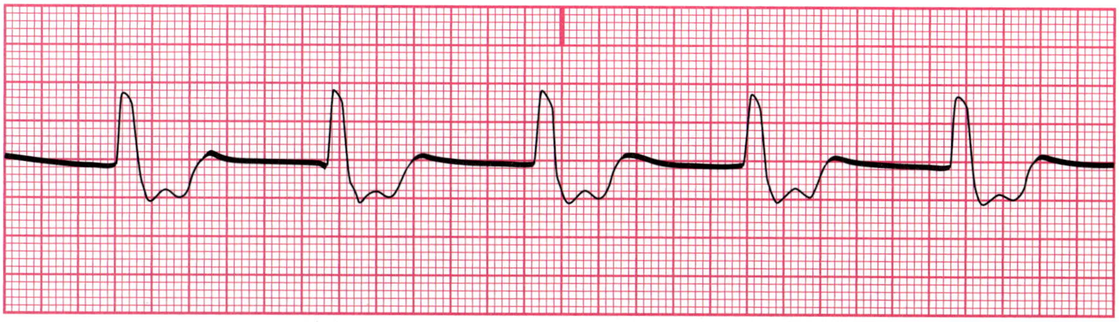

How the Patient Is Affected and What You Should Know

The patient may or may not be able to tolerate this dysrhythmia due to the decrease of cardiac output as a result of the loss of atrial kick and the slower ventricular rate. The patient may or may not be conscious. You must notify a licensed healthcare practitioner immediately. This patient may require treatment with cardiac medications and/or pacing. ECG strips must be saved and mounted in the patient's medical record.

Checkpoint Question (LO 9.5)

Using the criteria for classification, select the rhythm that most closely resembles accelerated idioventricular rhythm.

A.

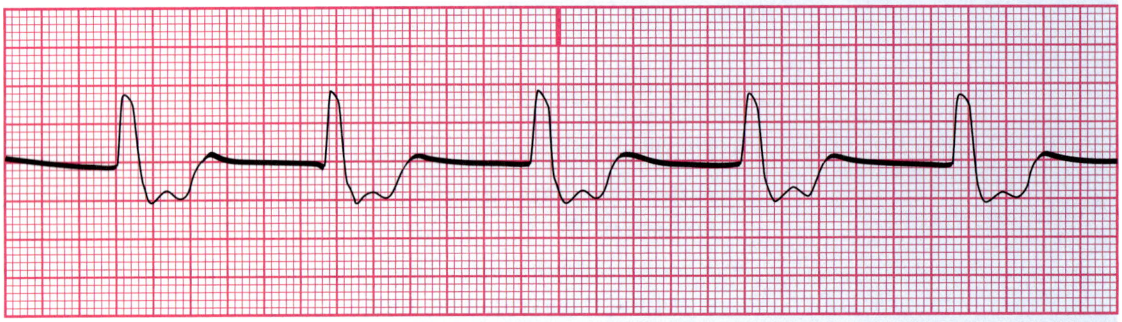

B.

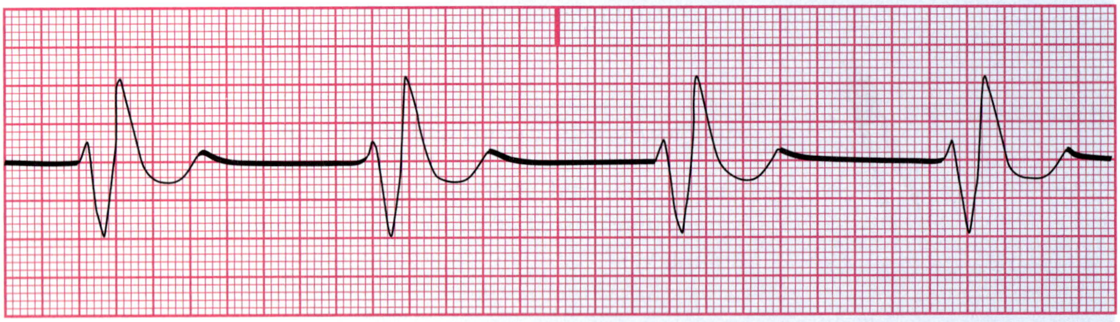

1. Which distinguishing feature(s) led you to make the selection?

____

____

____

9.6 Ventricular Tachycardia

Ventricular tachycardia occurs when three or more PVCs occur in a row and the ventricular rate is greater than 100 beats per minute (Figure 9-5). The ventricles are essentially in a continuous contraction-relaxation pattern and no period of delay exists between depolarizations (contractions).

Torsades de Pointes A type of ventricular tachycardia in which depolarization impulses move from one ventricle to the other, resulting in a "twisted ribbon" appearance on the ECG tracing.

Another type of ventricular tachycardia is called **Torsades de Pointes,** a French term meaning "twisting of the points." The difference between traditional ventricular tachycardia and Torsades de Pointes is in the morphology of the ventricular depolarization. Ventricular tachycardia has a consistent morphology. Torsades reflects changing voltages and durations due to the depolarization impulses in the ventricles moving to different locations in one ventricle, then the other. This tracing appears somewhat like party streamer paper as it twists and turns around the isoelectric line (Figure 9-6). This dysrhythmia usually occurs as a result of electrolyte deficiencies. The pharmacologic treatment of choice is magnesium sulfate. Other than this aspect of care, there is no change in patient management.

Criteria for Classification

- ***Rhythm:*** The P-P interval is usually not identifiable due to the large ventricular activity recorded. The R-R interval is usually regular, but it may be slightly irregular at times.
- ***Rate:*** Atrial rate cannot be determined because the P-P interval cannot be recognized. The ventricular rate is between 100 and 200 beats per minute.
- ***P wave morphology:*** The P wave is usually absent; therefore, no analysis of the P wave can be done.

Figure 9-5 Ventricular tachycardia.

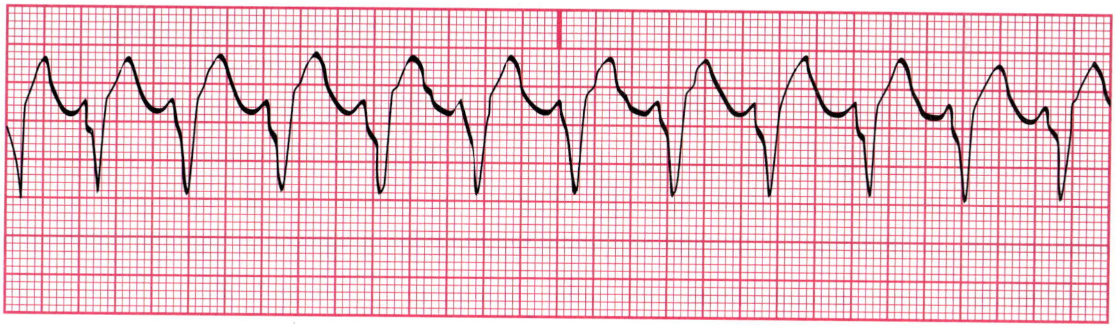

Figure 9-6 Torsades de Pointes.

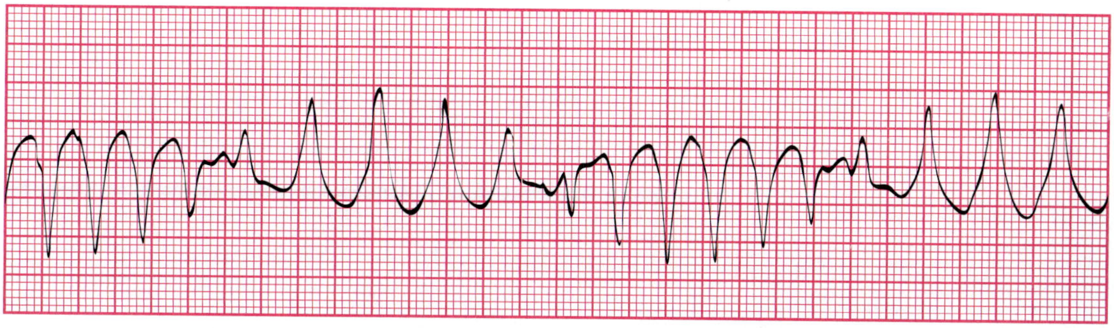

- ***PR interval:*** The PR interval cannot be measured because the P wave is not identifiable.
- ***QRS duration and morphology:*** The QRS duration and morphology measure greater than 0.12 second and have a wide and bizarre appearance with an increase in amplitude. The T wave is in the opposite direction (usually downward) from that of the QRS complex.

Interpret-TIP

Ventricular Tachycardia

Ventricular tachycardia has wide and bizarre QRS complexes with a classic "sawtooth" appearance, a rate in excess of 100 beats per minute, and no P waves.

How the Patient Is Affected and What You Should Know

The patient will have a decrease in cardiac output due to the decrease in ventricular filling time and the loss of the atrial kick. Some patients can tolerate the dysrhythmia for a short time—they have a pulse and remain conscious—whereas other patients will be unresponsive immediately. About 50% of patients become unconscious immediately, with no pulse or respiration.

As soon as you recognize ventricular tachycardia on the monitor or ECG equipment, you should notify a licensed practitioner because the patient needs to be assessed for unresponsiveness. If the patient is unresponsive, an emergency protocol or Code Blue is initiated, and CPR is begun. Emergency equipment such as a defibrillator, medications, and intubation equipment are necessary. Rhythm strips are saved to document the changes in rhythm that have occurred and should be mounted in the patient's medical record. If the patient is responsive, the licensed practitioner may initiate a treatment plan of medications and electrical treatments.

Troubleshooting

Escape Beats

PVCs, called "escape beats," can often occur when the heart rate is less than 60 beats per minute. This is the heart's effort to pick up the rate. PVCs may also occur because of hypoxia or abnormal lab values, such as an electrolyte imbalance.

What are likely causes of PVCs?

____

____

Checkpoint Question (LO 9.6)

Using the criteria for classification, select the rhythm that most closely resembles ventricular tachycardia.

A.

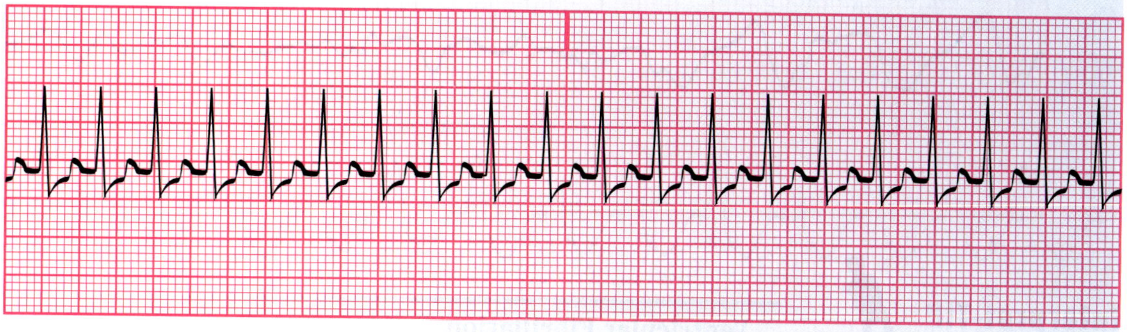

B.

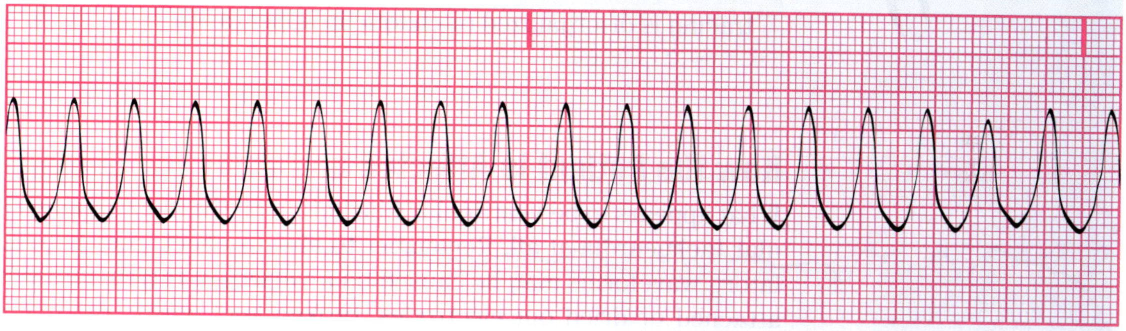

1. Which distinguishing feature(s) led you to make the selection?

____

____

____

9.7 Ventricular Fibrillation

Ventricular fibrillation is chaotic, asynchronous electrical activity within the ventricular tissue. The ventricle walls are quivering due to small, isolated portions of the ventricles depolarizing. There is no classic, uniform depolarization causing a true contraction. This prevents any ejection of blood out of the ventricles, so it results in no cardiac output (Figure 9-7). The entire myocardium is quivering similar to a bowl of Jell-O™ when shaken.

Criteria for Classification

- ***Rhythm:*** The P-P and R-R intervals cannot be determined because their waveforms are irregular and chaotic on the rhythm strips.
- ***Rate:*** The atrial and ventricular rates cannot be determined or identified.
- ***P wave morphology:*** The P wave morphology is not identifiable.
- ***PR interval:*** The PR interval cannot be identified.
- ***QRS duration and morphology:*** The QRS duration and morphology cannot be determined because only fibrillatory waves are present. No uniform depolarization of the ventricle occurs.

9.8 Asystole

Asystole is absence of ventricular activity and depolarization. Often this is called the "straight line" or "flat line" of rhythms. No electrical activity is present in the myocardium (Figure 9-8).

Note: Asystole is always confirmed in at least two different leads to rule out "fine" ventricular fibrillation.

Criteria for Classification

- ***Rhythm:*** Because no waveforms are present, there are no P-P or R-R intervals.
- ***Rate:*** No atrial or ventricular rates are present.
- ***P wave morphology:*** No P waves are present.
- ***PR interval:*** The PR interval cannot be measured because no waveforms are being recorded.
- ***QRS duration and morphology:*** The QRS duration and morphology are not measurable because no QRS waveform is observed.

How the Patient Is Affected and What You Should Know

This rhythm is associated with life-threatening conditions. The patient has no pulse and no cardiac output, as evidenced by unconsciousness and apnea. The patient is in cardiac arrest and emergency procedures must be initiated immediately. Emergency care includes immediate CPR and advanced cardiac life support measures.

Patient Education & Communication

Handling Emergency Situations

During an emergency, family, friends, and other patients will be apprehensive and curious regarding the situation. You should calmly explain that there is an emergency and escort individuals out of the immediate area and view of the situation. Explain to any family members that a licensed practitioner will speak to them concerning their loved one as soon as possible.

Your local protocol may be different. Remember to follow the rules of your organization.

Figure 9-8 Asystole.

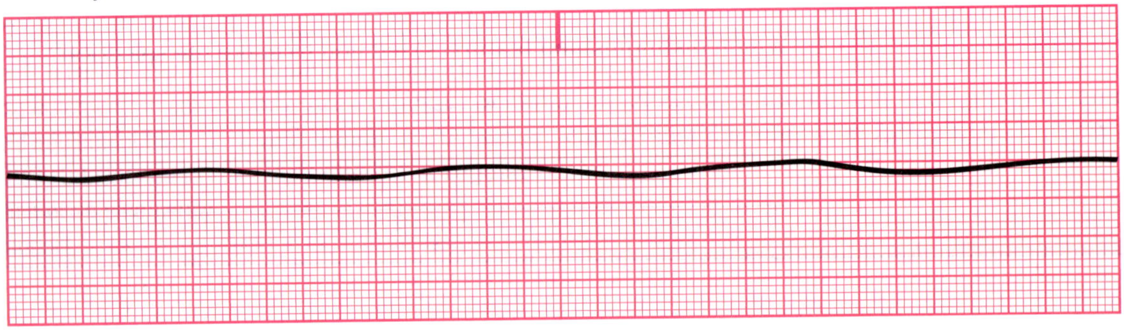

Checkpoint Question (LO 9.8)

Using the criteria for classification, select the rhythm strip that most closely resembles asystole.

A.

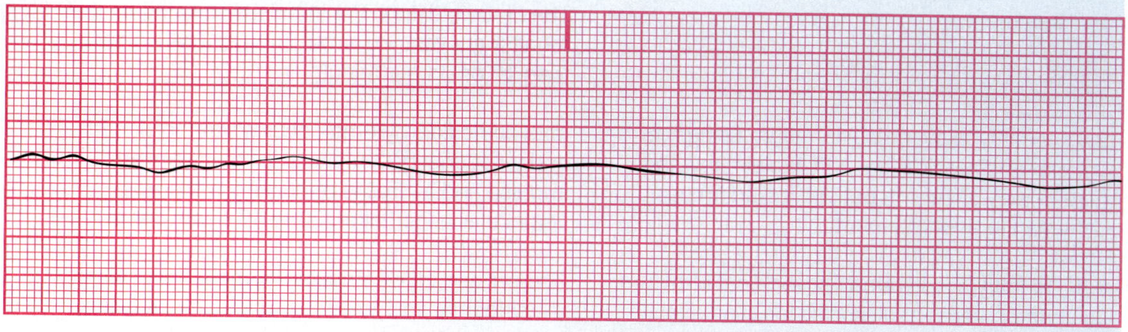

B.

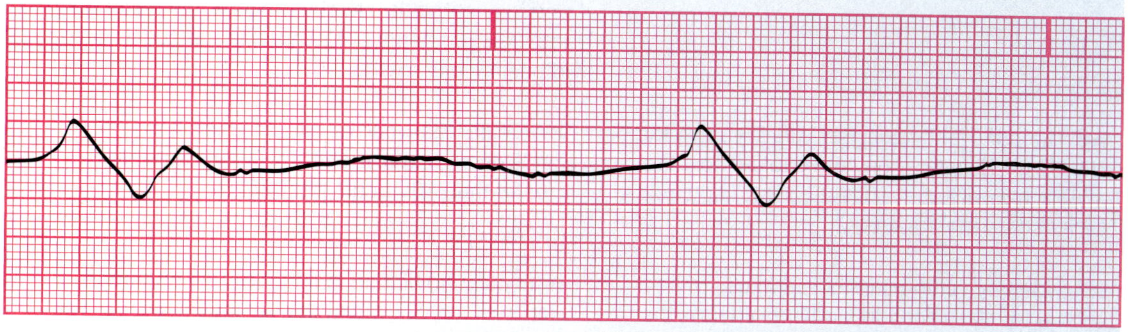

1. Which distinguishing feature(s) led you to make the selection?

____

____

____

Chapter Summary

Learning Outcomes	Summary	Pages
9.1 Describe the various ventricular dysrhythmias.	Ventricular complexes and rhythms share a conspicuous morphologic similarity: missing P waves and wide and bizarre QRS complexes (0.12 second or greater).	205
9.2 Identify premature ventricular complexes (PVCs) using the criteria for classification, and explain how the rhythm may affect the patient, including basic patient care and treatment.	A premature ventricular complex (PVC) is caused by an ectopic impulse that occurs early in the cycle and originates from the ventricles.	205–209

(Continued)

Learning Outcomes	Summary	Pages
9.3 Identify agonal rhythm using the criteria for classification, and explain how the rhythm may affect the patient, including basic patient care and treatment.	Agonal rhythms occur when essentially all of the pacemakers in the heart have failed. This is the last semblance of ordered electrical activity in the heart. The heart is dying. The impulses showing on the monitor are ventricular but firing at a rate of less than 20 beats per minute.	210–211
9.4 Identify idioventricular rhythm using the criteria for classification, and explain how the rhythm may affect the patient, including basic patient care and treatment.	Idioventricular rhythms occur when the sinoatrial and junctional pacemakers fail to initiate an impulse and all that is remaining is the slow ventricular pacemaker (20 to 40 beats per minute).	211–213
9.5 Identify accelerated idioventricular rhythm using the criteria for classification, and explain how the rhythm may affect the patient, including basic patient care and treatment.	Accelerated idioventricular rhythms occur when the sinoatrial and junctional pacemakers fail to initiate an impulse and all that is remaining is the slow ventricular pacemaker. The primary difference between accelerated idioventricular and idioventricular dysrhythmias is the faster heart rate (40–100 beats per minute) in the accelerated idioventricular rhythm.	213–214
9.6 Identify ventricular tachycardia using the criteria for classification, and explain how the rhythm may affect the patient, including basic patient care and treatment.	Ventricular tachycardia occurs when three or more PVCs occur in a row and the ventricular rate is greater than 100 beats per minute.	215–217
9.7 Identify ventricular fibrillation using the criteria for classification, and explain how the rhythm may affect the patient, including basic patient care and treatment.	Ventricular fibrillation is chaotic, asynchronous electrical activity within the ventricular tissue. The ventricle walls are quivering due to small, isolated portions of the ventricles depolarizing. P-P and R-R intervals cannot be determined because only chaotic waveforms are recorded on the rhythm strips.	217–219
9.8 Identify asystole using the criteria for classification, and explain how the rhythm may affect the patient, including basic patient care and treatment.	Asystole is absence of ventricular activity and depolarization. Often this is called the "straight line" or "flat line" of rhythms. No electrical activity is present in the myocardium.	220–221

Chapter Review

Multiple Choice

Circle the correct answer.

1. Which ventricular dysrhythmia has no P waves? (LO 9.2–9.8)
   a. Accelerated idioventricular
   b. Idioventricular
   c. Accelerated idioventricular
   d. Ventricular tachycardia
   e. Ventricular fibrillation
   f. All of the answers are correct

2. Which ventricular dysrhythmia has a heart rate between 40 and 100 beats per minute? (LO 9.5)
   a. Asystole
   b. Idioventricular
   c. Accelerated idioventricular
   d. Ventricular tachycardia
   e. Ventricular fibrillation
   f. Agonal

3. Which ventricular dysrhythmia has a heart rate less than 20 beats per minute? (LO 9.3)
   a. Idioventricular
   b. Accelerated idioventricular
   c. Ventricular tachycardia
   d. Ventricular fibrillation
   e. Agonal

4. Which ventricular dysrhythmia has a heart rate between 20 and 40 beats per minute? (LO 9.4)
   a. Asystole
   b. Idioventricular
   c. Accelerated idioventricular
   d. Ventricular tachycardia
   e. Ventricular fibrillation
   f. Agonal

5. What is unique about ventricular dysrhythmias with regard to the P-P intervals? (LO 9.1)
   a. They are irregular.
   b. They are biphasic.
   c. They are regular.
   d. There are no P waves, so the P-P interval cannot be measured.

6. QRS complexes that measure 0.12 second or greater with a rate between 20 and 40 beats per minute indicate that the impulses causing ventricular depolarization are coming from the ____________________. (LO 9.1)
   a. SA node
   b. interatrial pathways
   c. AV node
   d. Purkinje fibers (ventricles)

7. Ventricular fibrillation is typically described as "____________________." (LO 9.7)
   a. regular
   b. absent
   c. chaotic
   d. none of the answers are correct

8. Which of the following dysrhythmias is *not* considered to be a medical emergency? (LO 9.2)
   a. Agonal
   b. Asystole
   c. Ventricular fibrillation
   d. Occasional PVCs

Short Answer

9. What is the difference between idioventricular rhythm and accelerated idioventricular rhythm? (LO 9.4, 9.5)

   ____

   ____

10. How are agonal rhythm and asystole the same? (LO 9.3, 9.8)

   ____

   ____

11. What is the difference between ventricular tachycardia and ventricular fibrillation? (LO 9.6, 9.7)

   ____

   ____

Matching

Match the predominant type or pattern of premature complex with each of the images below. (LO 9.1, 9.2)

_______ **12.** bigeminy

_______ **13.** coupling

_______ **14.** interpolated PVC

_______ **15.** multifocal PVCs

_______ **16.** occasional PVC

_______ **17.** quadgeminy

_______ **18.** R-on-T PVCs

_______ **19.** trigeminy

_______ **20.** unifocal PVCs

_______ **21.** run of ventricular tachycardia

_______ **22.** paroxysmal event

a

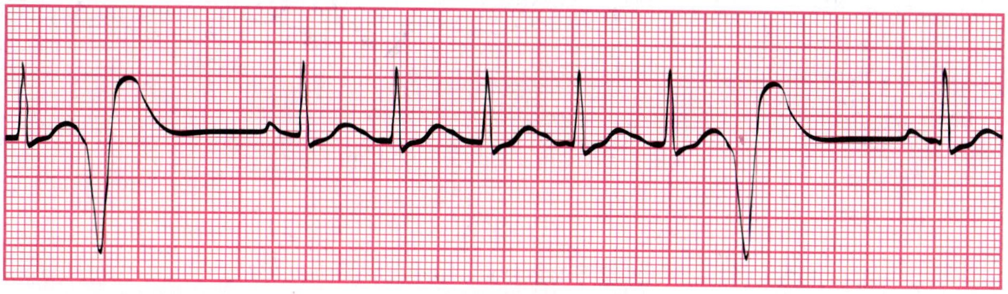

b

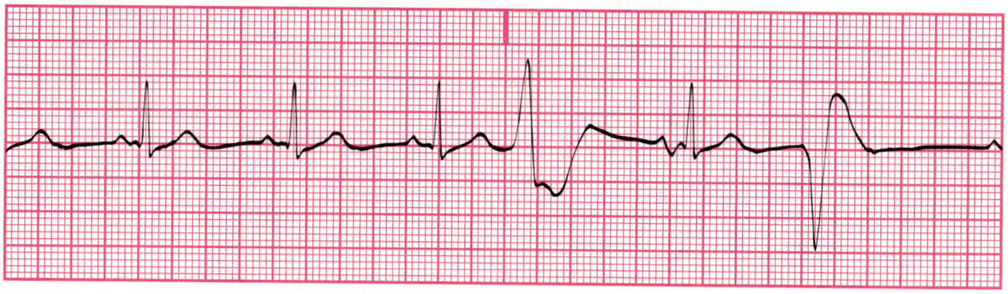

c

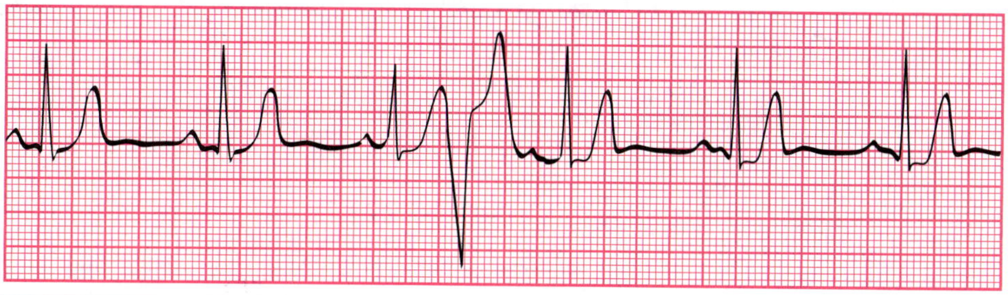

d

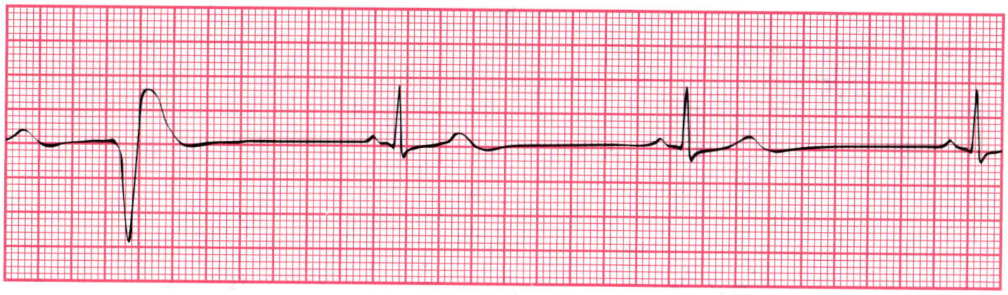

e

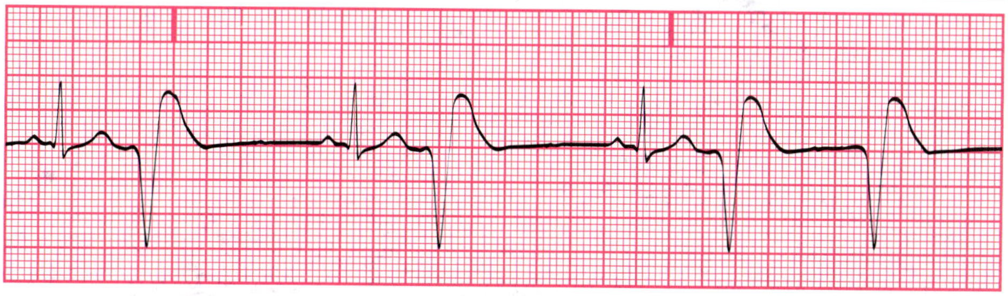

f

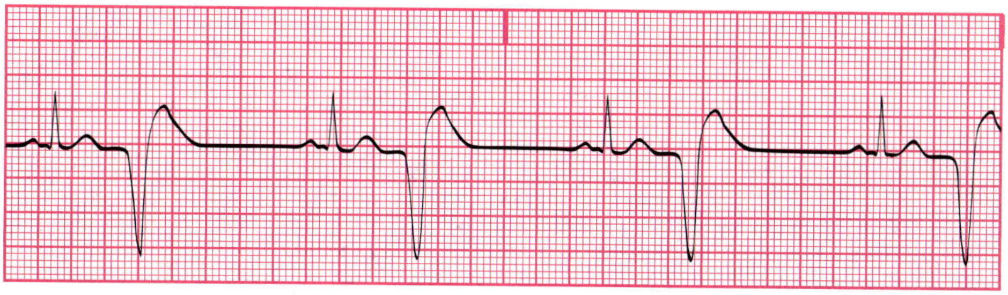

g

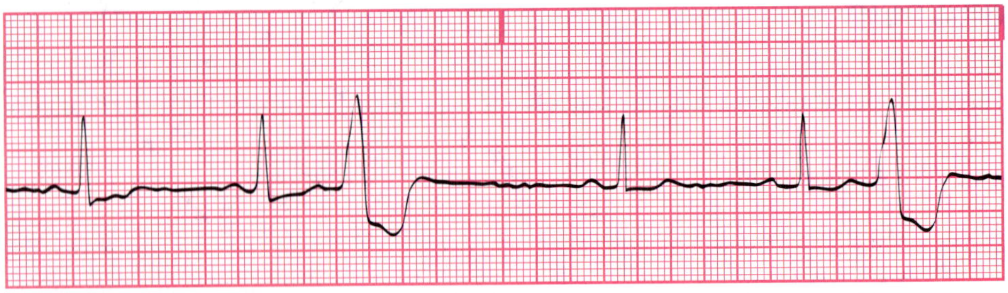

h

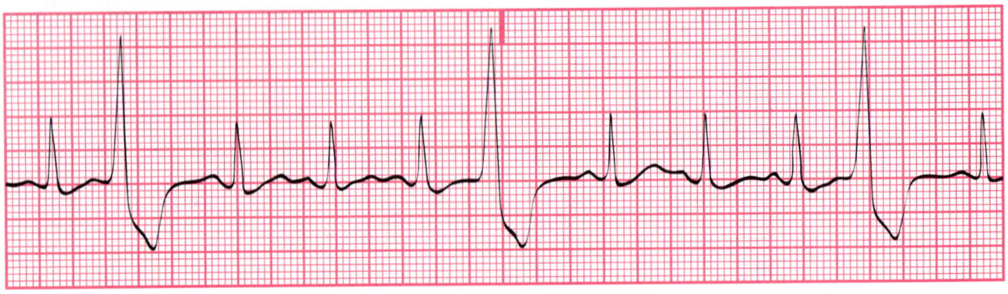

i

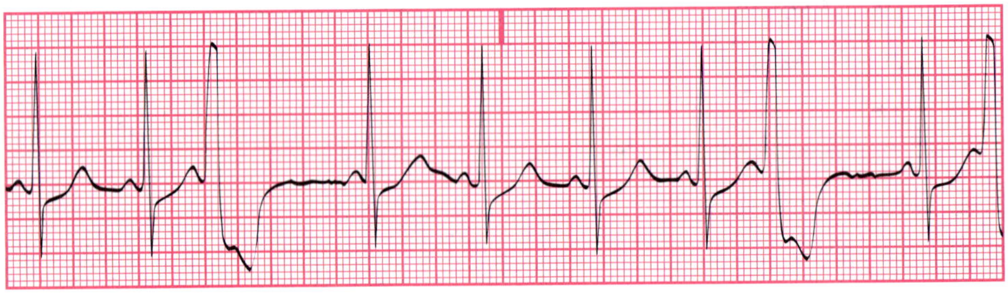

j

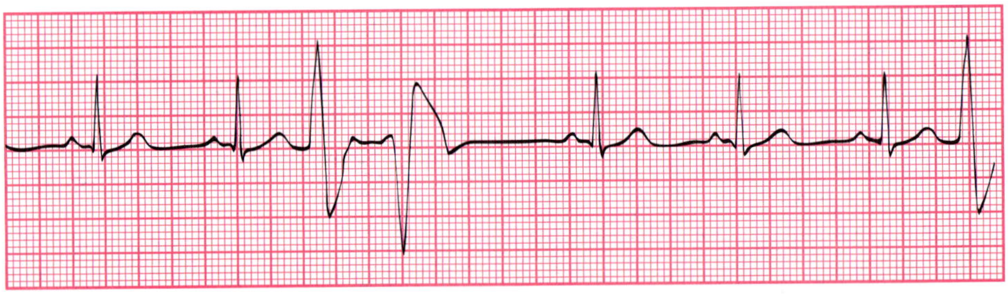

k

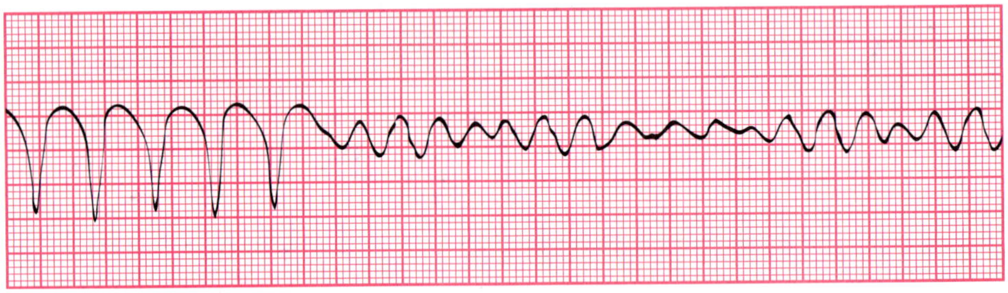

l

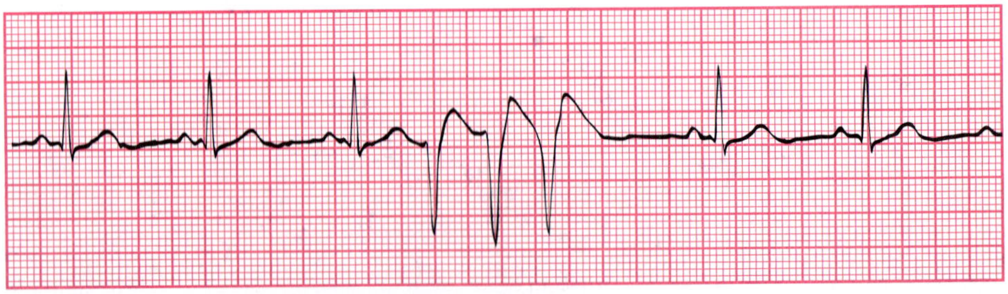

Critical Thinking Applications *Rhythm Identification*

Review the dysrhythmias pictured here. Using the criteria for classification provided in the chapter as clues, identify each rhythm, and provide the information you used to make your decision. (LO 9.2–9.8)

23.

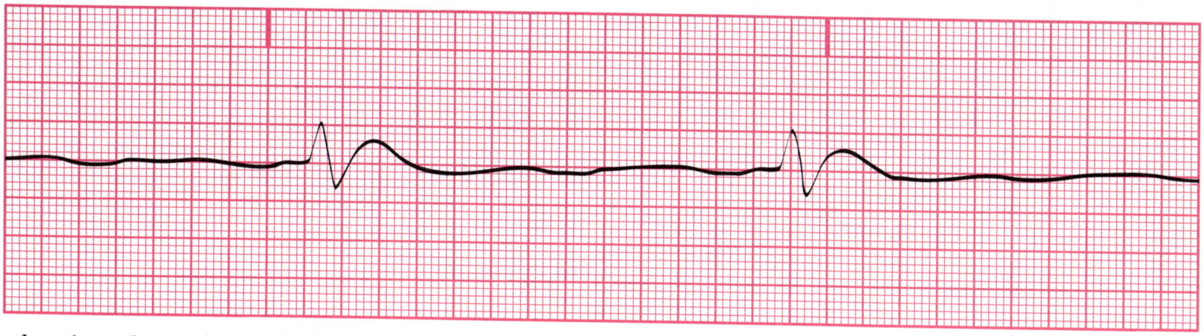

Rhythm (regular or irregular): ____________________ PR interval: ____________________

Rate: ____________________ QRS: ____________________

P wave: ____________________ Interpretation: ____________________

24.

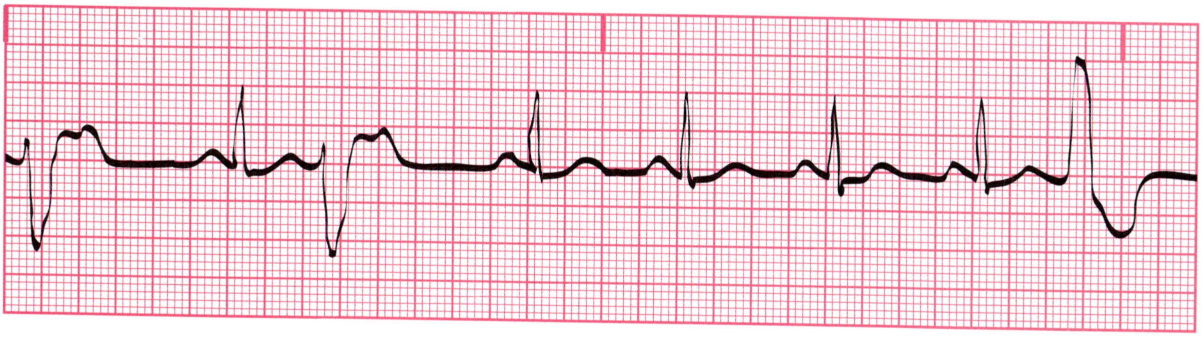

Rhythm (regular or irregular): ____________________ PR interval: ____________________

Rate: ____________________ QRS: ____________________

P wave: ____________________ Interpretation: ____________________

25.

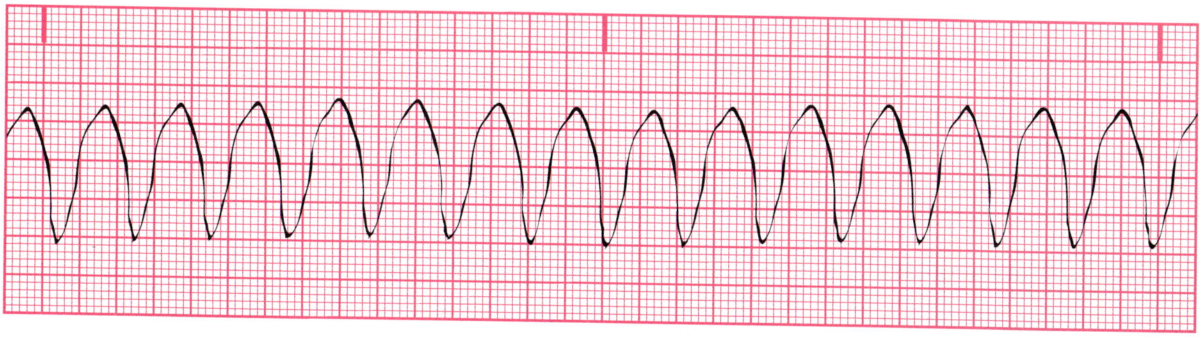

Rhythm (regular or irregular): ____________________ PR interval: ____________________

Rate: ____________________ QRS: ____________________

P wave: ____________________ Interpretation: ____________________

26.

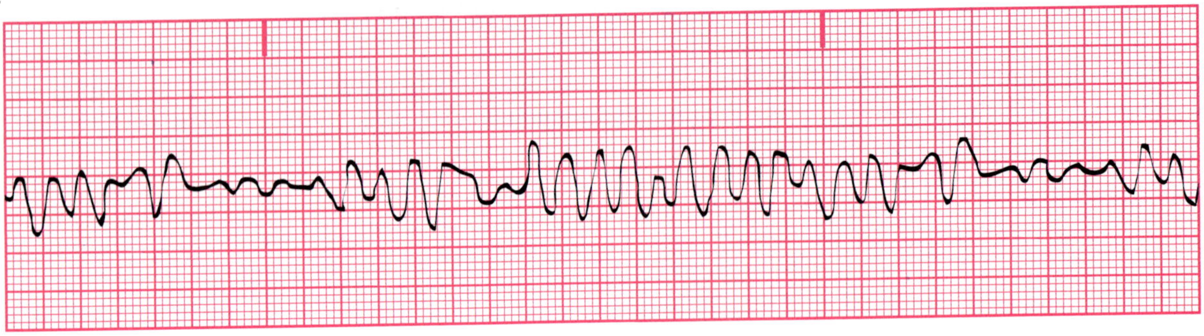

Rhythm (regular or irregular): ____________ PR interval: ____________

Rate: ____________ QRS: ____________

P wave: ____________ Interpretation: ____________

27.

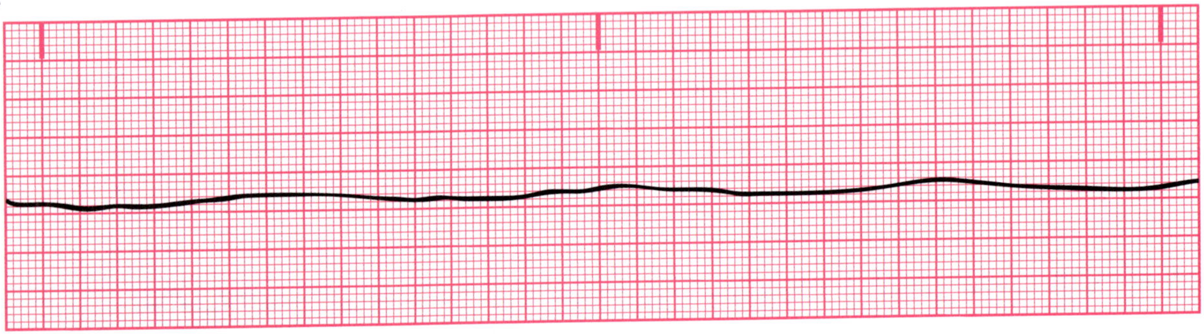

Rhythm (regular or irregular): ____________ PR interval: ____________

Rate: ____________ QRS: ____________

P wave: ____________ Interpretation: ____________

28.

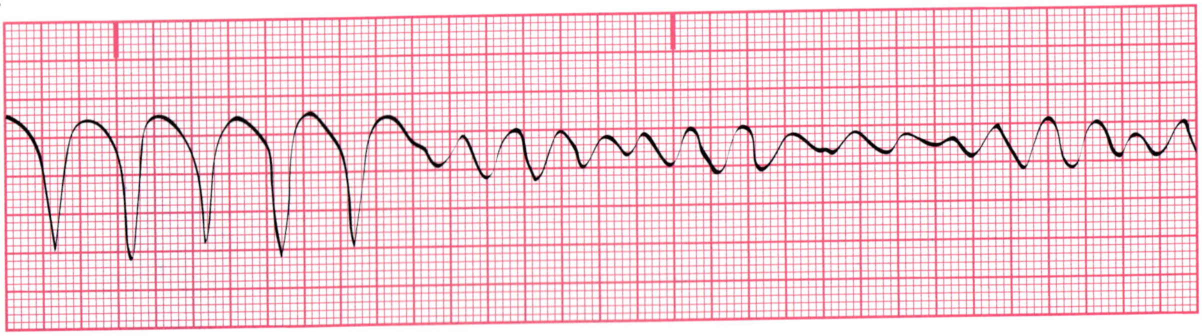

Rhythm (regular or irregular): ____________ PR interval: ____________

Rate: ____________ QRS: ____________

P wave: ____________ Interpretation: ____________

29.

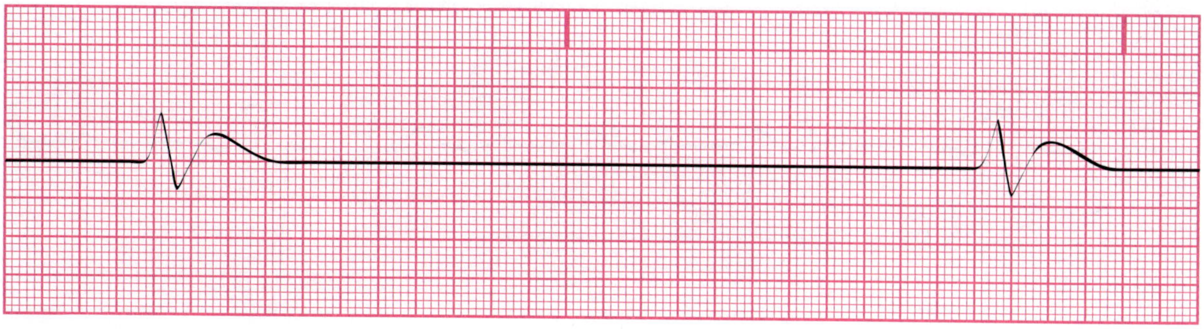

Rhythm (regular or irregular): ____________ PR interval: ____________

Rate: ____________ QRS: ____________

P wave: ____________ Interpretation: ____________

30.

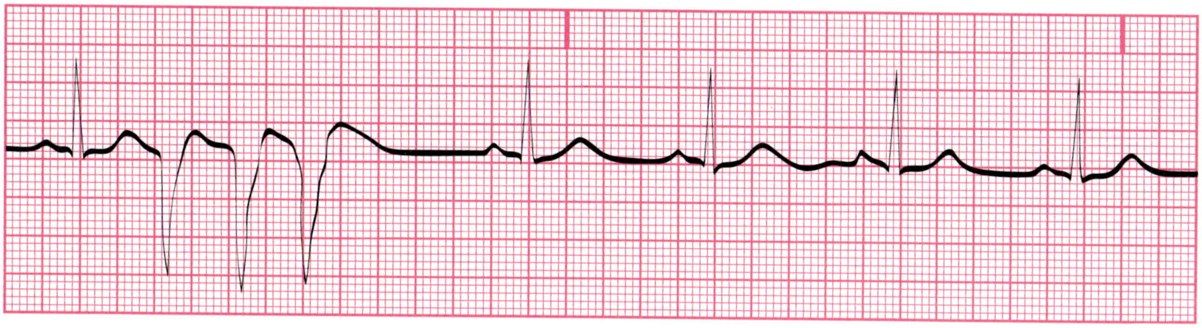

Rhythm (regular or irregular): ____________ PR interval: ____________

Rate: ____________ QRS: ____________

P wave: ____________ Interpretation: ____________

31.

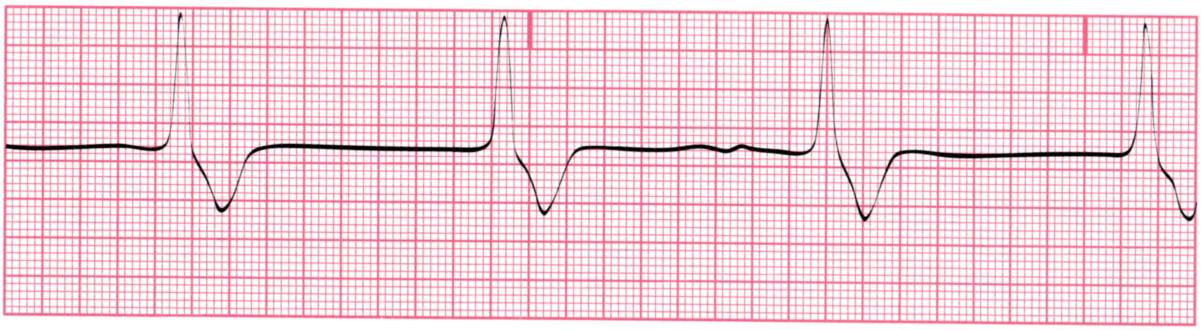

Rhythm (regular or irregular): ____________ PR interval: ____________

Rate: ____________ QRS: ____________

P wave: ____________ Interpretation: ____________

32.

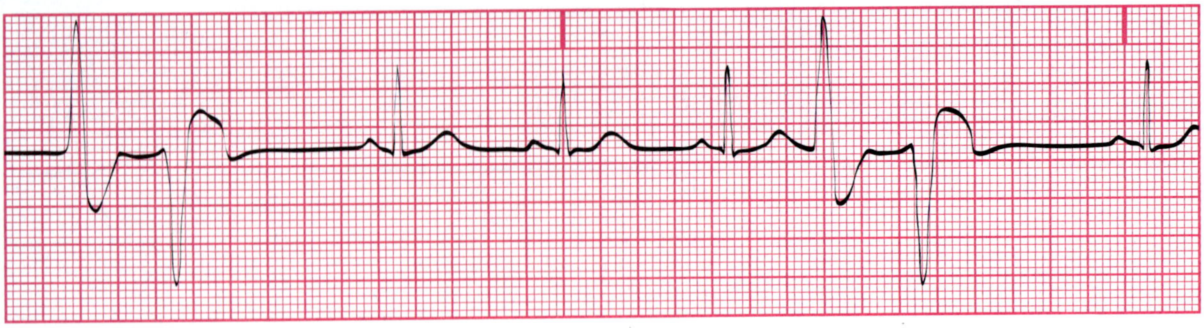

Rhythm (regular or irregular): ______ PR interval: ______

Rate: ______ QRS: ______

P wave: ______ Interpretation: ______

33.

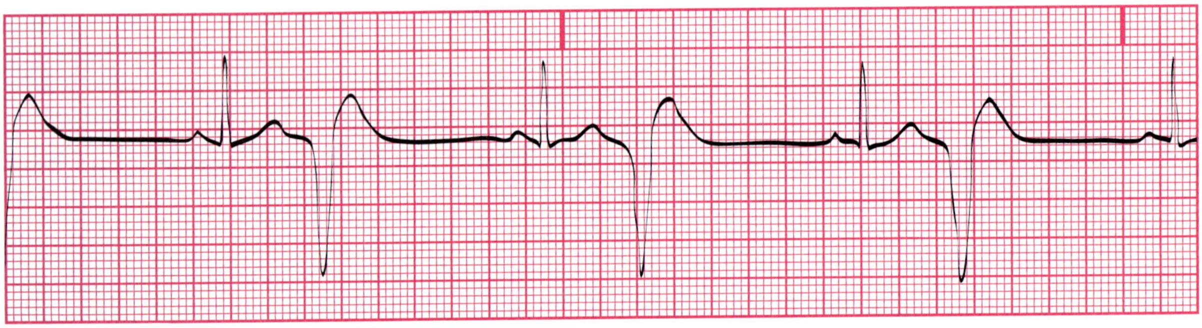

Rhythm (regular or irregular): ______ PR interval: ______

Rate: ______ QRS: ______

P wave: ______ Interpretation: ______

34.

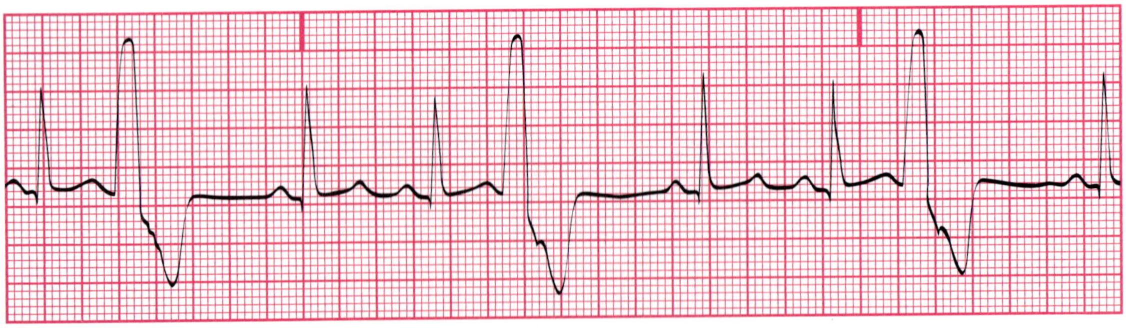

Rhythm (regular or irregular): ______ PR interval: ______

Rate: ______ QRS: ______

P wave: ______ Interpretation: ______

35.

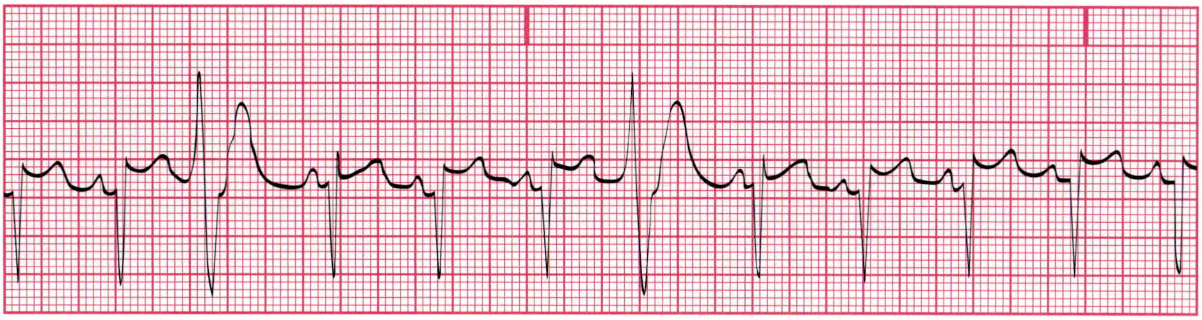

Rhythm (regular or irregular): ______________ PR interval: ______________

Rate: ______________ QRS: ______________

P wave: ______________ Interpretation: ______________

36.

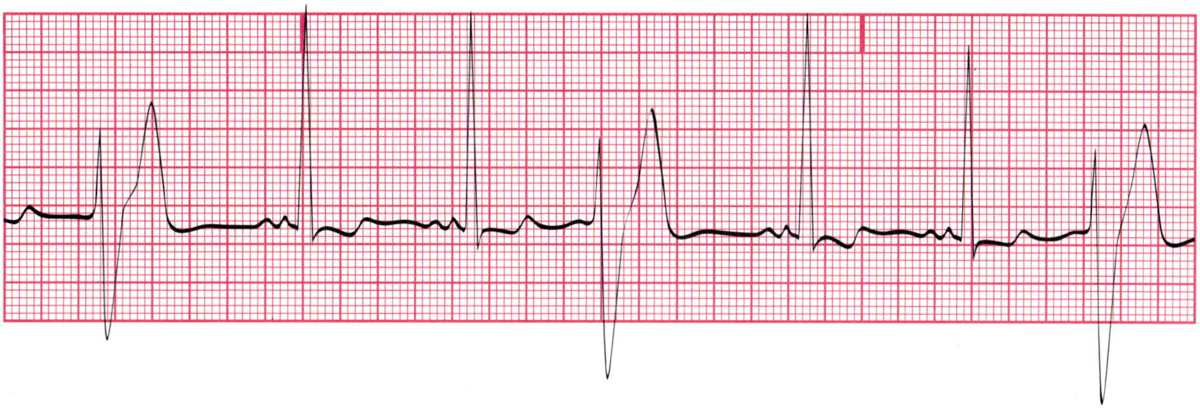

Rhythm (regular or irregular): ______________ PR interval: ______________

Rate: ______________ QRS: ______________

P wave: ______________ Interpretation: ______________

37.

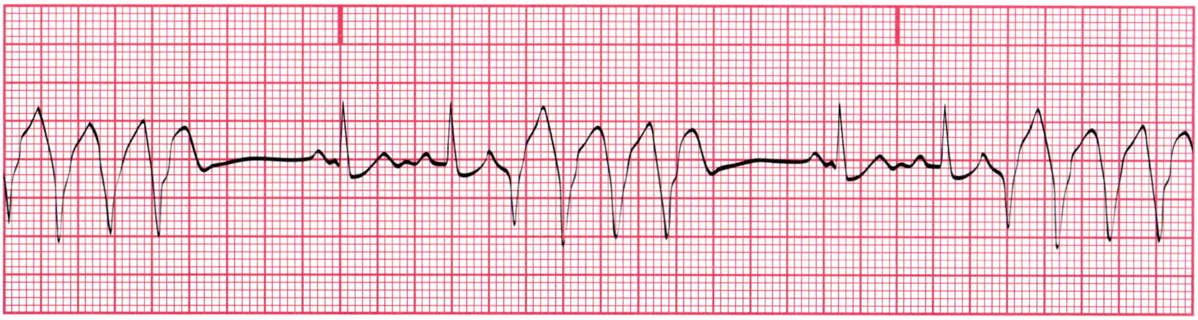

Rhythm (regular or irregular): ______________ PR interval: ______________

Rate: ______________ QRS: ______________

P wave: ______________ Interpretation: ______________

38.

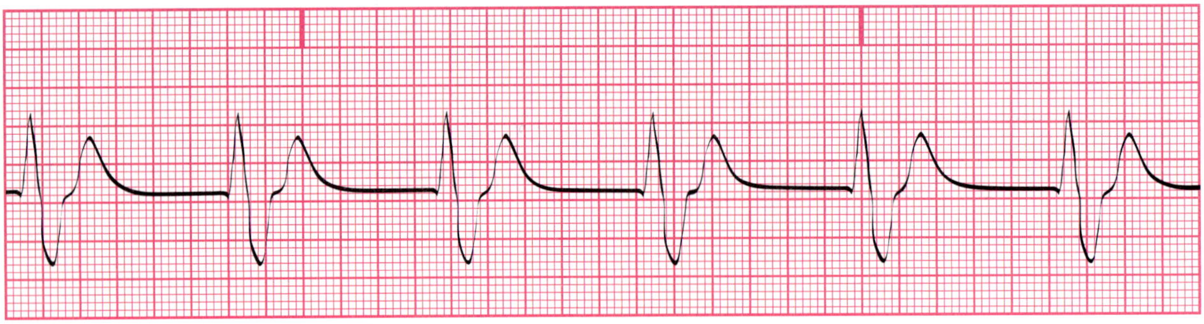

Rhythm (regular or irregular): ________ PR interval: ________

Rate: ________ QRS: ________

P wave: ________ Interpretation: ________

39.

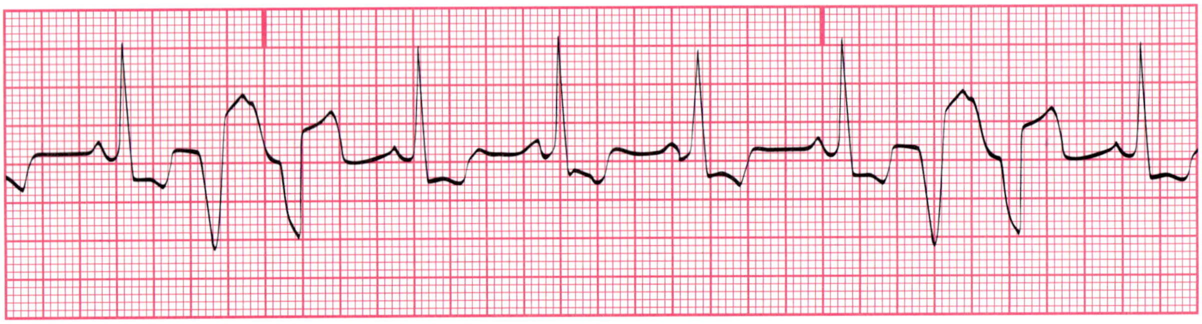

Rhythm (regular or irregular): ________ PR interval: ________

Rate: ________ QRS: ________

P wave: ________ Interpretation: ________

40.

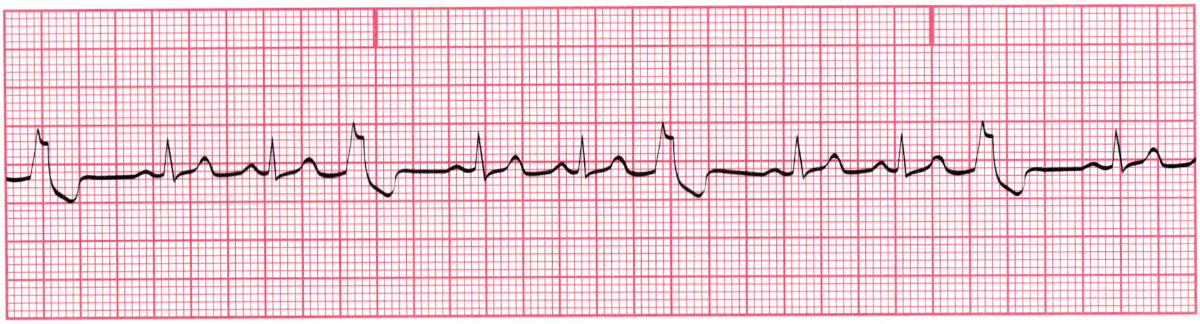

Rhythm (regular or irregular): ________ PR interval: ________

Rate: ________ QRS: ________

P wave: ________ Interpretation: ________

41.

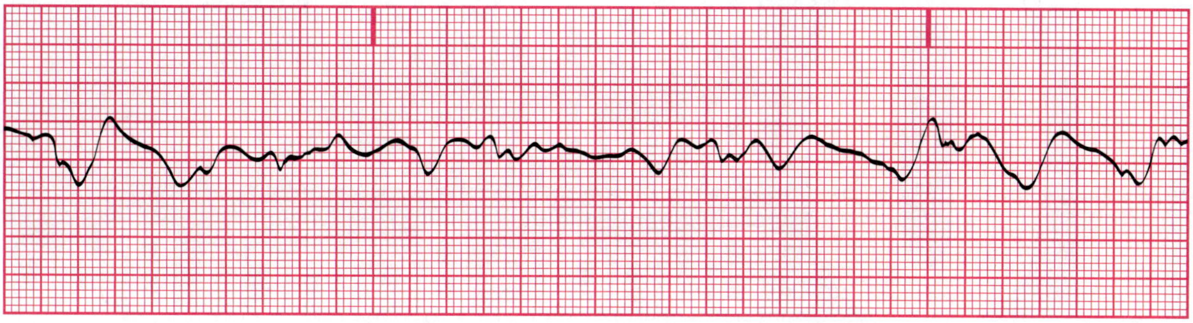

Rhythm (regular or irregular): ______ PR interval: ______

Rate: ______ QRS: ______

P wave: ______ Interpretation: ______

42.

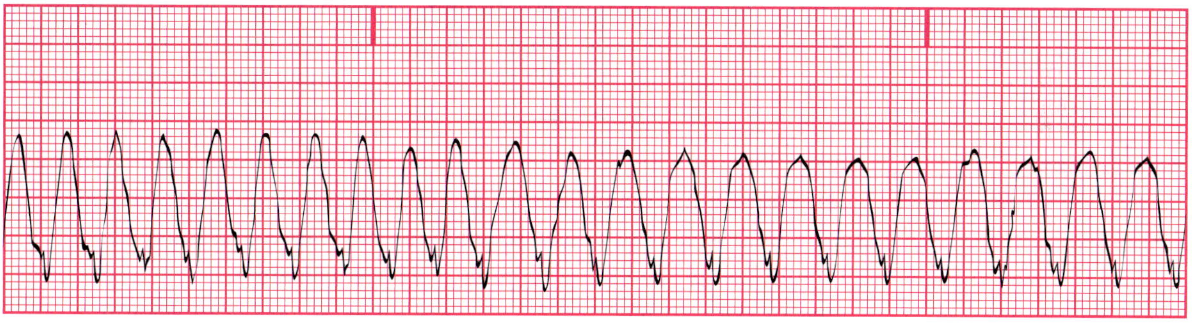

Rhythm (regular or irregular): ______ PR interval: ______

Rate: ______ QRS: ______

P wave: ______ Interpretation: ______

connect® Now that you have completed the material in the chapter text, go to Connect and complete any chapter activities you have not yet done.

10 Pacemaker Rhythms and Bundle Branch Block

Learning Outcomes

10.1 Describe the various pacemaker rhythms.

10.2 Identify pacemaker rhythms using the criteria for classification, and explain how the rhythm may affect the patient, including basic patient care and treatment.

10.3 Summarize pacemaker complications relative to the ECG tracing.

10.4 Identify bundle branch block using the criteria for classification, and explain how the rhythm occurs and may affect the patient.

Key Terms

atriobiventricular pacing
atrioventricular delay
atrioventricular sequential pacing
bundle branch block
electrical capture
electronic pacemaker
inherent rhythm
loss of capture (failure to depolarize)
malfunctioning (failure to pace)
malsensing (failure to sense)
mechanical capture
oversensing
pacemaker competition
pacing spike
triggered
undersensing

10.1 Introduction to Pacemaker Rhythms

electronic pacemaker A synthetic source of electrical current causing depolarization of the myocardium; artificial pacemakers are electronic.

Electronic pacemakers, also known as *artificial pacemakers,* are devices that deliver an electrical impulse to the myocardium to cause the cells to depolarize. This electrical generator provides small amounts of electrical current at predetermined intervals to mimic the normal pacemaker of the heart. Pacemakers can be used to pace the atria, ventricles, or both sets of chambers. They are sometimes temporary but are usually implanted under the skin (Figure 10-1) to correct dysrhythmias. Although many different types of electronic pacemakers are implanted, the mode in which they function varies in only a few ways. Because of the variety of pacemakers available on the market, it is recommended that you check in advance regarding the proper procedure for performing an ECG on a patient with a pacemaker.

Figure 10-1 Implanted pacemaker.

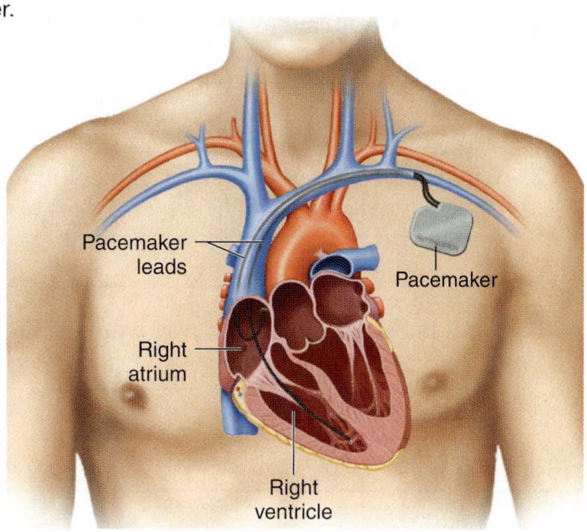

Safety & Infection Control

Pacemaker

The pacemaker's electrical current is not dangerous to you or other people who encounter the patient. The skin does not conduct electricity, so current will not be transmitted to another person from the pacemaker.

The fastest pacemaker in the heart controls the heartbeat, whether it is an inherent pacemaker, such as the SA node, or an artificial one. Electronic pacemakers work based on this principle. For example, when a patient is experiencing a bradycardic dysrhythmia, an artificial pacemaker is used and typically set at a rate of between 70 and 72 beats per minute. This artificial pacemaker becomes the fastest pacemaker in the heart and thus controls the heart rate.

The function of a pacemaker is to stimulate a contraction. Pacemakers can be inserted in the atria, the ventricles, or both, depending on the patient's needs. For example, if the patient is experiencing problems with the conduction system in the ventricles, a ventricular pacemaker is inserted to deliver direct stimulation to the ventricles and produce a ventricular contraction. Atrial pacing is used alone when the conduction system from the atrioventricular node through the ventricles is intact and functioning.

atrioventricular sequential pacing A pacemaker stimulation of the atria and then the lower part of the right ventricle in a sequence that mimics the normal cardiac conduction system and allows for atrial kick.

atriobiventricular pacing A sequential pacemaker stimulation of the atria and then both ventricles, rather than just the lower right ventricle.

Atrioventricular pacing provides direct stimulation of the atria and ventricles in a sequence pattern known as **atrioventricular sequential pacing.** This pacing option mimics the normal cardiac conduction system. It allows the atria to contract completely prior to the ventricles to allow an atrial kick. (Remember that the atrial kick provides the extra blood supply needed for approximately 10% to 30% of the normal cardiac output.) This pacing function is being used more when pacemakers are inserted because it mimics normal cardiac function and provides the atrial kick needed. A newer type of atrioventricular sequential pacing is atriobiventricular pacing, which is used commonly in patients with heart failure. **Atriobiventricular pacing** stimulates both ventricles to contract instead of the typical stimulation of only the lower portion of the right ventricle.

Checkpoint Questions (LO 10.1)

1. When is a ventricular pacemaker used?

2. When is an atrial pacemaker used alone?

3. What is the advantage of atrioventricular pacing?

10.2 Evaluating Pacemaker Function

Pacemaker function can be evaluated based on the ECG tracings. Several different ECG characteristics must be identified prior to evaluating the pacemaker function. The most important aspect of care is to verify the effectiveness of the pacemaker and determine the presence of a pulse with each captured beat. The term *capture* is used to mean two different things. **Electrical capture** refers to the evidence we see when viewing the cardiac tracing on the heart monitor or ECG machine (the spacing of spikes and waveforms). **Mechanical capture** refers to the heart's ability to respond to the electrical impulses that are being delivered to the heart. It is important to note that just because we see electrical evidence on a heart monitor, it does not mean that the heart is actually pumping well enough to sustain life. *Always remember to check the patient!*

electrical capture Evidence on an ECG tracing, including the spacing of spikes and waveforms.

mechanical capture The heart's ability to respond to electrical impulses delivered by a natural or electronic pacemaker.

pacing spike A thin spike on the ECG tracing that results from the pacemaker stimulation impulse.

Pacing Spike

The **pacing spike** denotes the discharge of electric current from the pacemaker, producing a spike on the ECG tracing. The current is a quick delivery and is reflected as a thin spike on the ECG tracing (Figure 10-2). After the pacing spike, a tracing of a P wave or a wide QRS complex or both will appear, depending on which chamber is being paced.

Interpret-TIP

Pacemaker Rhythms

Pacemaker rhythms are distinguished by the conspicuous presence of a spike prior to the waveform of the portion of the heart that is being paced. For example, a spike before the P wave indicates that the pacemaker is pacing the atrial portion of the depolarization.

Figure 10-2 The pacing spike is atrial, ventricular, or both depending on the type of pacemaker.

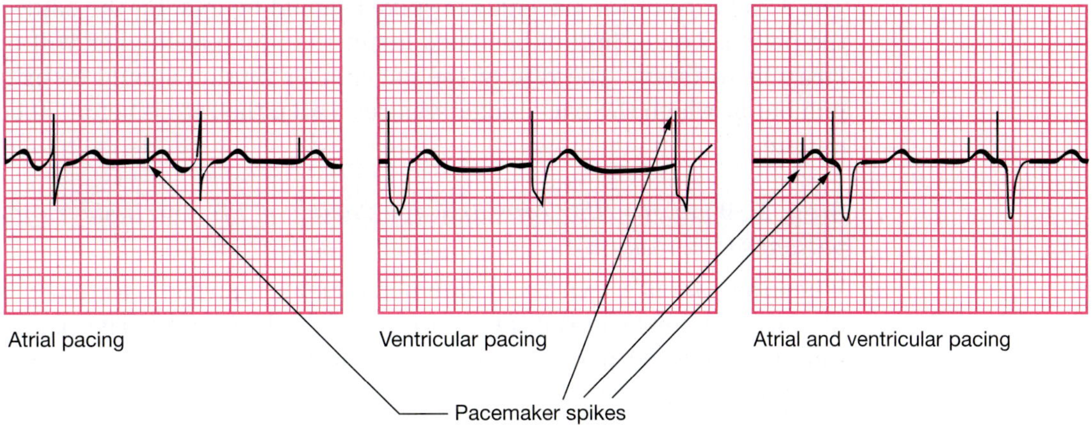

Chamber Depolarization Characteristics

If the pacemaker delivers atrial pacing, the pacing spike will be followed by a P wave. When the pacemaker delivers ventricular pacing, the pacing spike will be followed by a wide QRS complex, which looks similar to a left bundle branch block (LBBB) pattern. The ventricles are stimulated low in the right ventricle, causing the myocardium to depolarize slowly. The complex is wide and shaped differently from a natural QRS complex. It is similar to the LBBB because the left ventricle takes longer than the right to depolarize due to its size.

AV Delay

atrioventricular delay The measurement from the atrial spike to the ventricular spike, or from the beginning of the P wave to the ventricular spike on a pacemaker tracing.

The AV sequential pacemaker tracing has an **atrioventricular delay.** An atrioventricular delay is similar to the measurement of the PR interval on a normal rhythm tracing. It is measured from the atrial spike to the ventricular spike. Usually this programmed time frame is somewhere between 0.12 and 0.20 second, similar to a normal PR interval.

If the patient has a normal P wave and a pacer-induced ventricular complex, the atrioventricular delay is determined from the beginning of the P wave to the ventricular spike. If the patient has a pacer-induced atrial complex and a normal QRS measurement, the measurement from the pacing spike to the beginning of the QRS complex should be less than the set atrioventricular delay time frame.

Evaluating a Pacemaker ECG Tracing

inherent rhythm The patient's own heart rhythm.

Evaluating a pacemaker rhythm involves seven steps, which are similar to those used to evaluate a nonpaced rhythm. In addition, it is important to estimate the frequency of the pacemaker initiating the rhythm compared to the patient's **inherent rhythm.** The estimates are usually referred to in 25% intervals. If the entire rhythm strip displays an atrioventricular paced rhythm, it is referred to as 100% atrioventricular pacing (1:1). (When less than 100% paced rhythm occurs, identify the patient's inherent rhythm, and then include the estimate of paced beats and the type of pacing function as seen on the rhythm strip.)

Step 1. *What are the rate and regularity of the paced rhythm?*

The regularity of the pacemaker spikes should be exactly the same. Only if the patient's own rhythm becomes faster than the pacemaker will the regularity be different. The rate of the pacemaker rhythm should be exactly the number at which the pacemaker was set. Often the rate is set at 70 beats per minute.

Step 2. *What are the rate and regularity of the intrinsic rhythm (the patient's own rhythm)?*

When the patient's own heart rate beats faster than the pacemaker rhythm, the patient's intrinsic rhythm will control the heart rate. The patient's own rhythm should be noted on the ECG tracing. The rate and regularity will depend on the patient's inherent rhythm.

Step 3. (for AV sequential pacemakers only) *Is the atrial lead sensing appropriate?*

Evaluate the ECG tracing for the presence of atrial spikes with the P wave following the spike. Occasionally, the patient's own SA node or an atrial ectopic focus will initiate atrial contraction as evidenced by a P wave without an atrial spike.

Step 4. (for atrial, AV sequential, and atriobiventricular pacemakers) *Is atrial capture present?*

Every atrial spike should have a P wave after it to indicate that the electrical current is causing the atrial cells to depolarize. The P wave after the spike indicates that the atrial capture occurred.

Step 5. (for AV sequential and atriobiventricular pacemakers) *Is atrioventricular delay appropriate?*

Measuring from the atrial spike to the ventricular spike, or from the beginning of the P wave to the ventricular spike, will give you the atrioventricular delay interval. This time frame should be the same as the atrioventricular delay set on the pacemaker program. This information should be available on the patient's medical record or pacemaker information card.

Step 6. *Is ventricular sensing appropriate?*

The ECG tracing needs to be evaluated for the presence of ventricular spikes with the wide QRS complex following the spike. Occasionally the patient's own conduction system will work appropriately, as evidenced by a normal P wave and/or QRS complex. If the ventricular contraction occurs normally before the pacemaker sends a ventricular impulse, the pacemaker generator is inhibited, or stopped. This is evidenced by the absence of a ventricular spike.

Step 7. *Is ventricular capture present?*

Every ventricular spike should have a wide QRS complex after it to indicate that the electrical current caused the ventricular cells to depolarize. Appearance of the QRS complex after the spike indicates that ventricular capture occurred.

Checkpoint Questions (LO 10.2)

1. Using the criteria for classification, select the rhythm that most closely resembles atrial pacemaker rhythm.

A.

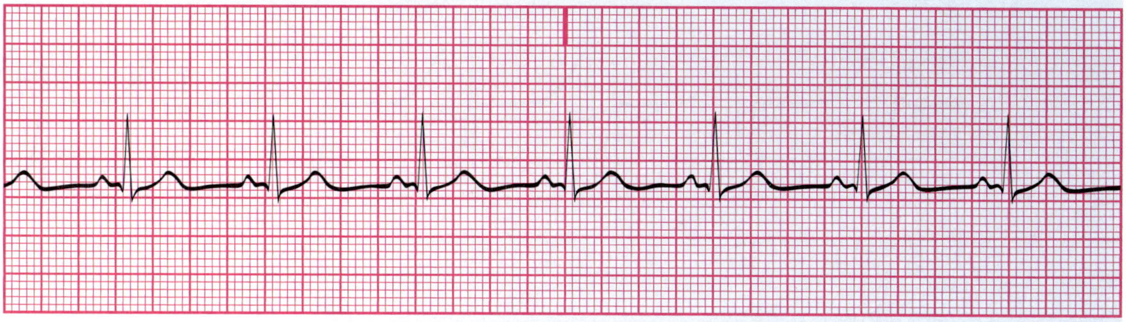

B.

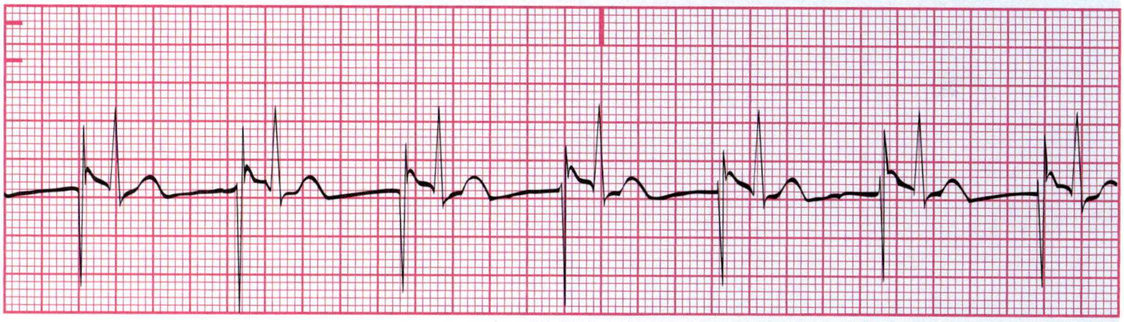

Which distinguishing feature(s) led you to make the selection?

____

____

____

(Continued)

2. Using the criteria for classification, select the rhythm that most closely resembles ventricular pacemaker rhythm.

A.

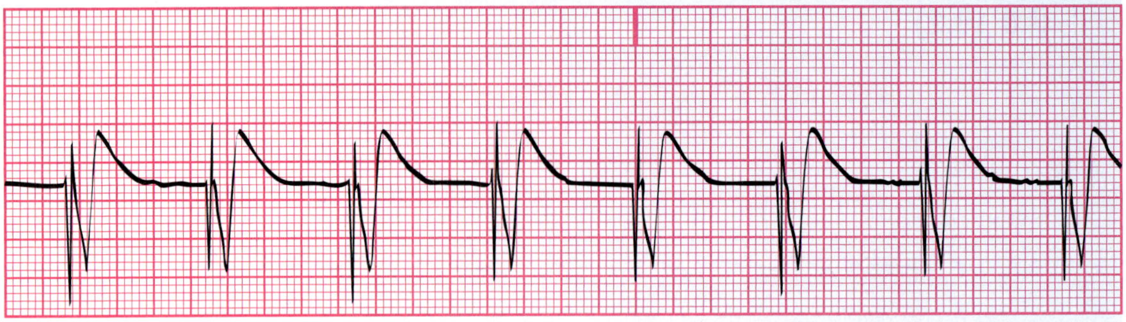

B.

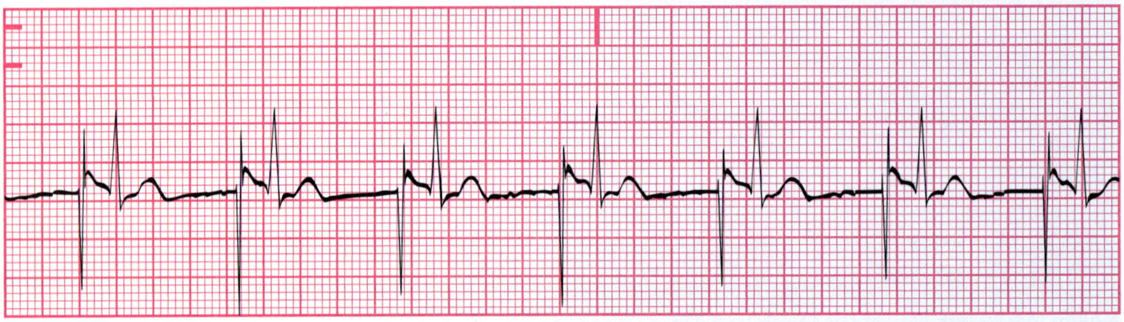

Which distinguishing feature(s) led you to make the selection?

____

____

____

3. Using the criteria for classification, select the rhythm that most closely resembles atrioventricular (AV sequential) pacemaker rhythm.

A.

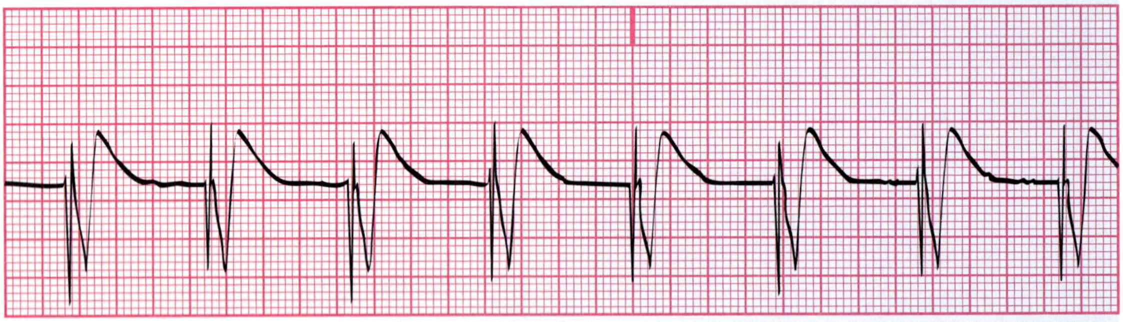

B.

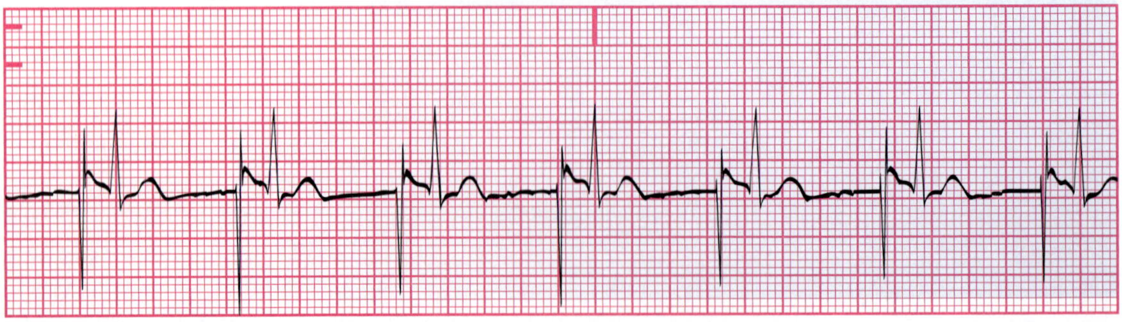

(*Continued*)

C.

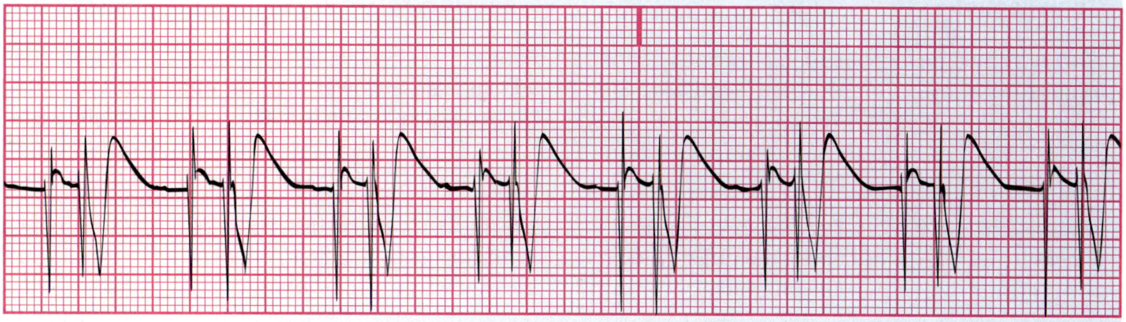

Which distinguishing feature(s) led you to make the selection?

____

____

____

triggered Caused to occur; in this case, the electrical impulses are caused to occur because the pacemaker fails to detect the normal contractions.

malfunctioning The pacemaker fails to send an electrical impulse to the myocardium.

malsensing The pacemaker does not recognize or sense the patient's own inherent cardiac electrical activity.

loss of capture The pacing activity continues to occur without evidence that the electrical activity has depolarized or captured the myocardium.

oversensing The pacemaker senses electrical current from other muscle movements or electrical activity outside of the body as the electrical current in the patient's heart.

undersensing The pacemaker is unable to detect any electrical activity and never turns off.

10.3 Pacemaker Complications Relative to the ECG Tracing

Pacemaker generators use lithium batteries to create an electrical impulse. As with any battery, the charge of the battery eventually decreases to the point at which the battery needs to be replaced. If a pacemaker is losing its ability to function properly, this failure will be evident on the ECG tracings. These changes in rhythms are often referred to as *complications* of the pacemaker. Complications include slower firing rates than set, less effective sensing capabilities, and lower electrical current than predetermined.

Another pacemaker complication is related to the functioning of the pacemaker generator when the sensing capability is too low. If sensing capability is low, the pacemaker will not be able to "see" the normal contractions occurring in the sensing chamber. Therefore, electrical impulses will not be inhibited but may actually be **triggered,** sending an impulse to the myocardium because the normal electrical current of the heart's conduction system was not "seen."

There are several different reasons for pacemaker complications, but only five basic changes are evident on the ECG tracing from these complications: **malfunctioning** (failure to pace), **malsensing** (failure to sense), **loss of capture** (failure to depolarize), **oversensing** (perceiving electrical current from sources other than the heart), and **undersensing** (unable to detect any electrical activity) (Table 10-1).

Responsibility in caring for patients with pacemakers requires recognizing normal pacemaker rhythms and possible complications. When you are performing an ECG or monitoring a patient with a pacemaker, you should be aware of the differences in the ECG waveforms, including the presence of a pacing spike, chamber depolarization characteristics, and atrioventricular delay. If you observe complications of a pacemaker rhythm, immediately notify licensed personnel for appropriate treatment and interventions.

TABLE 10-1 Pacemaker Complications

Complication	Cause	What Occurs	Patient Symptoms
Malfunctioning (failure to pace)	Pacemaker does not send electrical impulse to the myocardium.	Pacemaker intervals are irregular and impulse is slower than set rate. No pacemaker spike is seen.	Patient most often experiences hypotension, lightheadedness, and blackout periods due to bradycardic conditions.
Malsensing (failure to sense)	Pacemaker does not sense the patient's own inherent rate.	May send current to heart during relaxation (repolarization) phase; also known as **pacemaker competition** with the patient's own heart.	With atrial pacing, atrial fibrillation can occur; with ventricular pacing, ventricular tachycardia or ventricular fibrillation can occur.
Loss of capture (failure to depolarize)	Pacing activity occurs, but myocardium is not depolarized.	Pacing spikes will occur without a capture waveform, such as P wave or QRS complex (see first figure below).	Symptoms depend on the basic dysrhythmia and the patient's condition prior to the pacemaker insertion.
Oversensing	Pacemaker perceives electrical current from sources other than the heart.	Either (1) the patient's own heart rate is recorded and is slower than the set rate of the pacemaker or (2) the pacemaker spikes and captures at a slower rate than set (see second figure below).	Patient may have signs and symptoms of low cardiac output.
Undersensing	Pacemaker is unable to detect any electrical activity.	Pacemaker never turns off. Results in competition between the intrinsic and electronic pacemakers, which can lead to life-threatening complications, including cardiac arrest as a result of R-on-T pacing.	Patient may have signs and symptoms of low or no cardiac output, depending on the severity of the cardiac rhythm.

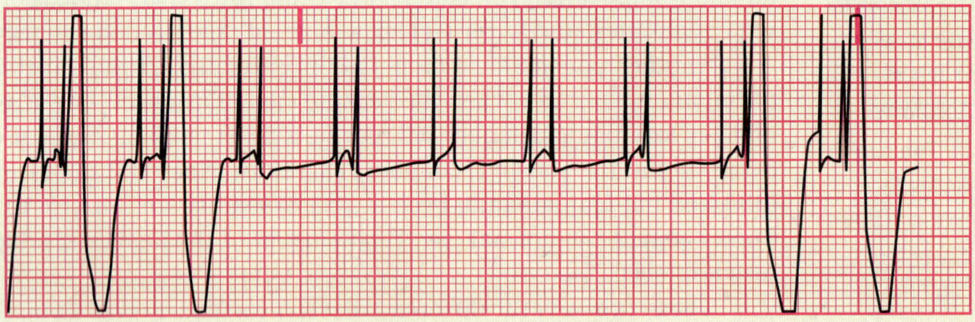

Loss of capture

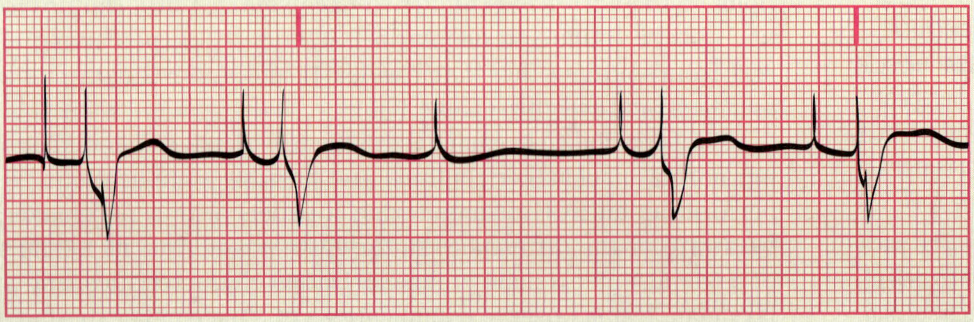

Oversensing

Checkpoint Question (LO 10.3)

1. Name and describe five different reasons for pacemaker complications.

___

___

___

10.4 Introduction to Bundle Branch Block Dysrhythmias

pacemaker competition Competition between the pacemaker generator and the heart's inherent rate over control of the myocardium.

bundle branch block Impulse is delayed or blocked within the bundle branches of the normal conduction pathway.

Bundle branch blocks occur when one or both of the ventricular pathways are damaged or the impulse is delayed due to cardiac disease, drugs, or other conditions. When an area of one of the bundle branches is damaged, electrical current cannot travel through that tissue to reach the myocardial tissue in its usual fashion. Current travels down the good bundle and activates the myocardial tissue in that corresponding ventricle only. The other ventricle must then receive the impulse as current travels from one cell to the next until the entire myocardial contraction occurs. It is similar to knocking down a line of dominoes, where each domino represents a cardiac cell. The cell will not contract until the next cell delivers the energy.

Current traveling via the abnormal pathways will take longer to achieve the full ventricular contraction. This longer time frame is similar to driving a car to a specific destination and having to find an alternate route or detour when the road is closed. This is what happens to the current traveling through the heart's conduction pathway when it has a blocked bundle branch. The increased length of time is reflected in a wider than normal QRS. Remember that the QRS duration is a measurement of how long it takes for current to travel through ventricular myocardial tissue.

When a patient has a right bundle branch block (RBBB), the impulse will travel down the conduction pathway normally until after the bundle of His. Because the right side of the conduction pathway is blocked, current must travel down the left bundle branch to activate the ventricles (Figure 10-3*A*).

In left bundle branch block (LBBB), the left conduction pathway is blocked. Current travels down the right bundle branch to cause the right ventricle, the septum, then the left ventricle to contract (Figure 10-3*B*).

The bundle branch block (BBB) classification provides additional information about another dysrhythmia. Information regarding a bundle branch block is extra data included with the basic rhythm classification. Typically the basic rhythm will be a rhythm that originates from above the ventricles. Any rhythm (sinus, atrial, junctional) that normally has a narrow QRS complex can be affected by BBB. The presence of BBB causes a widened QRS complex due to the delay of the electrical impulse as it spreads throughout the ventricles. The discovery of a wide QRS complex is the clue to further investigate for the bundle branch block. For example, the patient may be experiencing sinus rhythm with a left bundle branch block (SR with LBBB). The basic rhythm must always be determined with the distinction of a right bundle branch block or left bundle branch block present (see Figure 10-4).

Figure 10-3 Right and left bundle branch block ventricular conduction.

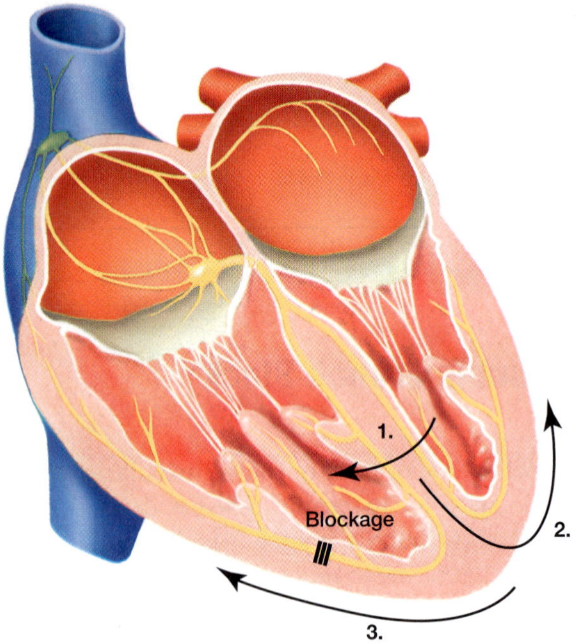

A. Ventricular conduction with RBBB

1. The septum is depolarized normally.
2. The left ventricle is activated.
3. The current travels to the right ventricle until there is complete ventricular contraction.

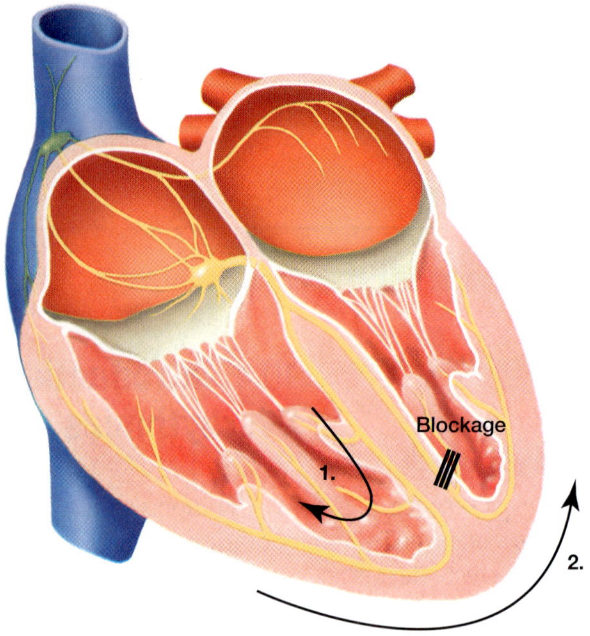

B. Ventricular conduction with LBBB

1. Current travels down the right bundle branch to cause right ventricle contraction.
2. The current moves to the left ventricle, causing the septum to be activated abnormally in a right-to-left fashion.

Figure 10-4 The presence of a P wave preceding each QRS complex indicates the rhythm is arising from the SA node. The wide QRS complexes result from a conduction defect through the ventricles, indicating a bundle branch block.

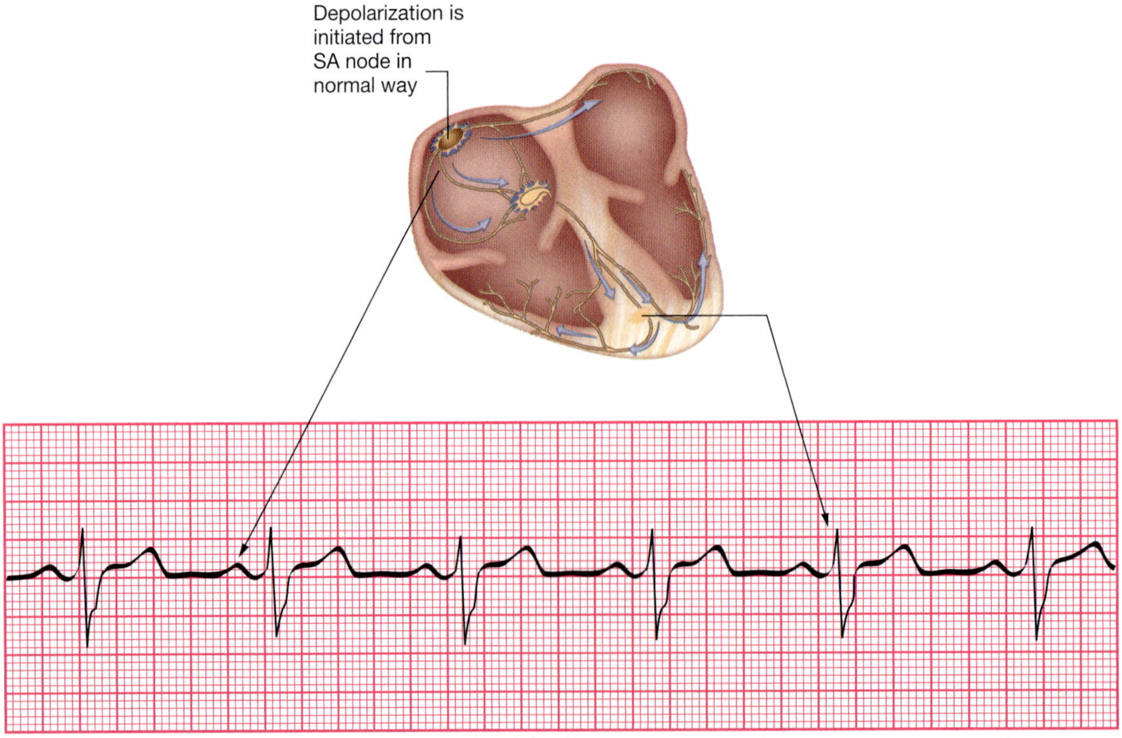

Interpret-TIP

Branch Bundle Blocks

The underlying rhythm has a P wave, and the QRS complex measures 0.12 second or greater.

Criteria for Classification

Characteristics of right and left bundle branch block will be similar over monitoring leads I, II, and III. Specific characteristics of the right or left bundle branch will be present when monitoring with leads V1 to V6. Although BBB is seen in the precordial leads, to distinguish RBBB from LBBB, lead V1 is referenced. If the QRS is positively deflected, it is RBBB. If the QRS is negative, it is LBBB.

- ***Rhythm:*** The regularity or irregularity depends on the underlying rhythm. Sinus or atrial is usually the underlying rhythm, with both regular and irregular rhythm patterns possible.
- ***Rate:*** The atrial and ventricular rates depend on the basic rhythm.
- ***P wave morphology:*** The morphology, deflection, and coordination with the QRS complex depend on the basic rhythm.
- ***PR interval:*** The PR interval has a normal measurement of 0.12 to 0.20 second.
- ***QRS duration and morphology:*** The QRS measurement is 0.12 second or greater in length. The widening of the QRS duration indicates the presence of a bundle branch block (see Figure 10-4).

How the Patient Is Affected and What You Should Know

The patient will exhibit the normal effects of the basic rhythm he or she is experiencing. For example, if the rhythm is sinus tachycardia, the patient will exhibit the signs and symptoms of a fast heart rate. A bundle branch block condition can further deteriorate to the development of another bundle branch block. If the current becomes totally blocked and current cannot reach the myocardium, this is considered a complete heart block.

Bundle branch block in and of itself is not considered to be life threatening, but what causes bundle branch block (e.g., a myocardial infarction) can be life threatening. Initially, you will observe a widening of the QRS complex, which indicates the presence of a bundle branch block. This should be reported to a licensed practitioner immediately. The patient will need to be monitored further by the licensed practitioner to determine whether RBBB or LBBB is present, and the patient's condition should be observed for deterioration. All patients must have a 12-lead ECG to document the bundle branch block. If further degeneration of the conduction system occurs, treatment may be a pacemaker. Pacemakers are applied to the external skin for a temporary condition for only 24 hours at a time. The patient may end up requiring emergency cardiac care and/or needing a permanent pacemaker.

Checkpoint Questions (LO 10.4)

1. What happens when one or both of the ventricular pathways are not functioning properly due to damage or a delay from cardiac disease, drugs, or other conditions?

___

___

2. Describe the electrical conduction for RBBB and LBBB.

___

___

3. Using the criteria for classification, select the rhythm that most closely resembles a rhythm containing bundle branch block.

A.

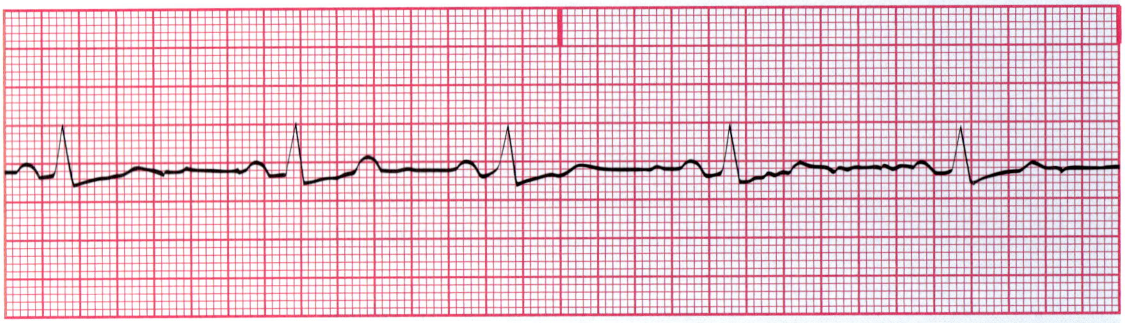

B.

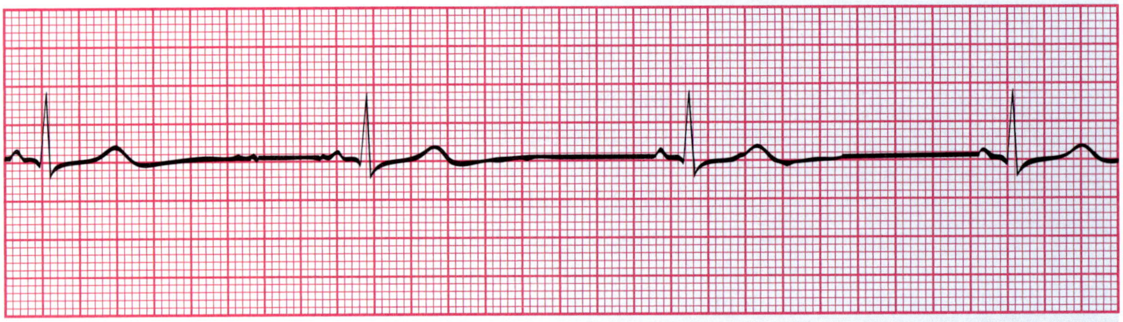

Which distinguishing feature(s) led you to make the selection?

___

___

___

Chapter Summary

Learning Outcomes	Summary	Pages
10.1 Describe the various pacemaker rhythms.	Electronic pacemakers, also known as artificial pacemakers, are devices that deliver an electrical impulse to the myocardium to cause the cells to depolarize. Pacemakers can be used to stimulate the atria, the ventricles, or both. Atrial pacing is used alone when the conduction system from the atrioventricular node through the ventricles is intact and functioning. Ventricular pacemakers are inserted to deliver direct stimulation to the ventricles and produce a ventricular contraction. Atrioventricular pacing provides direct stimulation of the atria and ventricles and mimics the normal cardiac conduction system.	234–236
10.2 Identify pacemaker rhythms using the criteria for classification, and explain how the rhythm may affect the patient, including basic patient care and treatment.	Pacemaker function can be evaluated based on the ECG tracings. The most important aspect of care is to verify the effectiveness of the pacemaker and determine the presence of a pulse with each captured beat. If a pacemaker is losing its ability to function properly, this failure will be evident on the ECG tracings.	236–241
10.3 Summarize pacemaker complications relative to the ECG tracing.	Caring for patients with pacemakers requires recognizing normal pacemaker rhythms and possible complications. When performing an ECG or monitoring a patient with a pacemaker, you should be aware of the differences in the ECG waveforms, including the presence of a pacing spike, chamber depolarization characteristics, and atrioventricular delay.	241–243
10.4 Identify bundle branch block using the criteria for classification, and explain how the rhythm occurs and may affect the patient.	Bundle branch blocks occur when one or both of the ventricular pathways are damaged or delayed due to cardiac disease, drugs, or other conditions. Current will travel down the good bundle and will activate the myocardial tissue in that corresponding ventricle only. An increased length of time of cell-to-cell conduction is reflected in a wider-than-normal QRS complex. The rhythm has all the basic properties of sinus rhythms, atrial dysrhythmias, or junctional dysrhythmias with the exception of a wide QRS complex. The patient will exhibit the normal effects of the basic rhythm he or she is experiencing. BBB should be reported to a licensed practitioner immediately. The patient will need to be monitored further to determine whether RBBB or LBBB is present, and the patient's condition should be observed for deterioration.	243–246

Chapter Review

Multiple Choice

Circle the correct answer(s). More than one can apply.

1. Which pacemaker rhythms have a pacing spike before P waves? (LO 10.1)
   - **a.** Atrial pacemaker rhythm
   - **b.** Ventricular pacemaker
   - **c.** Atrioventricular pacemaker
   - **d.** Normal sinus rhythm
2. Which pacemaker rhythms have a pacing spike before QRS complexes? (LO 10.1)
   - **a.** Atrial pacemaker rhythm
   - **b.** Ventricular pacemaker
   - **c.** Atrioventricular pacemaker
   - **d.** Normal sinus rhythm
3. Which pacemaker rhythm has a pacing spike before P waves and before QRS complexes? (LO 10.1)
   - **a.** Atrial pacemaker rhythm
   - **b.** Ventricular pacemaker
   - **c.** Atrioventricular pacemaker
   - **d.** Wandering atrial pacemaker
4. Which pacemaker complication shows a pacing spike but no waveform immediately following it? (LO 10.2)
   - **a.** Failure to sense
   - **b.** Failure to capture
   - **c.** Oversensing
   - **d.** Normal sinus rhythm
5. You observe a wide QRS complex while continuously monitoring a patient in lead II. Which lead placement is necessary to evaluate the location of blockage in the bundle branch system? (LO 10.4)
   - **a.** Lead I
   - **b.** Lead V4
   - **c.** Lead III
   - **d.** Lead V1
6. The labeling of the ECG rhythm strip for documentation of the bundle branch block should include what other information besides which bundle is being blocked? (LO 10.4)
   - **a.** Symptoms the patient is experiencing
   - **b.** Blood pressure reading
   - **c.** Presence of an MI diagnosis
   - **d.** Patient's inherent rhythm pattern

7. When the QRS complex measures ________, bundle branch block must be considered. (LO 10.3)
   - **a.** 0.06 to 0.10 second
   - **b.** 0.04 to 0.08 second
   - **c.** Less than 0.06 second
   - **d.** 0.12 second or greater

8. Which of the following is *not* one of the components to be evaluated on a pacemaker tracing? (LO 10.2)
   - **a.** The presence of atrial and/or ventricular spikes
   - **b.** The QT interval
   - **c.** The characteristic patterns of the chambers captured after the spikes
   - **d.** The atrioventricular delay period

Matching

Match the terms related to electronic (artificial) pacemakers on the left with their definitions on the right. (LO 10.2)

_______ **9.** pacemaker competition

_______ **10.** pacemaker (electronic)

_______ **11.** loss of capture

_______ **12.** undersensing

_______ **13.** malsensing

_______ **14.** malfunctioning

_______ **15.** oversensing

_______ **16.** triggered

_______ **17.** capture

a. electrical current causes the myocardial tissue to depolarize (contract)

b. heart muscle responds to electrical stimulation and depolarizes (contracts)

c. device that delivers electrical energy to cause depolarization (contractions)

d. pacing activity occurs but is not captured by the myocardium

e. pacemaker does not recognize the patient's inherent heart rate

f. electrical current from muscle movements or other activities are sensed by the pacemaker

g. pacemaker fails to send electrical impulse to the heart

h. pacemaker fails to detect any intrinsic electrical activity

i. rivalry between the intrinsic and electronic pacemakers, which can lead to life-threatening complications

Critical Thinking Application *Rhythm Identification*

Review the dysrhythmias pictured next and, using the criteria for classification provided in the chapter as clues, identify each rhythm and provide what information you used to make your decision. (LO 10.2, 10.4)

18.

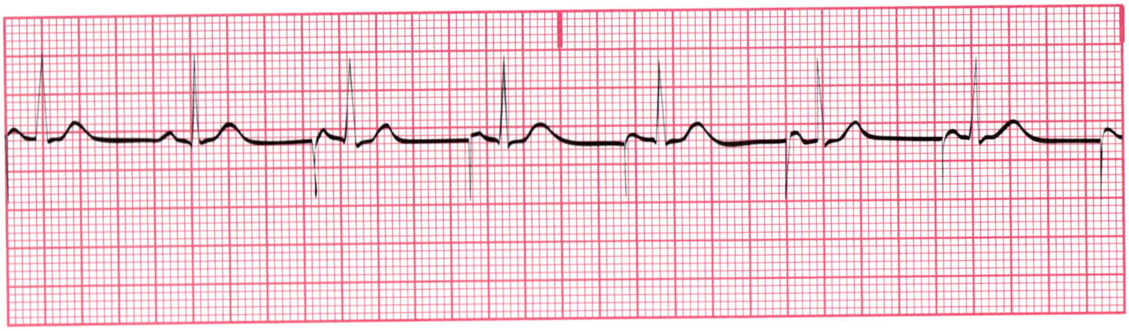

Rhythm (regular or irregular): ______________ PR interval: ______________

Rate: ______________ QRS: ______________

P wave: ______________ Interpretation: ______________

19.

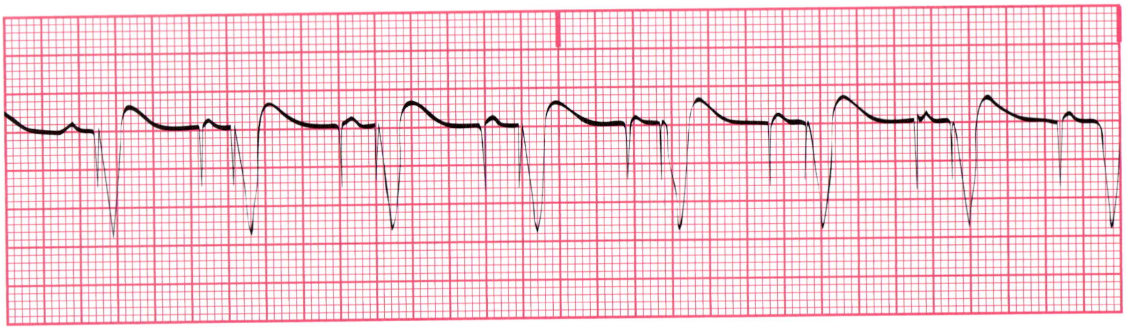

Rhythm (regular or irregular): ______________ PR interval: ______________

Rate: ______________ QRS: ______________

P wave: ______________ Interpretation: ______________

20.

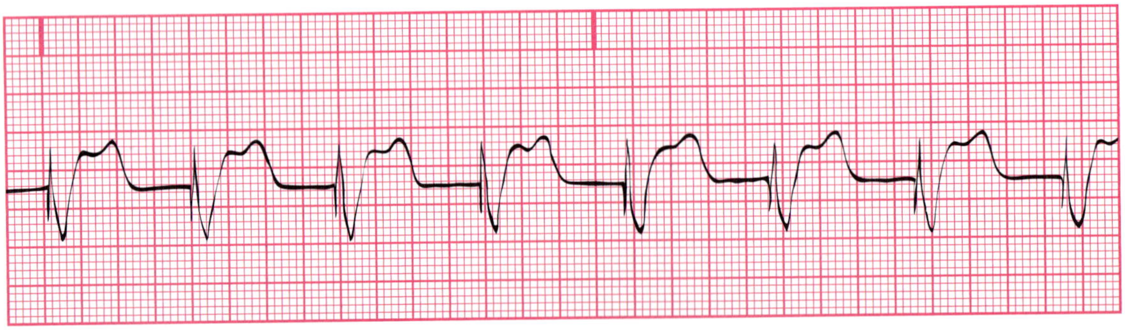

Rhythm (regular or irregular): ______________ PR interval: ______________

Rate: ______________ QRS: ______________

P wave: ______________ Interpretation: ______________

21.

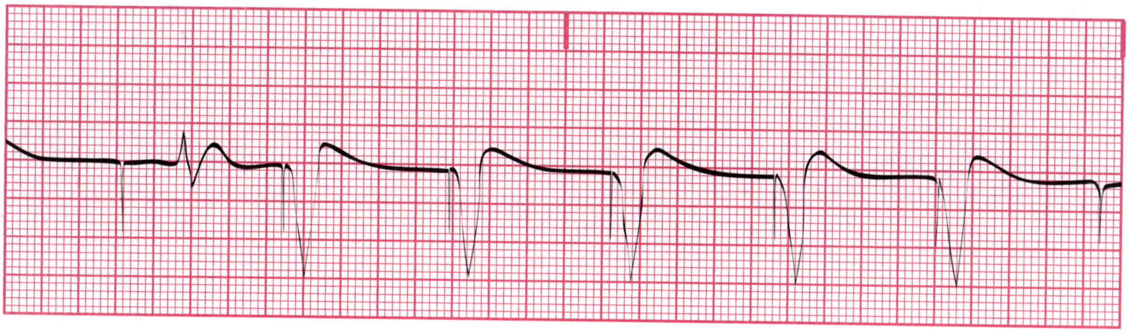

Rhythm (regular or irregular): ______________ PR interval: ______________

Rate: ______________ QRS: ______________

P wave: ______________ Interpretation: ______________

22.

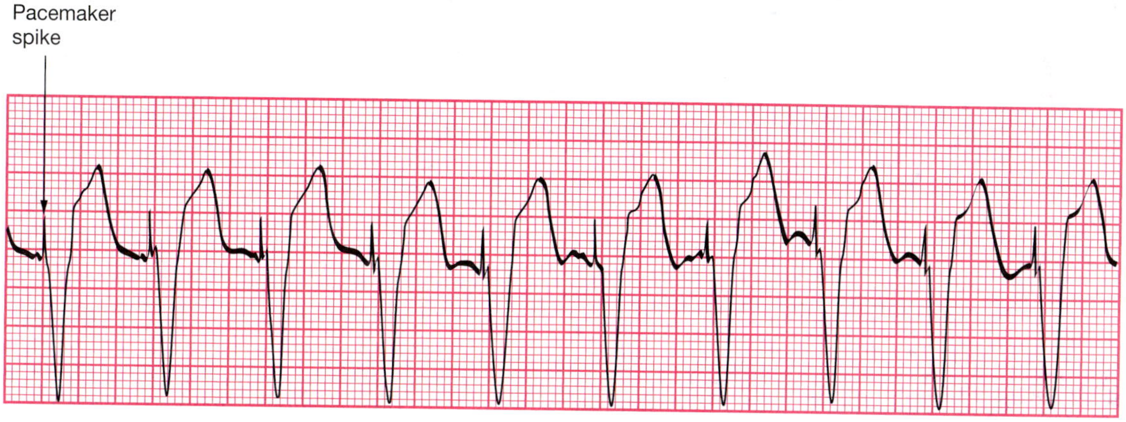

Rhythm (regular or irregular): ______________ PR interval: ______________

Rate: ______________ QRS: ______________

P wave: ______________ Interpretation: ______________

23.

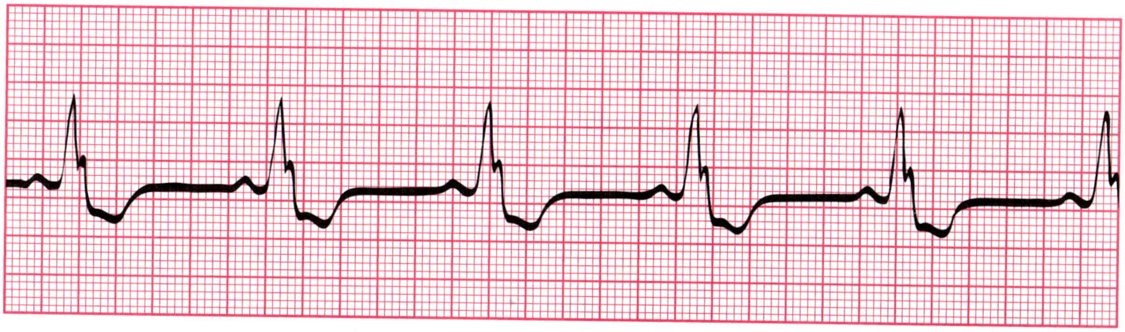

Rhythm (regular or irregular): ______________ PR interval: ______________

Rate: ______________ QRS: ______________

P wave: ______________ Interpretation: ______________

24.

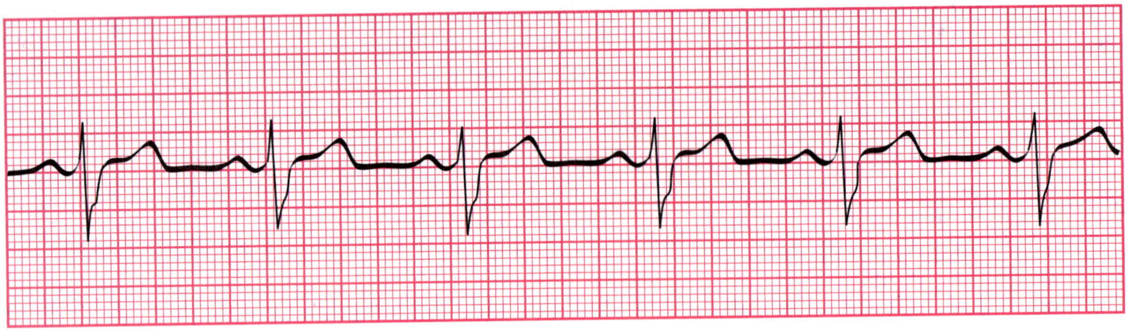

Rhythm (regular or irregular): ______________ PR interval: ______________

Rate: ______________ QRS: ______________

P wave: ______________ Interpretation: ______________

connect® Now that you have completed the material in the chapter text, go to Connect and complete any chapter activities you have not yet done.

11 Exercise Electrocardiography

Learning Outcomes

11.1 Describe exercise electrocardiography and identify its other names.
11.2 Identify uses of exercise electrocardiography.
11.3 Describe variations of exercise electrocardiography.
11.4 Prepare a patient for exercise electrocardiography.
11.5 Summarize safety measures that are used before, during, and after exercise electrocardiography.
11.6 Explain the responsibilities of a healthcare professional during exercise electrocardiography.
11.7 Compare common protocols followed in exercise electrocardiography.
11.8 Explain the responsibilities of a healthcare professional after exercise electrocardiography.

Key Terms

angina
beta blockers
cardiologist
chemical stress echocardiogram
chemical stress test
congestive heart failure (CHF)
coronary vascular disease (CVD)
echocardiogram
false positive
gamma camera
gate
hypertension
hyperventilation
maximal exercise
noninvasive
nuclear stress test
radiologist
rate pressure product (RPP)
skin rasp
stress echocardiogram
submaximal exercise
target heart rate (THR)

11.1 What Is Exercise Electrocardiography?

Often a patient has symptoms of cardiac problems that do not show up on a resting ECG. In order to determine the problems and to obtain an accurate diagnosis, the physician may order an exercise electrocardiograph. Exercise electrocardiography has been used for more than 50 years. This test is known by many names, such as an exercise tolerance test, a treadmill stress test, a cardiac stress test, a stress ECG, or an exercise treadmill test. It is most commonly known as a treadmill stress test because the blood to provide oxygen to the myocardium (heart muscle). The exercise increases the myocardial oxygen demand. If a patient has narrowed or obstructed arteries due to CVD, blood flow to the heart will not increase in response to the exercise. This additional workload may change the ECG tracing. One such change in the ECG tracing is ST segment depression, as shown in Figure 11-3. ST depression may indicate myocardial ischemia. Certain medications, such as digitalis, may also cause ST segment depression. The exercise may also produce symptoms of **angina** (chest pain) weakness, shortness of breath, palpitations, or dizziness.

angina An oppressive pain or pressure in the chest when the heart muscle does not receive enough oxygen due to partial or complete blockage of a coronary artery.

Exercise electrocardiography is used for other reasons as well. The physician may want to assess how well the patient's blood pressure is maintained during exercise. Exercise electrocardiography may be used to evaluate exercise-induced symptoms such as palpitations or angina or to determine the patient's risk of a myocardial infarction. After an MI or cardiac surgery, the treadmill stress test is frequently used to evaluate the functioning of the heart. It may be used to evaluate the effectiveness of cardiac medications, identify dysrhythmias that occur during exercise, and aid in the development of an exercise program. The following is a list of uses for exercise electrocardiography.

- Helps diagnose cause of chest pain
- Determines functional capacity of the heart after surgery or myocardial infarction
- Screens for heart disease (particularly in men over age 35) when no symptoms are present
- Helps set limitations for an exercise program
- Identifies cause of abnormal heart rhythms that develop during physical exercise
- Evaluates effectiveness of heart medications

Figure 11-3 ST segment depression is depression of the ST segment below the normal baseline of the ECG. It may indicate myocardial ischemia, which can occur during exercise electrocardiography.

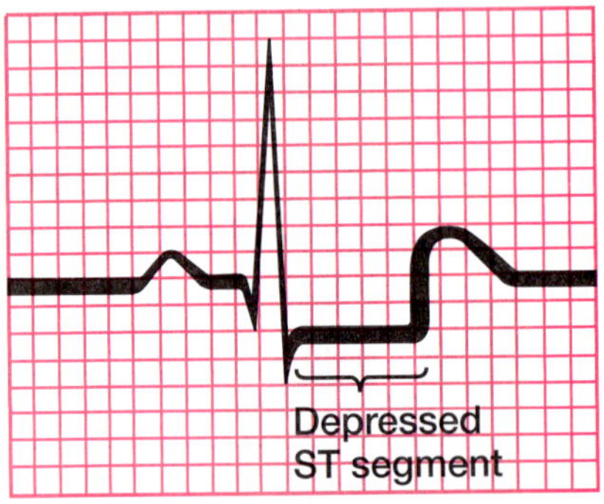

Checkpoint Question (LO 11.2)

1. What does exercise electrocardiography help identify?

____

____

11.3 Variations of Exercise Electrocardiography

One variation of exercise electrocardiography is a **chemical stress test.** This test is used when the patient is unable to run or walk on a treadmill or use an exercise bike due to age, injury, or physical defect. Chemical stress tests can be conducted using nuclear testing or in combination with echocardiography. Under the guidance of a **cardiologist** or **radiologist,** depending on the test, the patient is monitored in the same way as for a regular exercise stress test. However, instead of using a treadmill, a chemical stress test requires one or more IVs for the introduction of a stressing chemical such as adenosine, Persantine, dobutamine, or Lexiscan (Table 11-1). These drugs mimic the stresses placed on the heart during exercise. The physician determines whether the patient requires a regular stress test or a chemical stress test prior to the patient's arrival in the stress lab.

For a **nuclear stress test,** a nuclear medicine technologist first injects the patient with a stressing chemical. Then, prior to the completion of the stressing cycle, the technologist injects a radioactive tracer. The patient is then scanned using a **gamma camera.** This procedure involves the patient lying on his or her back, or in some cases sitting upright, with arms above the head while the camera rotates around the patient to produce a multidimensional image. An additional feature of the nuclear testing is that a three-lead electrocardiogram can be used to **gate** the study, triggering the camera to record at specific points during the cardiac cycle. This produces not only the multidimensional image, but also an image in which the heart beats, so heart wall motion can be evaluated. Depending on the protocol used, the patient can be scanned prior to stressing or 3 to 24 hours after stressing to provide a resting image series for a comparison. This can help minimize false positives caused by stress-induced ischemia.

Actual scan times can vary from 15 minutes to an hour for each phase, with gated studies on patients who have an irregular heart rate taking the longest time. As in other testing procedures, the female breast can cause imaging defects. Another consideration is the patient's diet until completion of the test, because the increased blood flow through the stomach after eating reduces the concentration of the radionuclide in the heart tissue.

An **echocardiogram** uses sound to study the heart, its valves, and the major blood vessels surrounding the heart. See Figure 11-4. The **stress echocardiogram** combines an exercise stress test or chemical stress test with an echocardiogram to assess left ventricular wall motion, both before and immediately after exercise. A stress echocardiogram is considered normal if left ventricular wall motion is normal both at rest and poststress. Ischemia is suspected when a change is seen in left ventricular wall shape or contractility with exercise.

The stress echocardiogram is divided into a resting echocardiogram phase, an immediate postexercise scan, and a recovery phase scan. All three phases require an experienced sonographer with a high level of skill and speed to obtain these images within a specific time frame. During the resting phase, the sonographer acquires four specific left ventricular wall motion images with the patient lying on his or her left side, with the head slightly elevated. The resting phase is then followed by either the regular stress test or chemical stress test.

As soon as the patient achieves 85% to 100% of the target heart rate during the exercise portion, the treadmill is stopped. The patient immediately and

chemical stress test Stress test performed after administering medications that cause the heart rate to increase or the coronary blood vessels to dilate; performed on patients who cannot perform the exercise required in a regular stress test.

cardiologist A physician who specializes in the study of the heart.

radiologist A physician who specializes in the use of radioactive substances to diagnose and treat disease.

nuclear stress test A stress test in which radionuclides (radioactive tracers) are administered to trace the path of blood through the heart.

gamma camera A camera that records the gamma radiation emitted by the radioactive tracers in a patient's blood.

gate A selective technique in which a gamma camera is triggered by specific events captured by a three-lead ECG monitor.

echocardiogram Noninvasive diagnostic test that uses sound to study the heart, heart valves, and blood vessels.

stress echocardiogram A test that combines an exercise stress test with an echocardiogram to assess left ventricular wall motion both before and immediately after exercise.

TABLE 11-1 **Common Cardioactive Medications***

Medication	Effect	Contraindications
Adenosine	Cardiac vasodilator Causes dilation of coronary vessels, which results in increased blood velocity and flow rate in normal vessels and less of a response in stenotic (narrowed) vessels	• Allergy to any ingredient in adenosine. • Second or third degree heart block in patients who do not have an artificial pacemaker. • Sinus node disease, such as sick sinus syndrome, in patients who do not have an artificial pacemaker. • Breathing problems, such as asthma.
Persantine (dipyridamole)	Cardiac vasodilator Causes dilation of coronary vessels, which results in increased blood velocity and flow rate in normal vessels and less of a response in stenotic (narrowed) vessels	• Patients with active bronchospasm or patients being treated for reactive airway disease. • Patients with more than first degree heart block (without a ventricular demand pacemaker) should not undergo dipyridamole infusion because this may lead to worsening of the heart block. • Patients with a systolic blood pressure of less than 90 mmHg should not undergo dipyridamole stress testing because of the potential for further lowering of the blood pressure. • Patients with a history of reactive airway disease (COPD/asthma).
Dobutamine	Cardiac inotrope (force of contractions) and chronotrope (speed of contractions); the heart responds to dobutamine similarly to the way it responds to exercise	• Patients with recent (1 week) myocardial infarction; unstable angina; significant aortic stenosis or obstructive cardiomyopathy; atrial tachydysrhythmias with uncontrolled ventricular response; history of ventricular tachycardia, uncontrolled hypertension, or thoracic aortic aneurysm; or left bundle branch block should not undergo dobutamine stress testing.
Lexiscan (regadenoson)	Cardiac vasodilator Causes dilation of coronary vessels, which results in increased blood velocity and flow rate in normal vessels and less of a response in stenotic (narrowed) vessels	• Regadenoson should not be administered to patients with second degree atrioventricular block or sinus node dysfunction, unless these patients have a functioning artificial pacemaker.

*Information adapted from www.medscape.com and www.drugs.com

safely moves from the treadmill to the echo bed while still attached to the ECG leads. The sonographer then has 45 to 60 seconds to obtain the same four left ventricular images as in the resting phase. This is the postexercise scan. A nurse, stress technician, or physician is present to perform the stress test and assess ischemic changes on the ECG during the postexercise and recovery phases.

chemical stress echocardiogram A stress echocardiogram in which the heart is stressed by chemicals, rather than physical exercise.

If a **chemical stress echocardiogram** is ordered, the patient remains on the echo table, on the left side with head slightly elevated, for all three phases of the stress echocardiogram. While a nurse infuses the stress chemical according to the specific protocol for the medication, the sonographer obtains the same four left ventricular wall motion images at specific intervals throughout the infusion.

Figure 11-4 Echocardiography of the heart showing hypertrophy of the left ventricle. Echocardiography directs beams of ultrasonic waves through the chest wall, which are echoed by the heart tissues providing motion pictures of the heart.

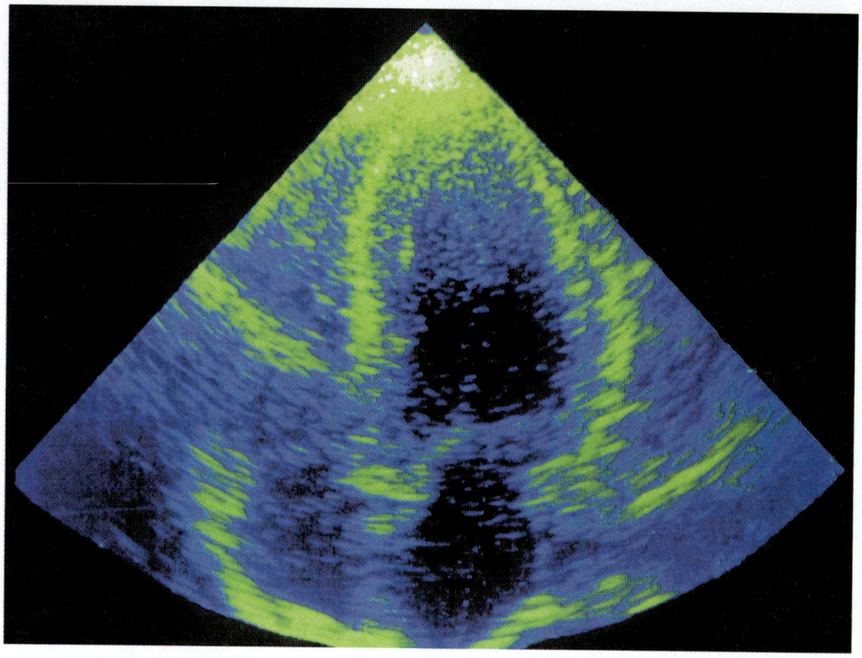

When the patient's heart rate returns close to the resting heart rate, the same four left ventricular wall motion images are acquired to complete the recovery phase. The test is terminated after the recovery scan is completed, when the ECG shows no ischemic changes and the patient's blood pressure and heart rate have returned to resting levels.

The cardiologist then views the side-by-side images of the resting, postexercise, and recovery images. The cardiologist assesses for changes in left ventricular motion and contractility, which can predict the presence of ischemia in one or more coronary arteries.

Patient Education & Communication

Complete Explanation Is Necessary

Patient education brochures are valuable to help the patient understand the procedure. However, they may not be enough. The physician should explain the purpose for the test, but it is your responsibility to ensure that the patient understands what will occur during the test and what the patient should report to the physician while the test is in progress.

Checkpoint Question (LO 11.3)

1. Why would it be necessary to use chemical stress testing?

____

____

11.4 Preparing the Patient for Exercise Electrocardiography

When scheduling a patient for exercise electrocardiography, you will need to make sure the patient comes prepared for the test (Table 11-2). Describe the procedure, and ensure that the patient understands what will happen. The patient should not use tobacco products or consume alcohol or caffeine 3 hours prior to the test. He or she should also be advised not to eat for at least 2 hours before the test. The patient should be instructed to bring or wear comfortable clothing and shoes. Tennis shoes and loose pants will make the exercise portion of the test easier for the patient.

TABLE 11-2 The Stress Test Procedure

Before the Test

- Verify that the medical history is complete.
- Explain the procedure, including the reason for the test, possible complications, and safety measures that will be followed during the procedure.
- Explain "informed consent," and ask the patient to sign the consent form.
- Inform patients that on the day of the test they should wear comfortable clothing (shorts, tennis shoes, etc.). Female patients should not wear an underwire bra. The patient should eat a light meal 2 hours prior to the test but should refrain from using tobacco, caffeine, or alcohol for *at least 3 hours* prior to test.
- Check the physician's orders against the patient's medication list to provide information as to what medications the patient should *not* take the day of the test.
- Go over all instructions and information with the patient. Encourage questions; make sure the patient fully understands the procedure.
- Provide a detailed list of instructions, making sure that your facility telephone number and your name appear on the list. Encourage patients to call if they have any questions prior to test day.

Day of Appointment

- Verify that equipment is in working order and supplies are on hand. (Ensure that plenty of tracing paper is available, inspect cables, check that the treadmill is working, and verify the computer setup and correct protocol.)
- Gather supplies—electrodes, alcohol, gauze sponges, razor, adhesive tape, blood pressure cuff, and so on.
- Check that the crash cart is ready and fully supplied and the defibrillator is working.
- Verify the physician's order, that the medical history is complete, and that the informed consent is signed.
- Bring the patient into the room.
- Verify with the patient that he or she has complied with all instructions.
- Provide the patient with privacy to change into a gown with the opening to the front unless the patient needs assistance. Female patients should not wear an underwire bra.
- *Remember: During all aspects of the procedure, always provide for the safety of the patient!*
- Assist the patient to lie down on the table. Prep the patient's skin and apply electrodes as indicated by the protocol of the facility or the equipment manual.
- Connect cables, apply the blood pressure cuff, and check the ECG tracing for artifact. Check and set the artifact filters as necessary.
- Obtain the patient's blood pressure and ECG in the following positions (assist the patient as necessary and provide for safety):
  - Supine
  - Sitting
  - Sitting, post 30-second hyperventilation
  - Standing

(Make sure you change the screen label to reflect the position of the patient for the pre-procedure assessment of blood pressure and 12-lead ECG.)

(Continued)

(*Continued*)

- Demonstrate the treadmill (posture, hand grip, etc.).
- Explain the test protocol, making sure the patient understands that the speed and incline will increase every 3 minutes during the test phase.
- *Be sure the patient understands that he or she is to report any pain, shortness of breath, faintness, tingling sensations, numbness, or extreme fatigue immediately. Monitor the patient closely during the test looking for visual signs of any of the above. Ask the patient repeatedly during the procedure how he or she feels. Providing for patient safety is your number one priority.*
- Explain again that the test will be completed when the target heart rate is reached [(220 − age) × 0.85] or when the patient cannot continue due to fatigue or other symptoms.
- Inform the physician that the patient is ready to begin the test. The physician should be present and immediately available.
- When the physician is in the room, assist the patient to the treadmill, making sure the patient's feet are not on the belt. Start the belt; tell the patient to get used to the speed and then to step onto the belt. Ask the patient if he or she is ready to begin, explaining again that the belt speed and incline will increase. Begin the test phase.
- At the 2½-minute mark of each phase, a blood pressure is taken and recorded. Remind the patient before every transition to a new phase. Be ready to assist the patient as needed.
- When the treadmill phase of the test is complete (the target heart rate is reached or the patient cannot continue), assist the patient to a waiting chair.

Posttest

- Continue to monitor and observe the patient's condition closely, taking the patient's blood pressure, entering data, and then taking an ECG tracing every 3 to 5 minutes for 10 to 15 minutes.
- When the cooldown period is completed, remove the cables and electrodes; wipe off any remaining gel or adhesive.
- Allow the patient to dress (assist if needed).
- Explain to the patient that he or she should avoid tobacco, caffeine, and alcohol for at least 3 hours. The patient should avoid extreme temperature changes, including hot showers or baths, for 2 hours. The patient should rest and recuperate after the test.
- Explain that the physician will have the results of the test in 10 days (refer to local policy for the specific turnaround time of your organization). Thank the patient for his or her cooperation.
- File your report per the protocol of the facility.
- Make sure all information from the patient chart is maintained confidentially within the medical record.
- Prepare for the next patient.

Law & Ethics

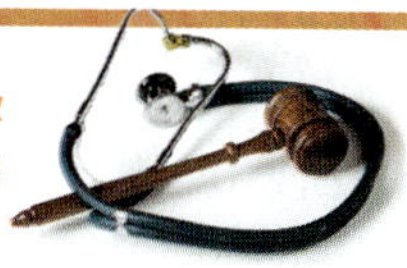

Informed Consent

Informed consent is required for surgery, HIV testing, and other procedures, including exercise electrocardiography. Informed consent affirms that the patient understands the treatment, why it is being performed, any risks to the patient, alternative treatments and their risks, and the risk involved if the patient refuses treatment. Table 11-3 lists the typical reasons patients refuse the test and suggestions for resolving the problem.

What happens when you ask the patient to sign an informed consent form and he or she refuses?

____

____

TABLE 11-3 Handling a Patient's Refusal to Grant Consent

Reason for Refusal	Possible Solution
Patient does not understand why the consent form is necessary.	Explain the legal requirement of an informed consent, and refer the patient to the physician for questions, if necessary.
Patient does not understand the procedure.	Notify the physician, and provide a brochure for the patient to review while he or she is waiting for the physician to explain the procedure.
Patient is illiterate and unable to sign his or her name.	Have a witness present (preferably a family member), and have the consent form marked with an *X* by the patient and signed by the witness and yourself.
Patient is unable to sign because glasses are not available or because the patient is blind.	Make every attempt to obtain the glasses and then have the patient sign; if this is not possible, have the patient sign to the best of his or her ability. Be certain to have a witness (preferably a family member) sign the form as well.

beta blockers Drugs used to treat hypertension.

Sometimes certain medications should not be taken prior to the test. The patient may need instruction regarding medications that can affect the test results and should not be taken. Always check the physician's order. If it is not written on the chart or order, ask the physician. When asking, have a list of the patient's current medications or the patient's chart available for the physician to review. Medications commonly known as **beta blockers**—drugs used to treat hypertension—are frequently stopped prior to an exercise electrocardiography test because this type of medication could affect the test results or delay the test. See the appendix *Cardiovascular Medications* for more information. Remember, it is your responsibility to ensure that the patient comes to the office or clinic properly prepared for the exercise electrocardiography test.

A complete history of the patient may need to be recorded before beginning the test. A standard form should be used. The information you need to obtain from the patient includes the medical history, medications currently being taken, cardiovascular risk factors (see the chapter *Electrocardiography*), and the reason for this examination. Much of this information may already be on the patient's chart. In addition, an informed consent form must be signed and witnessed (Figure 11-5). The patient should understand the procedure, its risks, and the reason the test has been ordered before signing the informed consent form.

The patient should be informed that exercise electrocardiography is not a "timed" test. The length of time the test takes depends on several factors, including the patient's age, degree of conditioning or health status, other medical problems, and medications. You should inform the patient that the test will take approximately 45 minutes up to three hours depending on the type of test being done. Carefully explain the safety precautions provided during the procedure to help alleviate any fears the patient may have.

Figure 11-5 Your patient must sign an informed consent for exercise electrocardiography. Most facilities use a standardized form such as the one pictured here.

Consent Form for Exercise/Chemical Stress Testing

A stress test is being performed to provide information about the blood supply to your heart, as well as to assess your ability to do various activities.

The information obtained will help your physician recommend treatment options regarding your cardiovascular health. The test that you will undergo will be performed on a treadmill with the amount of effort increasing gradually as the test progresses. This increase in effort will continue until either a predetermined heart rate is achieved or symptoms such as fatigue, shortness of breath, or chest discomfort appear, which indicate to you to stop. An alternative type of stress test may be administered in which a medication may be used to "stress" or exercise the heart. During the performance of the test, trained staff will closely monitor your pulse, blood pressure, and electrocardiogram.

If performed as part of a nuclear myocardial perfusion study, a small amount of radioactive material (thallium) will be injected followed by imaging of the heart. The amount of radioactivity you will be exposed to is about equivalent to a chest x-ray.

There is always the possibility of certain changes occurring during the test. They include abnormal blood pressure, fainting, shortness of breath, abnormal heart rhythms (too rapid, too slow, or ineffective), and very rare instances of heart attack. Every effort will be made to minimize them by the preliminary examination and by observations during and immediately after testing. Emergency equipment and highly trained personnel are available to manage any unusual situations that may arise.

- -

In order to determine an appropriate plan of medical management, I hereby consent to voluntarily engage in a myocardial stress test to determine the state of my heart and circulation.

I have read the above information and understand the procedures, as well as any possible complications or risks. I understand that in rare instances, heart attack or stroke has been reported. I acknowledge that my physician has explained my condition and the nature and purpose of this test, as well as alternative tests, and that all questions asked about my care and its attendant risks have been answered in a satisfactory manner. I understand that any question(s) I still may have can be answered by my physician or clinic staff members at any time. I hereby accept the risk of harm, if any, in hopes of obtaining the desired beneficial diagnostic information.

Signed:

______________________________ ________________
Patient Date

______________________________ ________________
Patient Name Printed Witness

____
Physician Supervising Test

Checkpoint Questions (LO 11.4)

1. Stress testing is a noninvasive procedure. Why is informed consent necessary?

____

____

2. Why should you obtain a list of the current medications the patient is taking before the stress test procedure?

____

____

11.5 **Providing Safety**

Exercise electrocardiography is done on patients who are already at risk. At-risk patients may have just recently had a myocardial infarction (MI) or may currently be experiencing some type of chest pain or other symptoms, or they may have a history of coronary vascular disease. Exercise electrocardiography does place stress on the patient's heart. There is some risk of an MI or cerebrovascular accident (CVA) during the procedure that should be considered. You should follow the safety measures and be prepared for emergencies (Table 11-4).

In order to provide for safety, certain rules must be followed. A physician should always be present during the procedure. Emergency equipment should be in the room or nearby, including a crash cart with emergency medications and supplies. You must know the location of this equipment. In addition, the patient should be monitored at all times, and he or she must understand the need to report any abnormal symptoms when they occur.

Some health conditions prevent patients from participating in exercise electrocardiography. These conditions include but are not limited to:

- A change in the resting ECG
- Abnormal heart rhythms, including uncontrolled ventricular or atrial dysrhythmia or a third degree AV block
- Recent myocardial infarction or unstable angina
- Inflammation surrounding the heart or heart muscle (pericarditis or myocarditis)
- Uncontrolled **hypertension** (high blood pressure)
- Certain cardiovascular conditions such as severe aortic stenosis, aneurysm, thrombophlebitis, and systemic or pulmonary embolism
- **Congestive heart failure (CHF)** (the heart's failure to pump an adequate volume of blood)
- Acute infection
- Significant emotional stress (psychosis)

hypertension High blood pressure.

congestive heart failure (CHF) Failure of the heart to pump an adequate amount of blood to the body tissues.

The physician should be aware of any of these conditions. Make sure that the health history is current and complete for the physician to review.

TABLE 11-4 **Preparing for Emergencies During Exercise Electrocardiography**

• Inform the patient of how he or she can expect to feel during the test, including mild fatigue, increased heart rate, perspiration, and increased respiratory rate.
• Explain to the patient the need to report signs and symptoms such as chest or other pain, dizziness, weakness, or extreme fatigue.
• Make sure the patient knows to stop the exercise if any pain or extreme fatigue is felt.
• *Make sure the physician is present during the entire procedure.*
• Check to see that emergency equipment is close by, including a code or crash cart with defibrillator.
• Observe and monitor the patient, and report any symptoms to the physician immediately.

Safety & Infection Control

hyperventilation Breathing at an increased rate and depth of inspiration and expiration.

Observe Patients Carefully

Observe your patient carefully when he or she changes position and during **hyperventilation** for dizziness and potential for a syncopal (fainting) episode. Many patients will have cardiac and/or vascular disease that increases the chances for these symptoms.

Checkpoint Question (LO 11.5)

1. Can everyone have a standard stress test? Why or why not?

____

____

11.6 Performing Exercise Electrocardiography

Assemble and prepare the equipment before the patient's arrival. You will need:

- Blood pressure equipment
- Shaving equipment, abrasive skin cleaner, skin rasp
- Skin prep solution
- 2×2 or 4×4 gauze
- Chest electrodes
- Stress test unit
- Lead wires
- Treadmill or cycle ergometer
- Adhesive tape belt (used to attach monitoring unit) or mesh vest
- Crash cart

Safety & Infection Control

CPR Required

As a healthcare professional you should know cardiopulmonary resuscitation (CPR) and be prepared to respond to cardiac or respiratory emergencies.

skin rasp A rough piece of material used to abrade (scrape) the skin prior to electrode placement.

When the patient arrives for the test, you should verify that he or she has come properly prepared by making sure the patient has not had alcohol, caffeine, or tobacco for at least 3 hours or food for 2 hours prior to the test. Verify that medications were stopped, if required. Complete the patient's medical history, and make sure the informed consent form has been signed.

Next, prepare the electrode sites for placement. If the sites are hairy, dry shave the skin. Rub the site with skin prep solution, and let it dry. Abrade the skin using a special prep pad, dry 4×4 gauze, **skin rasp,** or other type of abrasive cleaner. Abrading the skin consists of rubbing firmly and briskly at each of the sites where the electrodes will be placed to ensure that they will adhere better to the skin.

Attach the blood pressure cuff and electrodes. Check the manufacturer's instructions for the system you are using and the policy at your facility for correct placement of the electrodes (Figure 11-6). Typical placement of precordial leads for stress testing is almost the same as for the traditional 12-lead ECG. The difference is that the limb sensors must be moved from the arms and legs to the upper chest and torso because of the exercise component. *Note:* In order to minimize artifact, avoid placing the leg sensors in a location on the abdomen where they will contact the belt that is placed around the patient's waist. This placement also increases safety by reducing the chance of tripping and falling over the lead wires. This placement technique is referred to as the Mason-Likar attachment. Many exercise electrocardiography monitors include leads for both chest and back.

Check and set the artifact filters before running the stress test. These filters help reduce small signals caused by muscle movements from the ECG tracing during the test. Review the manufacturer's instructions to ensure the proper setting.

Prior to the exercise test, a series of blood pressures and 12-lead ECGs will be obtained with the patient in different positions. The following is a common example. Your facility may or may not use each of these pretest steps. Check the policy where you are employed.

First: A resting ECG and blood pressure are obtained while the patient is supine.

Second: The patient is asked to sit up, and another blood pressure and ECG are obtained.

Third: The patient is asked to breathe quickly and deeply to produce a state of hyperventilation for about 30 seconds. Then another blood pressure and ECG are taken. This ECG is done to identify ECG changes caused by breathing. These changes could be misinterpreted as being related to heart disease if they occurred during the stress test.

Fourth: The patient is asked to stand, and the final pre-exercise blood pressure and ECG are obtained.

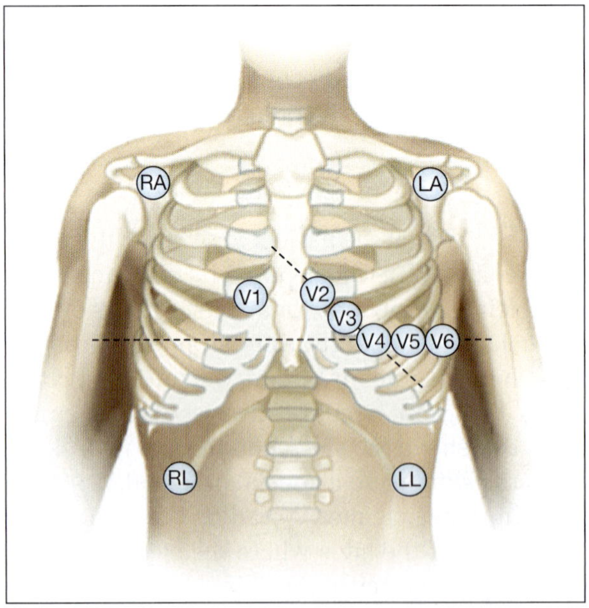

Figure 11-6 Because machines may vary, check the manufacturer's instructions for proper placement of the electrodes for the exercise electrocardiograph machine you are using.

Troubleshooting

Reporting Problems

If your patient has any complaints or problems during exercise electrocardiography, you should be prepared to respond. Keep in mind that while the physician should be in the room, he or she may not always be aware of the patient's complaints or problems. Any symptom that the patient reports, such as extreme fatigue, dizziness, shortness of breath, or chest pain, should be immediately reported to the physician.

What should you do if the patient collapses?

____

____

Checkpoint Question (LO 11.6)

1. What equipment must be assembled before exercise electrocardiography can be performed?

____

____

11.7 Common Protocols

The stress test is divided into stages of 2 or 3 minutes each. Each stage is based on stress test protocols. The protocols include the length of time of exercise and the incline of the treadmill. The physician determines the protocol or length and incline of each stage of exercise (Table 11-5 and Figure 11-7).

Patient Education & Communication

Reducing the Patient's Fears

You can help reduce the patient's fears by maintaining a sense of confidence, answering questions, and following safety precautions during exercise electrocardiography.

The entire exercise period lasts up to 15 minutes. The time may vary based on the patient's cardiac risk factors and ability. Toward the end of each stage, the patient's blood pressure is checked, the ECG is repeated, and the level of exercise is increased.

Most people exercise to the point of fatigue or symptoms of chest discomfort or shortness of breath. The supervising physician may halt the test because of blood pressure, ECG, or heart rhythm changes that are not perceived by the patient. In other words, though the patient may not complain

TABLE 11-5 **Common Stress Testing Protocols**

Bruce Protocol: Most commonly utilized stress test. Uses 3-minute stages.

Stage	Speed (mph)	Grade (%)
1	1.7	10
2	2.5	12
3	3.4	14
4	4.2	16
5	5.0	18
6	5.5	20
7	6.0	22

"Modified" Bruce Protocol: Most often used in older individuals or those whose exercise capacity is limited by cardiac disease. Uses 3-minute stages.

Stage	Speed (mph)	Grade (%)
1	1.7	0
2	1.7	5
3	1.7	10
4	2.5	12
5	3.4	14
6	4.2	16
7	5.0	18
8	5.5	20

Naughton Protocol: Better suited for sicker patients; more gradual increase in intensity. Speed stays at 2 mph. Uses 2-minute stages.

Stage	Grade (%)
1	0.0
2	3.5
3	7.0
4	10.5
5	14.0
6	17.5
7	21.0

Figure 11-7 During a Bruce protocol stress test, ECG recordings are made continuously during and after exercise. This image shows ST segment depression and depicts a positive test (identifies a problem). This result coupled with any patient complaints would support the diagnosis.

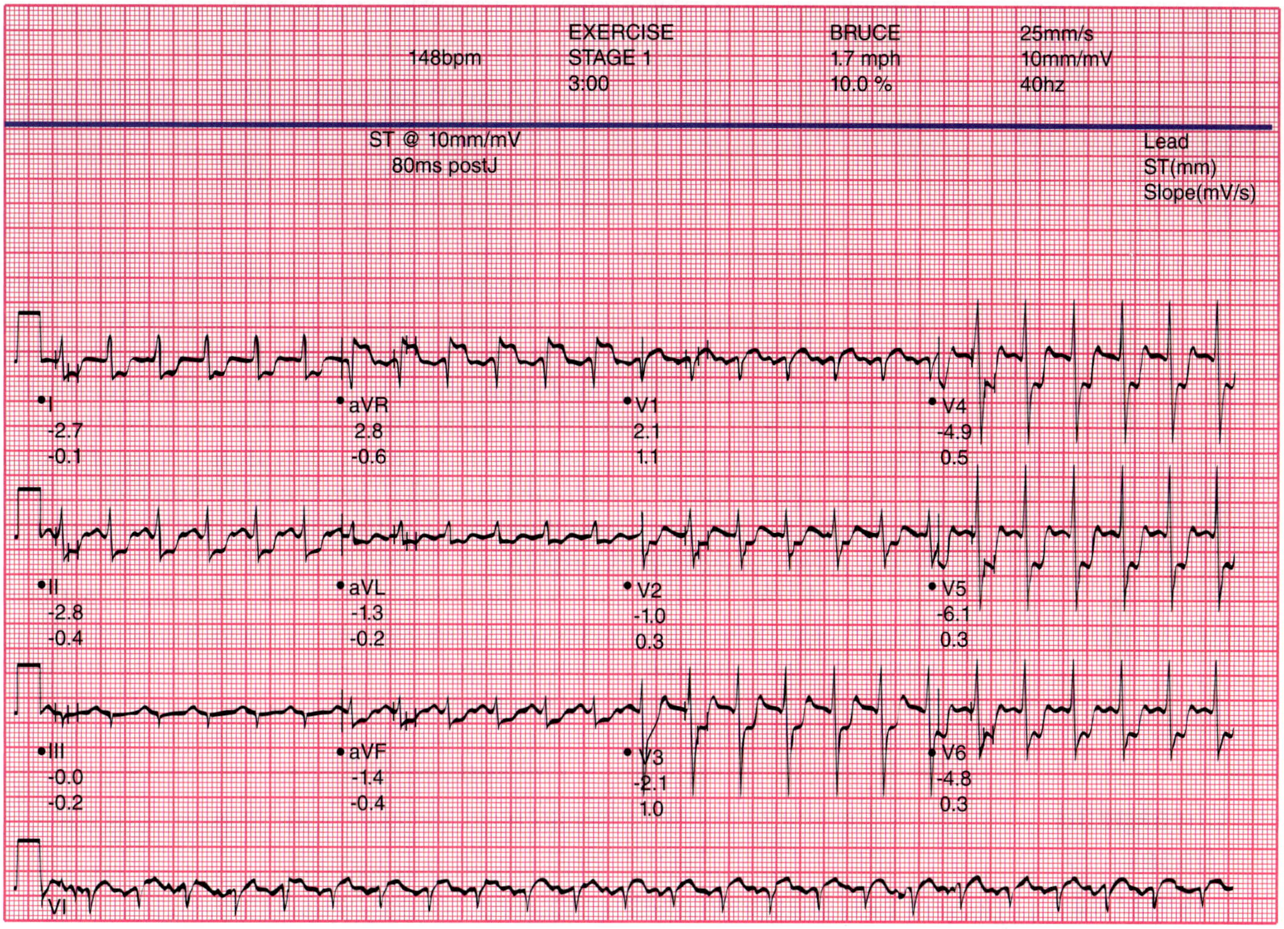

of any symptoms, the physician may identify changes in the blood pressure, heart rate, or ECG tracing that may lead to complications and may order that the test be stopped.

target heart rate (THR) Heart rate measurement needed to truly exercise the heart.

submaximal exercise Target heart rate of 220 minus the age multiplied by a percentage between 60 and 85.

maximal exercise Target heart rate of 220 minus the age of the patient.

During the test, the goal is to achieve the **target heart rate (THR)** without symptoms or complications such as a dysrhythmia. The target heart rate is 220 minus the patient's age multiplied by a percentage that ranges between 60 and 85, depending on which testing protocol is being followed (often referred to as **submaximal exercise**). This is different from the target heart rate for aerobic exercise, which is simply 220 minus the age of the person without using an additional multiplier (often referred to as **maximal exercise**).

The THR is the rate that the patient should not be allowed to exceed during the test. Achieving the THR without symptoms or abnormalities is a good indication that the heart is functioning well. Generally, the closer the patient is to the target heart rate, the more reliable the test results.

Instruct the patient to report any symptoms—such as shortness of breath, chest pain, dizziness, or weakness—he or she experiences during the procedure because you are responsible for monitoring and recording this information. You will need to monitor blood pressure, pulse, and any signs of cardiac distress. You may also be monitoring the patient's blood oxygen level on the monitor screen.

rate pressure product (RPP) Systolic blood pressure multiplied by the heart rate; also known as *double product.*

Rate pressure product (RPP) or *double product* is a measurement that may be asked for by the doctor. To find the RPP, multiply the systolic blood pressure by the patient's heart rate. This is one technique used to estimate oxygen utilization or myocardial work. For example:

$$\begin{aligned} \text{Systolic blood pressure (SYS BP)} &= 118 \\ \text{Heart rate (HR)} &= 88 \\ \text{SYS BP} \times \text{HR} &= \text{RPP} \\ 118 \times 88 &= \text{RPP} \\ 10{,}384 &= \text{RPP} \end{aligned}$$

During exercise, the heart rate and systolic blood pressure are the two main factors determining the workload on the heart. If these factors increase, the heart has to work harder and requires more oxygen and nutrients to keep going, thus putting stress on the heart. The response of the heart rate and blood pressure to a fixed level of exercise tends to decrease with regular exercise. So a person with good blood supply and a strong heart muscle should have a lower RPP than a person who has a disruption of the blood supply to the heart muscle and a weaker heart muscle. Thus the RPP is an index of the myocardial oxygen requirement and helps determine the work placed on the heart, as well as the heart's response.

Watch the patient closely, including skin color, breathing pattern, amount of perspiration, and facial expressions. Many times a patient is hesitant to report a symptom. If you suspect a problem, ask the patient and then report your suspicion to the supervising physician.

Checkpoint Questions (LO 11.7)

1. Identify which stress-test protocol would most likely be used for each of the following patients.
   a. A 76-year-old, 285-pound man who has recently had a heart attack
   b. A 46-year-old airline pilot during a yearly physical
   c. A 65-year-old patient with hypertension and complaints of chest pain
2. What is the target heart rate of a patient who is 49 years old?

   ____

   ____

11.8 After Exercise Electrocardiography

When the patient has completed the exercise portion of the test, monitoring will continue during a "cooling-off" period. This will last from 6 to 15 minutes, depending on the protocol at your place of employment and the physician's preference. You will need to stay with the patient and continue to monitor the patient for any changes.

Many factors are used to interpret the results of exercise electrocardiography. The most important factors are the presence of ECG changes and symptoms. Other factors include heart rate and rhythm, blood pressure, and changes in oxygen saturation. If a patient has no abnormal ECG changes or unusual elevations in blood pressure, this usually means the risk for coronary vascular

Patient Education & Communication

Exercise Electrocardiography Results

As a healthcare professional, you are not responsible for reporting the results of exercise electrocardiography to the patient. If the patient asks you about the results, refer the patient to the physician.

Law & Ethics

Secure Patient Testing Information

Remember to save and secure all patient testing information upon completion.

disease is low. If the test is stopped early because of ECG or blood pressure changes or patient symptoms, this is a sign of abnormal test results. When the results of the test are inconclusive or abnormal, additional tests may be performed. An inconclusive test is one with questionable results, meaning it does not necessarily show an abnormality or eliminate the potential for an abnormality. Additional testing is needed to either identify or eliminate any abnormalities.

After exercise electrocardiography, the patient should be given some instructions. These include the following:

- Rest for several hours.
- Avoid extreme temperature changes.
- Avoid stimulants, such as caffeine, tobacco, or alcohol, for at least 3 hours.
- Do not take a hot shower or bath for at least 2 hours.
- When to expect the test results.
- The results should be discussed with the physician.

Stress testing is considered a good method to detect early coronary vascular disease. However, it is interesting to note that approximately 5% of healthy adults may have **false positive** results, meaning that the test may indicate that disease is present when it is not. Research has shown that false positives occur more frequently in females than in males, though researchers are not sure why. False positives can cause unnecessary fears and the need for additional expensive tests. As a healthcare professional you should be aware of this problem and be sensitive to the patient when concerns arise. However, the physician is responsible for providing additional information to the patient regarding false positive test results and any additional testing that may be required.

false positive When a diagnostic test indicates that disease is present, but in reality, no disease is present. A false positive is never considered a negative result. It is a positive result, albeit a falsely positive one.

Checkpoint Question (LO 11.8)

1. Name at least three instructions you would give a patient after exercise electrocardiograpy.

____

____

Chapter Summary

Learning Outcome	Summary	Pages
11.1 Describe exercise electrocardiography and identify its other names.	Exercise electrocardiography is the recording of an ECG and monitoring of a patient during active or medication-induced exercise to diagnose problems that do not occur when the patient is at rest.	253–255
11.2 Identify uses of exercise electrocardiography.	Exercise electrocardiography is used to screen for heart disease, assist in diagnosing the cause of chest pain, and determine the functional capacity of the heart (ability to respond to physical stress) after MI or heart surgery.	255–256
11.3 Describe variations of exercise electrocardiography.	Chemical stress tests are variations of exercise electrocardiography that include the injection of medications before the procedure. A stress echocardiogram combines an exercise or chemical stress test with an echocardiogram to assess left ventricular wall motion before and after exercise.	257–259
11.4 Prepare a patient for exercise electrocardiography.	To prepare a patient for exercise electrocardiography, you must schedule the appointment, prepare the patient, obtain a consent form, and document what you have completed. The patient needs to be taught about the procedure, its complications, what to wear, what medications or other substances can and cannot be taken, and what to report during the procedure itself.	260–263
11.5 Summarize safety measures that are used before, during, and after exercise electrocardiography.	Providing for safety before, during, and after exercise electrocardiography includes following standard precautions, preparing the crash cart, monitoring the patient, providing complete patient instructions, and making sure the physician is present during the entire exercise portion of the procedure.	264–265
11.6 Explain the responsibilities of a healthcare professional during exercise electrocardiography.	As an assistant during the procedure, you may be responsible for safety, education, and preparation of the patient; attachment of the electrodes; instructions on reporting symptoms; and monitoring the patient, including taking the blood pressure.	265–267
11.7 Compare common protocols followed in exercise electrocardiography.	Common protocols for exercise electrocardiography include Bruce, modified Bruce, and Naughton.	267–270
11.8 Explain the responsibilities of a healthcare professional after exercise electrocardiography.	After exercise electrocardiography, the patient will need to be monitored during the cooling-off period and provided with additional education and information about when the results will be ready.	270–271

Chapter Review

Multiple Choice

Circle the correct answer.

1. What is your most important responsibility during exercise electrocardiography? (LO 11.5)
   - **a.** Providing for safety
   - **b.** Applying the leads
   - **c.** Monitoring the ECG tracing
   - **d.** Taking the patient's blood pressure
2. Which of the following conditions would be a reason that a patient should *not* perform exercise electrocardiography? (LO 11.5)
   - **a.** Coronary vascular disease
   - **b.** Previous heart attack
   - **c.** Congestive heart failure
   - **d.** Previous symptoms of angina
3. What type of test would be performed on a patient who is unable to stand or exercise? (LO 11.3)
   - **a.** Chemical stress test
   - **b.** Blood pressure test
   - **c.** Treadmill stress test
   - **d.** Stress echocardiogram
4. During exercise electrocardiography, your patient appears to be short of breath. After informing the physician of your suspicions, what would you do? (LO 11.6)
   - **a.** Continue the test.
   - **b.** Take the patient's blood pressure.
   - **c.** Ask the patient to stop the exercise portion of the test.
   - **d.** Without the patient's knowledge, count the respiratory rate and compare to the previous rate.
5. Mr. Jones is on several medications and is scheduled for an exercise electrocardiography test tomorrow. What should you do first to determine if he should take his medications prior to the test? (LO 11.5)
   - **a.** Check the chart or order.
   - **b.** Ask the physician.
   - **c.** Instruct the patient not to take his beta blocker medications.
   - **d.** Mr. Jones should take all of his medications because they are necessary for his treatment.
6. A beta blocker is (LO 11.5)
   - **a.** a protocol for exercise electrocardiography.
   - **b.** a medication for hypertension.
   - **c.** necessary when performing exercise electrocardiography.
   - **d.** a type of ultrasound.

7. Which of the following is measured during exercise electrocardiography? (LO 11.6)
   a. Blood pressure and temperature
   b. Blood pressure and weight
   c. 12-lead ECG and weight
   d. 12-lead ECG and blood pressure

8. When educating the female patient for exercise electrocardiography, you should instruct her *not* to wear (LO 11.4)
   a. shorts.
   b. tennis shoes.
   c. an underwire bra.
   d. comfortable clothing.

Patient Education

You are assigned to teach Mr. Hussein about exercise electrocardiography. From the following list, determine which are correct patient instructions for exercise electrocardiography and which are not. Place a *C* beside the correct statements and an *I* beside the incorrect statements. For each of the incorrect (*I*) statements, write the correct instructions for the patient.

_______ **9.** Patients should avoid alcohol, tobacco, and caffeine for at least 8 hours prior to exercise electrocardiography. (LO 11.4)

____

____

_______ **10.** Patients should be encouraged to report any symptoms such as shortness of breath, weakness, dizziness, or fatigue during exercise electrocardiography. (LO 11.6)

____

____

_______ **11.** After exercise electrocardiography, the patient should not take a hot bath or shower for at least 2 hours. (LO 11.8)

____

____

_______ **12.** You should discuss the results of exercise electrocardiography with the patient as soon as the results are available. (LO 11.8)

____

____

_______ **13.** Patients should wear comfortable, casual clothing on the day of the test, including tennis shoes and loose-fitting pants. (LO 11.4)

____

____

_______ **14.** You should attach the leads to the chest at the same sites as you would for an ambulatory monitor. (LO 11.6)

____

____

_______ **15.** Emergency equipment should be available in the room or nearby during exercise electrocardiography. (LO 11.6)

____

____

Matching

Match the terms on the left with their definitions on the right.

_______ **16.** chemical stress test (LO 11.3)

_______ **17.** myocardium (LO 11.2)

_______ **18.** hypertension (LO 11.5)

_______ **19.** beta blocker (LO 11.4)

_______ **20.** nuclear stress test (LO 11.8)

_______ **21.** angina (LO 11.2)

_______ **22.** dysrhythmia (LO 11.7)

_______ **23.** cardiologist (LO 11.3)

_______ **24.** congestive heart failure (LO 11.5)

_______ **25.** coronary vascular disease (LO 11.2)

_______ **26.** echocardiogram (LO 11.8)

_______ **27.** false positive (LO 11.8)

_______ **28.** THR (LO 11.7)

a. medication used to treat hypertension

b. pain around the heart caused by lack of oxygen to the heart

c. failure of the heart to pump an adequate amount of blood to the tissue

d. loss of normal rhythm of the heart beat

e. a physician who specializes in the study of the heart

f. stress test in which radioactive tracers are administered to trace the path of blood through the heart

g. accumulation of plaque and fatty deposits in the coronary arteries

h. noninvasive diagnostic test that uses ultrasound to study the heart and blood vessels

i. a diagnostic test result that indicates that disease is present when in reality it is not

j. high blood pressure

k. middle layer of the heart, composed of muscle tissue

l. calculated by subtracting your age from 220

m. exercise electrocardiography that is invasive because of injection of a radiopaque substance to view the vessels around the heart

Lead Placement

29. Draw and label the electrodes for exercise electrocardiography in the figure below. (LO 11.6)

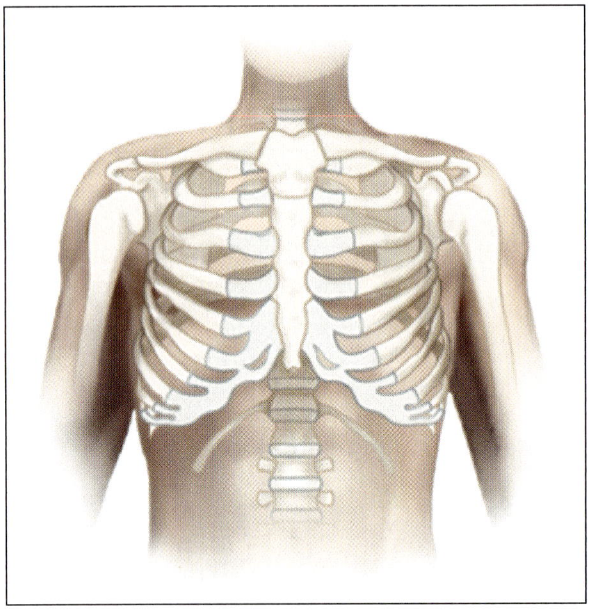

True/False

Read each statement and determine if it is true or false. Circle the T or F. For false (F) statements, correct them on the lines provided.

T F 30. A noninvasive procedure requires entrance into a body cavity, tissue, or blood vessel. (LO 11.1)

____

____

T F 31. A Naughton protocol is most commonly utilized for a stress test. (LO 11.7)

____

____

T F 32. A modified Bruce protocol is most often used during a stress test for patients with an exercise capacity limited by cardiac disease. (LO 11.7)

____

____

T F 33. A 12-lead ECG is obtained toward the beginning of each stage of exercise electrocardiography. (LO 11.7)

____

____

T F 34. After a stress test, the patient should avoid alcohol, tobacco, and caffeine for at least 3 hours. (LO 11.8)

____

____

T F 35. A patient should take all of his prescribed medications on the day of his stress test. (LO 11.1)

____

____

Critical Thinking Application *What Should You Do?*

Read the following situations, and use your critical thinking skills to determine how each should be handled. Write your answer in detail in the space provided.

36. A male patient is scheduled for an exercise electrocardiography test on Friday. When scheduling the appointment, you notice he is taking several heart medications, including atenolol. You check the patient's order, and it does not mention whether any of the medications should not be taken before the procedure. The patient is getting ready to leave. What should you do? (LO 11.4)

____

____

37. During an exercise electrocardiography procedure, your patient complains of weakness and shortness of breath. He suddenly collapses on the treadmill. What should you do? (LO 11.6)

____

____

38. A female patient just had an exercise electrocardiography procedure performed. You are responsible for providing instructions to her before she leaves. After you review the instructions, she tells you she is going to go for a walk to have a cigarette while she waits for her husband to pick her up. It is about 97 degrees Fahrenheit outside. What should you do? (LO 11.8)

____

____

39. A male patient is required to have a thallium stress test at the outpatient clinic where you are employed. He is a very busy business executive and requests to have the test during his lunch hour. What would be the best response? (LO 11.4)

____

____

connect® Now that you have completed the material in the chapter text, go to Connect and complete any chapter activities you have not yet done.

COMPETENCY CHECKLIST 11-1

Assisting with Exercise Electrocardiography (Stress Testing)

Procedure Steps (*Rationale*)	Practice Yes	Practice No	Practice Yes	Practice No	Performed Yes	Performed No	Mastered Date	Mastered Initials
Preprocedure								
1. Verify that the medical history is complete (to ensure safety and accurate testing).								
2. Explain the procedure, including the reason for the test, possible complications, and all safety measures that will be followed during the procedure.								
3. Explain "informed consent," and ask the patient to sign the consent form.								
4. Inform the patient that on the day of the test he or she should wear comfortable clothing (shorts or gym suit, tennis shoes). The patient should refrain from use of tobacco, caffeine, or alcohol for *at least 3 hours* prior to the test. The patient should eat a light meal 2 hours prior to the test. (The effects of tobacco, caffeine, or alcohol could affect the results of the test.)								
5. Check the physician's order against the patient's medication list to provide information as to what medications the patient should *not* take the day of the test. (Certain medications can affect the results of the test.)								
6. Go over all instructions and information with the patient. Encourage questions, and ask the patient to repeat important information back to you (to make sure the patient fully understands the procedure).								
7. Provide a copy of the detailed list of instructions, making sure the facility telephone number and your name appear on the list. Encourage the patient to call if he or she has any questions prior to test day.								
Procedure: Day of Appointment								
1. Verify that the equipment is in working order and supplies are on hand, including plenty of tracing paper. Be certain to inspect the cables; make sure the treadmill and computer are working and the correct protocol is determined (to prevent problems during the procedure when the patient and physician are present).								
2. Gather all supplies, including electrodes, alcohol, gauze sponges, razor, adhesive tape, and blood pressure cuff.								
3. Check that the crash cart is ready and fully supplied and that the defibrillator is working.								

Procedure Steps (*Rationale*)	Practice Yes	Practice No	Practice Yes	Practice No	Performed Yes	Performed No	Mastered Date	Mastered Initials
Procedure: Day of Appointment (*Continued*)								
4. Verify the physician's order, that the medical history is complete, and that the informed consent is signed.								
5. Bring the patient into the room.								
6. Verify with the patient that he or she has complied with all instructions.								
7. Provide the patient with privacy to change into the gown with the opening in the front. Assist if necessary. (The opening needs to be in the front in order to place leads.)								
8. Assist the patient onto the examination table (provides for patient safety).								
9. Prepare the skin, and apply electrodes as indicated by the protocol of the facility or equipment manual.								
10. Connect the cables, apply the blood pressure cuff, and check the ECG tracing for artifact (ensures proper results during the examination).								
11. Obtain the patient's blood pressure and ECG in the following positions. Assist as necessary (provides for patient safety). • Supine • Sitting • Sitting, post 30-second hyperventilation • Standing								
12. Change the resting position designation in the stress test machine, and enter the new blood pressure for each tracing.								
13. Demonstrate the treadmill, including the proper posture and holding the hand grip (prevents falls).								
14. Explain the test protocol, making sure the patient understands that the speed and incline will increase every 3 minutes during the test phase.								
15. Be sure the patient understands that he or she is to report any pain, shortness of breath, faintness, tingling sensations, numbness, or extreme fatigue immediately (provides for patient safety).								

Procedure Steps (*Rationale*)	Practice Yes	Practice No	Practice Yes	Practice No	Performed Yes	Performed No	Mastered Date	Mastered Initials
Procedure: Day of Appointment (*Continued*)								
16. Watch the patient closely during the test, looking for visual signs of any pain, shortness of breath, faintness, tingling sensations, numbness, or extreme fatigue (provides for patient safety).								
17. Ask the patient repeatedly during the procedure how he or she feels (provides for patient safety).								
18. Explain to the patient again that the test will be completed when the target heart rate (THR) is reached [THR = (220 − age) × 0.85] or when the patient cannot continue due to fatigue or other symptoms.								
19. Inform the physician that the patient is ready to begin the test. (The physician must be present during the procedure.)								
20. When the physician is in the room, assist the patient to the treadmill, making sure the patient's feet are not on the belt.								
21. Start the belt; tell the patient to get used to the speed and then to step onto the belt. Ask the patient if he or she is ready to begin, explaining again that the belt speed and incline will increase. Begin the test phase.								
22. At the two-and-one-half-minute mark of each phase, take the blood pressure, and enter the data into the computer. Remind the patient before every transition to a new phase, and be ready to assist the patient as needed (provides for patient safety).								
23. When the treadmill phase of the test is complete either because the THR has been reached or because the patient cannot continue, assist the patient to the waiting chair (provides for patient safety).								
Postprocedure								
1. Continue to monitor and observe the patient's condition closely, taking the blood pressure, entering the data, and then taking an ECG tracing every 3 to 5 minutes for 10 to 15 minutes (verifies the patient's condition and tolerance of the testing procedure).								
2. After the 10- to 15-minute cool-down period, remove the cables and electrodes and wipe off any remaining gel or adhesive.								

Procedure Steps (*Rationale*)	Practice Yes	Practice No	Practice Yes	Practice No	Performed Yes	Performed No	Mastered Date	Mastered Initials
Postprocedure (*Continued*)								
3. Allow the patient to dress (assist if needed).								
4. Explain to the patient that he or she should avoid tobacco, caffeine, and alcohol for at least 3 hours. The patient should avoid extreme temperature changes, including a shower or bath, for 2 hours. The patient should rest and recuperate after the test (provides for patient safety).								
5. Explain when the results will be available based on the facility's protocol. Thank the patient for his or her participation.								
6. File the results and report per the protocol of the facility.								
7. Make sure all information from the patient chart is returned to its proper place (maintains HIPAA).								

Comments: ______________________________

____

____

____

Signed

Evaluator: ______________________________

Student: ______________________________

12 Ambulatory Monitoring

Learning Outcomes

12.1 Identify the types of ambulatory monitors and their functions.

12.2 Explain why ambulatory monitoring is used in addition to the 12-lead ECG.

12.3 Summarize the common uses and variations of ambulatory monitoring.

12.4 Educate the patient about ambulatory monitoring.

12.5 Prepare a patient for application of an ambulatory monitor.

12.6 Describe the procedure for applying an ambulatory monitor correctly.

12.7 Describe the procedure for removing the ambulatory monitor and reporting the results.

Key Terms

ambulating
antidysrhythmic
Holter monitor
palpitations
stress ECG
syncope

12.1 What Is Ambulatory Monitoring?

ambulating Walking.

Holter monitor An instrument that records the electrical activity of the heart during a patient's normal daily activities; the Holter monitor is one type of ambulatory monitor.

Ambulatory monitoring is the process of recording an ECG tracing for an extended period of time while a patient goes about his or her daily activities, including walking or **ambulating.** A typical ambulatory monitor is a small box that is strapped to the patient's waist or shoulder to record an ECG over a set period of time (Figure 12-1). Inside the box is a recording device; the entire device weighs less than 2 pounds. The most common type looks like a small cell phone. Most ambulatory monitors are digital recorders, as seen in Figure 12-2. One type of ambulatory monitor is also known as a **Holter monitor,** named after its inventor, Norman Holter. The name "Holter" is often applied to any type of ambulatory monitor.

During ambulatory monitoring, the patient has three to five leads attached to his or her chest, depending on the type of monitor used. The patient may move around and is encouraged to maintain his or her normal daily activities. While the monitor is in place and recording, the patient is

Figure 12-1 An ambulatory monitor is attached to the shoulder or waist so the patient is free to move about during the 24- to 48-hour period while the electrical activity of the heart is being recorded.

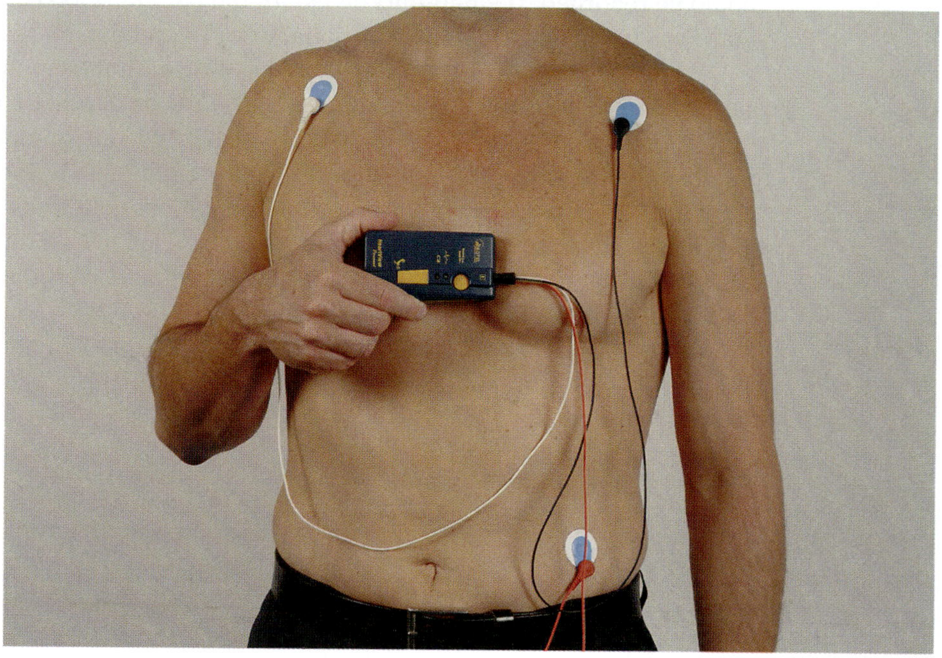

Figure 12-2 Digital ambulatory monitors record the electrical activity of the heart, which is transferred directly to a computer or over the Internet or phone line for interpretation.

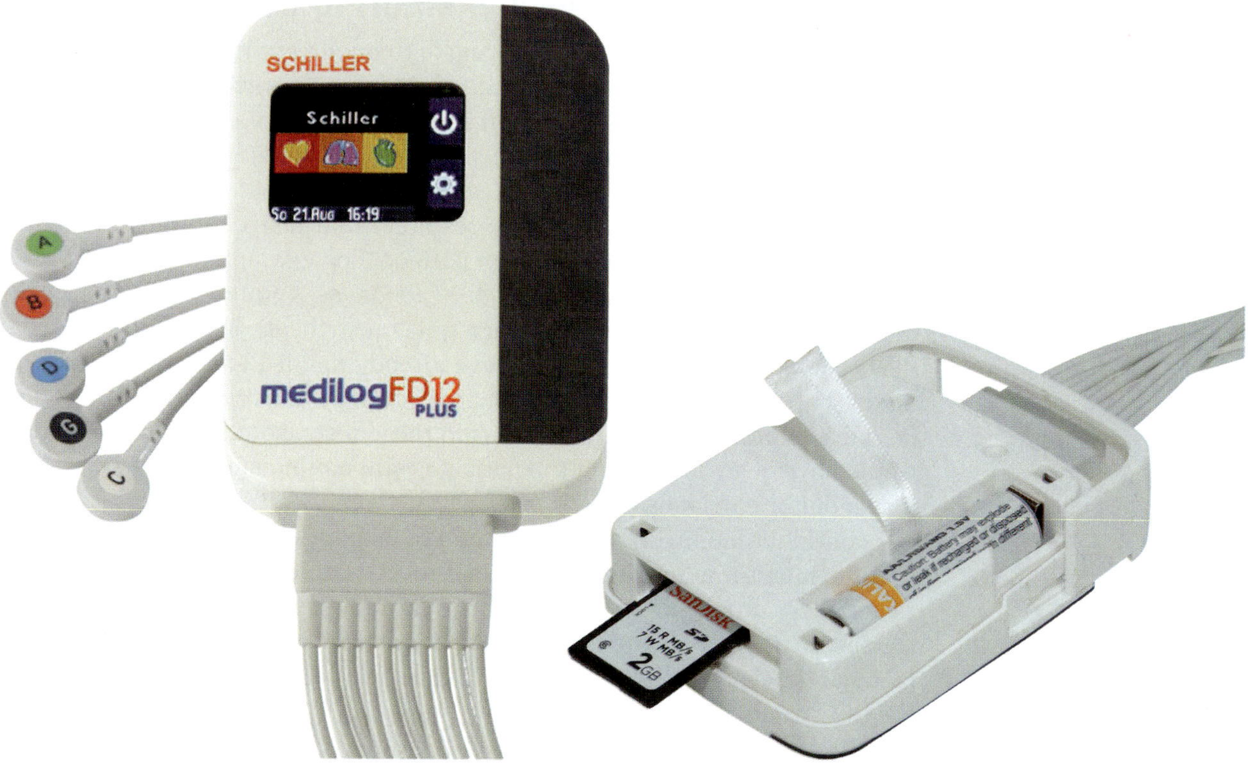

asked to keep a record, called a diary, of all usual and unusual activities. Any symptoms or abnormal sensations such as chest pain, indigestion, or dizziness should be recorded. If symptoms do occur, the patient is asked to monitor the symptoms and what he or she was doing prior to and during the symptoms.

When the monitoring is completed, the information from the monitor and diary must be interpreted. A computer is used to print and/or view the ECG tracing from the monitor. A computer may also be used to analyze the tracing.

As a healthcare professional, you may be responsible for applying and removing the ambulatory monitor, providing patient education, and ensuring that the results are placed in the patient's chart. Depending on your place of employment, you may also be responsible for transferring the content from the digital storage device. The computer or scanner will analyze the data, highlighting any irregularities, or provide a report for the physician to interpret. Part of your job may be to assist with distinguishing artifact from cardiac dysrhythmias.

Checkpoint Question (LO 12.1)

1. What responsibilities might you have for ambulatory (Holter) monitoring?

____

____

12.2 How Is Ambulatory Monitoring Used?

The purpose of ambulatory monitoring is to document the electrical activity in the heart and identify any abnormal heart behaviors such as dysrhythmias. Abnormal heart behaviors can occur randomly or spontaneously and may be sleep related, disease related, or diet or stress induced. Abnormal electrical behavior of the heart can be life threatening.

The ambulatory monitor captures abnormal heart rhythms and correlates symptoms experienced by the patient. For example, a typical patient may be experiencing chest pain, light-headedness, **syncope** (fainting spells), dizziness, or **palpitations** (rapid, irregular heartbeat). To find the cause of these symptoms, the patient may have already had a 12-lead ECG and a cardiac **stress ECG** (exercise electrocardiography). However, the patient may not have experienced symptoms during these tests, so no abnormal rhythms would have been detected. If the patient is still having symptoms, an ambulatory monitor can be used.

syncope Loss of consciousness (fainting).

palpitations Fast, irregular heartbeat sensation felt by the patient, which may or may not be associated with complaints of chest pain.

stress ECG Another name for exercise electrocardiography.

In Holter monitoring, during the 24 to 48 hours (or in some cases longer) that the monitor is in place, the patient records all daily activities, abnormal experiences, and symptoms in a diary. The Holter monitor provides an ECG tracing at the exact time the patient experiences any symptoms. The physician can interpret the results and evaluate the patient's symptoms based on the ECG tracing.

Ambulatory monitoring is used for other reasons as well. The physician may want to evaluate the effectiveness of cardiac medications such as **antidysrhythmic** drug therapy (medication given to prevent cardiac rhythm abnormalities). Ambulatory monitoring is also used to evaluate artificial

antidysrhythmic Type of medication given to prevent cardiac rhythm abnormalities. Also known as *antiarrhythmic.*

pacemaker functioning. Pacemaker functioning is evaluated after implantation or if problems arise. Ambulatory monitoring can also evaluate the function of the heart after a recent myocardial infarction.

As you can see, ambulatory monitoring is an effective tool to evaluate a wide variety of conditions and problems. However, the decision to use ambulatory monitoring does not come without problems. Patient education is essential, as discussed throughout this chapter. The patient must have the ability to understand the process. For example, a patient with dementia would not be a good candidate for ambulatory monitoring. Also, the equipment may fail; for example, a lead may fail or stop working during the monitoring process.

Checkpoint Question (LO 12.2)

1. Why is a diary a necessary part of Holter monitoring?

____

____

12.3 Functions and Variations

The two most common types of ambulatory monitoring are continuous and intermittent. Continuous monitoring provides a complete tracing of the ECG from the time the monitor is applied until it is removed. During continuous monitoring, the patient may be asked to press a button on the machine to mark the tracing whenever a symptom is felt. This is known as an *event marker.* The marker marks the tracing at the exact time the event occurs. The monitor has an accurate clock that indicates the time the marker is applied. The clock is necessary for the physician to be able to correlate the diary entries with what is happening on the ECG tracing.

Intermittent recording records only while the patient is experiencing symptoms. The patient is instructed to press a button on the machine when symptoms occur to start the ECG tracing. The results from this type of tracing are shorter and can be evaluated more quickly than continuous monitoring. However, intermittent monitoring shows the ECG tracing only during the symptoms. Some abnormal rhythms can occur prior to symptoms, and an intermittent recording may not show these abnormalities.

Some ambulatory monitors can be voice activated. When the patient experiences an unusual symptom or changes in activity, he or she can speak into the recorder to describe each event. The event is timed for comparison to the ECG tracing during continuous monitoring. During intermittent monitoring, the ECG tracing may also be activated by the voice. It is your responsibility to know the type and features of the monitor used in order to properly apply and remove the monitor and to instruct the patient.

Variations of ambulatory monitoring include telemetry monitoring and transtelephonic monitoring. One type of monitoring device even includes a wearable defibrillator (Figure 12-3). Telemetry monitoring is real-time monitoring for patients. Real-time monitoring means that someone is viewing the ECG tracing as it occurs. Telemetry is common within a healthcare facility. Transtelephonic monitoring may be sent when completed or can also be real-time monitoring.

Safety & Infection Control

Handle Monitors Carefully

Ambulatory monitors are sensitive and can be very expensive. Be careful when handling an ambulatory monitor. Dropping or hitting the machine against something could cause permanent damage.

Telemetry monitoring is done with a small transmitting device attached to the chest with three or five electrodes. A continuous ECG tracing of the heart is recorded and sent directly to a monitoring station. Telemetry monitors are only transmitting devices designed to send the electrical signal of the heart to a central location to be evaluated continuously. At this location, single or multiple patients may be monitored at the same time on multiple screens (Figure 12-4). There is no need for a diary if the patient is admitted to a healthcare facility because the patient will be observed and monitored at all times. In a cardiac intensive care unit, your role as a healthcare professional may include observing the ECG tracings for abnormalities on a computer-type screen (Figure 12-5). You will need to be familiar with the dysrhythmias (irregularities in heart rhythm). In addition, you may also be required to pass a certification examination to work as a telemetry monitoring technician.

Transtelephonic monitoring is used to evaluate pacemaker function but is also used for any patient requiring long-term monitoring. Patients with permanent pacemakers or certain cardiac dysrhythmias may require monitoring for 30 days or more. Transtelephonic monitors are small and portable. The information recorded is stored in the monitor and transmitted over a phone line, cell phone tower, or wifi in real-time or at the end of the monitoring period (Figure 12-6).

There are two types of transtelephonic monitors. One type is known as a postsymptom event monitor. This type is used when a patient is experiencing symptoms. It is worn like a wristwatch or it can be handheld. The

Figure 12-3 One type of monitor (A) is worn outside of a healthcare facility and even includes a wearable defibrillator (B).

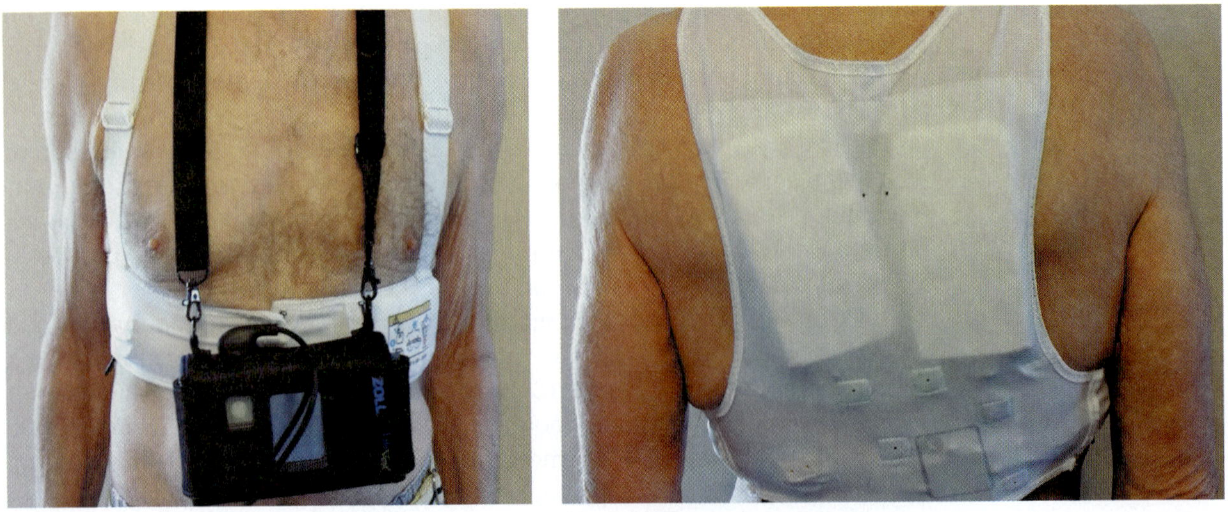

A. B.

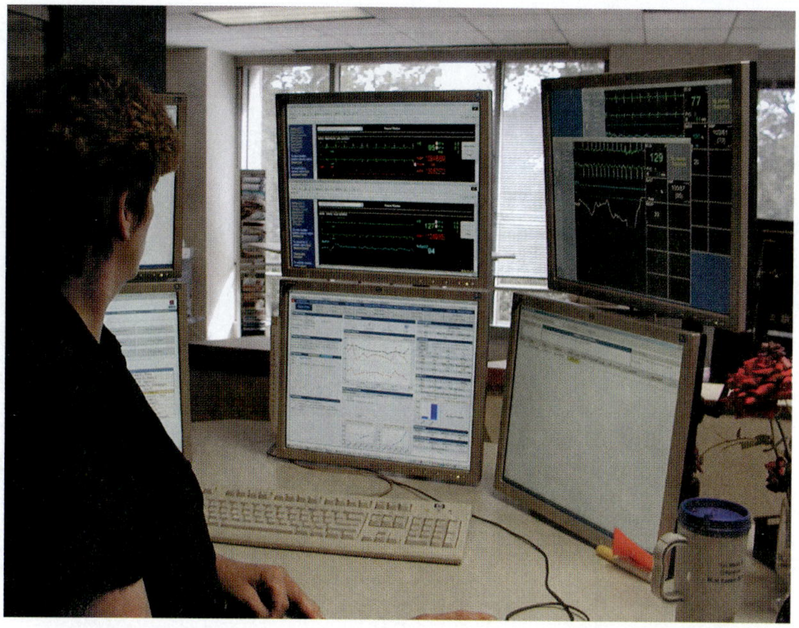

Figure 12-4 Several patients can be monitored simultaneously at a central patient care station. In this picture of an electronic Intensive Care Unit (eICU), the patients being monitored are in another building or even at home.

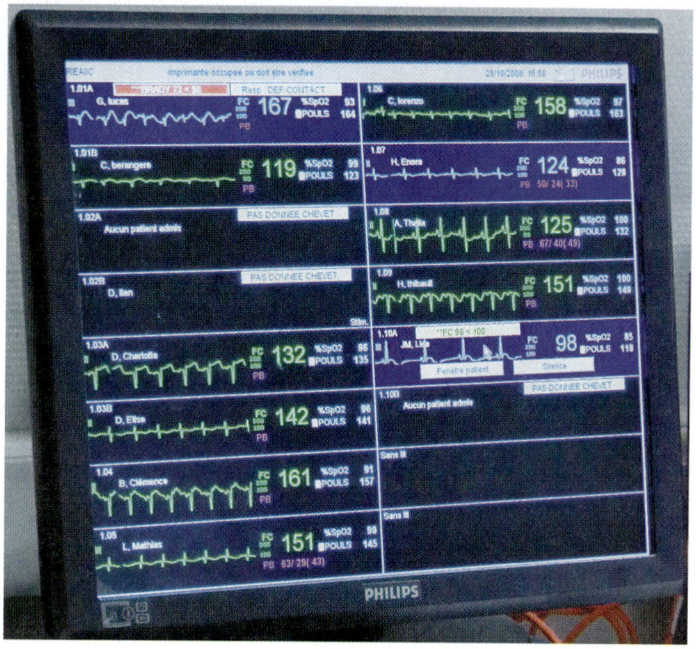

Figure 12-5 Multiple patients can be monitored on a single LCD display screen.

patient should keep the handheld type in a convenient place. It activates when pressed onto the patient's chest (Figure 12-7*A* and *B*). The patient should activate the monitor while experiencing symptoms. The electrode feet on the handheld monitor record a lead II tracing. The wristwatch type is worn at all times and records a two-directional or bipolar lead I tracing. Postsymptom event monitoring records the heart activity for short periods immediately after the patient experiences symptoms. It is used primarily to document dysrhythmias that last more than a few seconds, such as atrial fibrillation, atrial flutter, and supraventricular tachycardias.

Another type of transtelephonic monitor is a loop-memory monitor. This small device is attached to the chest with two lead wires. It remains in place continuously throughout the monitoring period, which may be 30 days or more.

Figure 12-6 Transtelephonic monitors such as this one include a transmitting device that is attached to the patient and also include a carrying case. A cellular phone device picks up the ECG tracing from the patient transmitter and sends it via cell phone to a monitoring location.

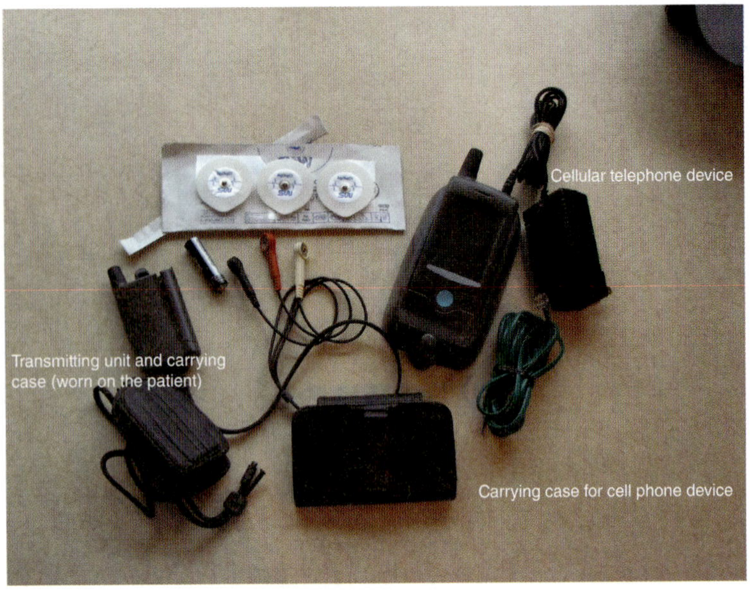

Figure 12-7 The small Heart Card monitor is activated by the patient when pressed onto the chest.

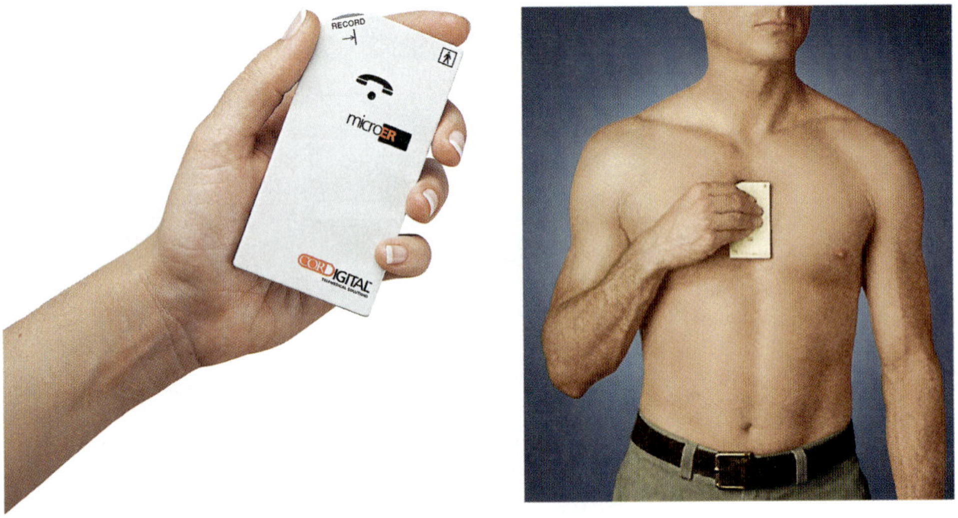

A.

B.

The memory on this monitor can hold up to 5 minutes of the ECG tracing and is programmed based on the patient's symptoms and complaints. For example, if a patient has a history of syncope (fainting spells), activating the monitor after an episode will lock the previous 5 minutes of ECG tracing into the memory for transmission over the telephone and evaluation. This provides the physician with an ECG tracing of the heart before, during, and after the episode and helps the physician determine the cause of the syncope (Figure 12-8).

A newer wireless capability is a 12-lead ECG. This 10-cable device is attached in the same manner and locations discussed in the chapter *Performing an ECG*. The difference is that the patient can activate this device any place at any time and send the data to the doctor's office or monitoring facility for immediate interpretation. Transtelephonic devices are small, lightweight, and portable. They also come in a variety of sizes depending on the manufacturer, model, and generation. As technology advances, this equipment is becoming smaller and lighter (Figure 12-9).

Figure 12-8 The patient presses a button once symptoms begin in order to record all pre- and post-ECG segments.

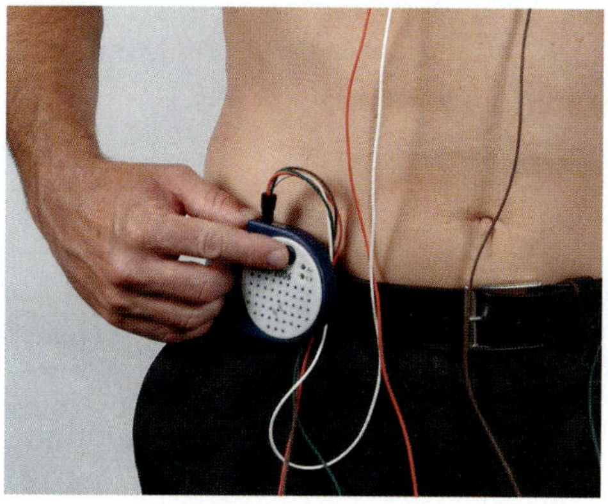

Figure 12-9 Twelve-lead transtelephonic monitor. A 12-lead ECG is produced with this 10-cable transtelephonic monitor.

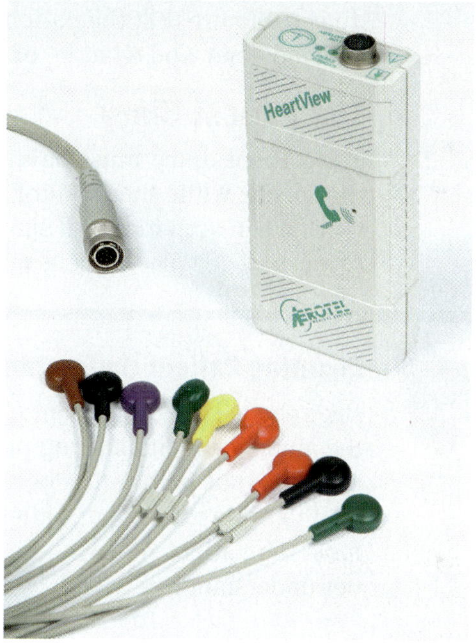

Troubleshooting

Patient Problems

Sometimes during ambulatory monitoring the electrodes may become loose or disconnected, and the patient will need to know how to handle this situation. Check the policy of the facility where you are employed to give the patient correct instructions. Usually patients are instructed to press loose electrodes in the center to reapply. However, if the electrode comes off completely, the patient will need to report this and return to the facility for replacement. Information about how and when to contact your place of employment should be provided to the patient.

A patient asks you what he should do if an electrode becomes loose. What should you do?

____

____

Checkpoint Question (LO 12.3)

1. What does real-time monitoring mean?

____

____

12.4 Educating the Patient

Prior to having a Holter monitor, the patient must be thoroughly instructed on its proper use. Maintaining a diary is vital for accurate interpretation and evaluation of the results of the ECG tracing. The ECG tracing alone is not helpful unless the physician can correlate the results with the activities and symptoms the patient was experiencing during the tracing. Your responsibility is to ensure that the patient understands the monitoring procedure, why it is being done, and what he or she must do while the monitor is in place.

The Patient Diary

The patient diary must be an accurate record of the events and symptoms that occur while the monitor is in place. Most diaries provide time blocks to mark when activities and symptoms occur, making entry easy for the patient (Figure 12-10). The patient must record *all* activities, including physical and

Patient Education & Communication

Ensuring Patient Understanding

Begin by asking the patient to tell you what he or she already knows about the ambulatory monitoring procedure. Based on the response, you can then explain what he or she does not know or understand. This is an effective way to ensure that your patient understands the procedure. You should also have the patient repeat the information back to you to demonstrate his or her understanding.

Figure 12-10 Note the sample entries in this Holter monitoring patient diary. The patient should make entries into the diary frequently throughout the Holter monitoring period.

Sample Diary

A portion of a sample diary is shown below. Remember that the more complete your diary, the more valuable it is for your doctor. If in doubt, write it down. Please print clearly so that your doctor or technician will understand your comments.

TIME	ACTIVITY	SYMPTOM
11:30 am	walking in hall	dizzy
1:45 pm	BM	
2:30 pm	exercise class began	
3:45 pm	sitting watching TV	flutter
11:30	Bed	

Patient Instructions

Carry this diary and a pencil with you at all times and enter your activities, symptoms, and times they occur. Generally you should record:

Time of Day: For every entry in the diary.

Activities: Routine and strenuous exercise, bowel movements, taking medication, or emotional upsets, such as anger.

Symptoms: Chest, neck, arm, or face pain; heart pounding; dizziness; nausea; shortness of breath; or any other—whether or not you feel they are important. If in doubt, write it down.

Important:
1. Do not tamper with the recorder, electrodes, or electrode leads.
2. Do not get the recorder wet.
3. Your recorder is equipped with a digital clock display and an event marker button; activate it when symptoms occur.

Patient Activity Diary

( )hr ( )12 hr ( )24 hr

Patient's Name______________

Patient's Addr.______________

____

Age:_____ Sex:_____

Phone:______________

Medication:______________

____

Date of Recording:__________

Started:__________a.m./p.m.

Connected By:__________

____

Ended:__________a.m./p.m.

Disconnected By:__________

____

emotional stress and all usual and unusual daily events, such as urinating, bowel movements, sexual activities, walking, emotional upset, eating, and sleeping. You should emphasize the need for an accurate and complete diary. Make sure the patient knows not to change diet or daily activity during Holter or any other type of ambulatory monitoring.

To ensure that the patient understands the diary recording procedure, have him or her repeat your instructions back to you. You may want the patient to demonstrate his or her understanding by placing a sample entry into the diary. Provide the patient with a complete set of instructions with your name and the facility phone number in the event the patient has any questions or problems. If the patient does not understand how to maintain the diary correctly, the monitoring procedure may have to be repeated. This unnecessary time and expense can be avoided by properly instructing the patient.

As previously mentioned, ambulatory monitoring may be done to evaluate the effectiveness of new cardiac medications or the patient's response to discontinuation of cardiac medications. In these circumstances, the physician may change the patient's heart medications prior to the monitoring, either adding a new medication or discontinuing one the patient is currently taking. It is your responsibility to remind the patient of medication changes prescribed by the physician.

Law & Ethics

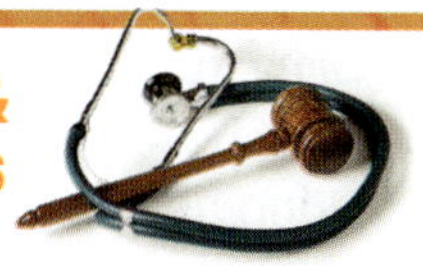

Scope of Practice

Licensed practitioners are responsible for educating the patient regarding actions, indications, side effects, and precautions of medications. When a question arises regarding this information, refer the patient to a licensed practitioner to avoid practicing outside the scope of your education and training.

Troubleshooting

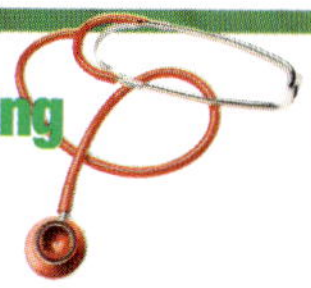

Patient Instructions

While you are reviewing the instructions for the diary with your patient, he asks you if he is allowed to do certain things during the monitoring, such as sleep on his stomach or dance at an upcoming dinner party. You should inform him that he is encouraged to participate in his normal daily activities during the monitoring, whatever they may be. Because there is a chance that some activities may cause the electrodes to become loose or disconnected, you should check to be sure he knows the procedure for correcting this situation. You should also explain that if the electrodes become loose or disconnected, it could interfere with the accuracy of the results.

Your patient wants to know if he can continue his daily bike ride while being monitored. What should you say?

____

____

It is best that the patient wear loose-fitting clothing during the monitoring procedure for comfort and convenience and to reduce artifact. A front-buttoning shirt is preferred because you can conveniently access the patient's chest and apply the electrodes. The patient must not tamper with the monitor or disconnect the lead wires or electrodes. While the monitor is in place, he or she may take only a sponge bath; no shower or tub bath is allowed during the monitoring because the equipment must not get wet. Patients may sleep in any position that does not apply tension on the lead wires or electrodes. Avoiding magnets, metal detectors, high-voltage areas, and electric blankets is necessary because these devices can interfere with the tracing. The patient should also know how the monitoring equipment works and be instructed to check that it is working properly during the procedure. Documentation of accurate patient education is necessary and must be included on the patient's chart. You may use a paper or electronic checklist similar to the one found in Table 12-1.

Checkpoint Question (LO 12.4)

1. Why should the patient wear loose-fitting clothing during ambulatory monitoring?

____

____

12.5 Preparing the Patient

Patients must be prepared for the ambulatory monitoring procedure both emotionally and physically. Many times the patient will be apprehensive. Children may be especially fearful. The first step in reducing the fear is to help them understand the procedure. Take time with the patient to explain each step of the procedure as you perform it. For children, be sure to explain in terms they can understand. Let the patient know it is normal to have some fear and allow the patient to express his or her feelings. Allow the patient to ask questions, and answer as completely as you can. If you do not know the answer, ask a licensed practitioner or your supervisor.

The patient should understand the physical requirements of the monitoring procedure. If the patient is male, he may have to have his chest shaved in order to place the electrodes. For both males and females, there may be some discomfort while the electrodes are in place. You should remind patients that during the procedure they should maintain all regular physical activities.

Patient Education & Communication

Pediatric Patients

Pediatric patients require special consideration when you are explaining the ambulatory monitoring procedure. Consider the child's age, and use terms that he or she will understand. To decrease the child's potential anxieties and fears, allow the patient to touch the equipment prior to applying it. Be sure to instruct the parent as well.

Checkpoint Question (LO 12.5)

1. While you are answering questions for a patient, she asks something and you do not know the answer. What would you say?

____

____

TABLE 12-1 **Ambulatory Monitoring Checklist**

A checklist such as this provides documentation for the medical record of patient instructions for the ambulatory monitoring procedure.		
Ambulatory Monitoring—Checklist for Patient Education		
Patient Name		
Patient was able to	**YES**	**NO**
• Describe ambulatory monitoring.		
• Explain why he or she is having the test performed.		
• Know the length of time the monitor will be on and when to return the monitor and diary.		
• State where the leads are placed and what they will feel like.		
• Adjust the shoulder strap or waist belt.		
• Wear loose-fitting clothing for comfort and convenience.		
• Operate the event marker.		
• Replace loose electrodes and report loose or removed electrodes.		
• Avoid metal detectors, electric blankets, high-voltage wires, and magnets.		
• State required physical restrictions such as bathing and swimming.		
• For Holter monitoring, log usual and unusual activities and symptoms experienced.		
• Contact the facility when necessary.		
Signature	**Date**	**Initials**

12.6 Applying an Ambulatory Monitor

Before the Procedure

Prepare for the procedure by gathering the necessary equipment (Figure 12-11). You will need the following:

- Monitor with holder and shoulder strap or belt
- New batteries and digital disk
- Electrodes (three to five, depending on the type of monitor used)
- Lead wires
- Alcohol and gauze
- Patient diary
- Skin preparation materials (prep pads, benzoin, abrasive cleaner, or skin rasp)
- Shaving equipment
- Tape
- Checklist for patient education
- Manufacturer's directions for specific monitor used
- Pen

Before entering the room to begin the procedure, you should prepare the monitor and review the manufacturer's instructions for the type of monitor you are using. Check to see that the monitor is adequately charged. You will need to insert new batteries to ensure that the monitor will not lose charge during the procedure. Insert a new blank digital disk if required.

Placing the Electrodes

Have the patient remove his or her clothing from the waist up so you can position the electrodes. You should provide a drape, especially for female patients. Have the patient sit or lie down in a comfortable position on the bed or examination table. The patient should be relaxed.

Prepare the sites for electrode placement. Rub the site with an alcohol swab and let it dry. If the sites are hairy, dry shave the skin. Wet shaving is not done because soap film will interfere with electrode adhesion. Use the adhesive side of tape to remove any shaved hair remaining. Abrade the skin using a special prep pad, a dry 4 × 4 gauze, a skin rasp, or another type of abrasive cleaner. Abrading the skin consists of rubbing firmly and briskly at each of the sites where the electrodes will be placed so they will adhere to the skin better. Preparation of the electrode sites may vary depending on the type of ambulatory monitoring performed. For telemetry monitoring, it is recommended that the chest hair be *clipped* and not shaved. This prevents irritation and keeps the patient from scratching, which can cause artifact on the tracing. Check the manufacturer's instructions and the policy of your facility for proper electrode placement.

Place the electrodes on the chest at the proper sites. Electrode placement depends on the number of lead wires, the type of monitor used, and the lead tracing to be produced. See Figure 12-12 for one example. Check the

Figure 12-11 Gather all the necessary equipment prior to applying the Holter monitor.

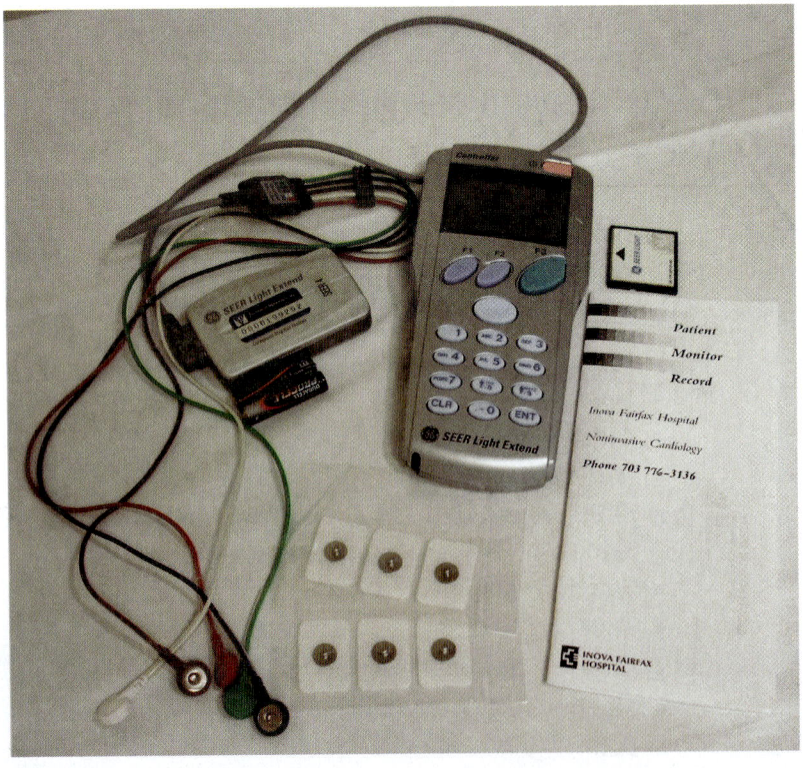

Safety & Infection Control

Elderly Patients

Elderly patients and patients taking certain medications may have very fragile, thin skin. Manipulate the electrodes as little as possible when applying and removing them, and use care to prevent skin damage or pain. You should apply less pressure when abrading the skin and avoid abrasive cleaners when preparing the sites.

manufacturer's instructions for accurate placement of the electrodes for the monitor you are using. If the lead wires are the "snap-on" type, you should attach the electrodes to the lead wires prior to placing them on the patient to reduce discomfort. Remove the backing from the adhesive, then apply each electrode to its proper position by pressing firmly at the center. Run your finger around the edge of each electrode to ensure firm attachment.

Attach the lead wires to the electrodes. Check the wire color and cable identification to ensure proper attachment to the electrode. Arrange the lead wires and cable comfortably on the patient. Tape each of the electrodes in place to reduce tugging and pulling on the electrodes during movement. Some electrodes include stress loops to reduce artifact (Figure 12-13).

Attach the cable to an electrocardiograph and run a baseline ECG tracing. Make sure the tracing is correct and that the machine is not malfunctioning. Have the patient put on his or her shirt and run the lead wire between the buttons or out the bottom of the shirt. Attach the cable to the monitor, place it in the carrying case, and attach it comfortably to the patient's waist or shoulder. Double-check the lead wires and electrodes to ensure that there is no tension on them.

Start the monitor and have the patient place the first entry into the diary. Make sure the beginning time is noted in the diary. Review all instructions with the patient, and set the date and time for him or her to return for removal. Make sure the patient knows how to get assistance in case problems arise.

Figure 12-12 This is one example of 5-lead electrode placement for ambulatory monitoring. Lead placement may vary, so check the manufacturer's instructions for the correct placement for the monitor you wil be using.

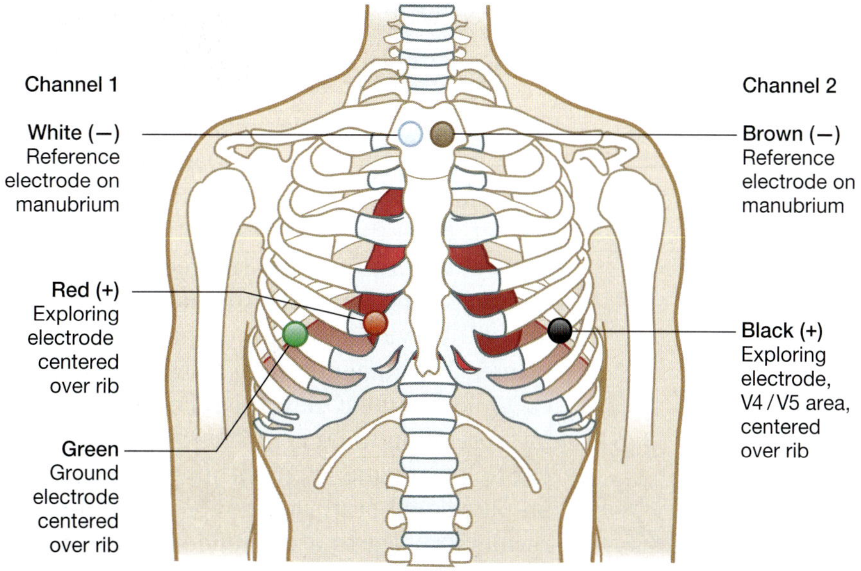

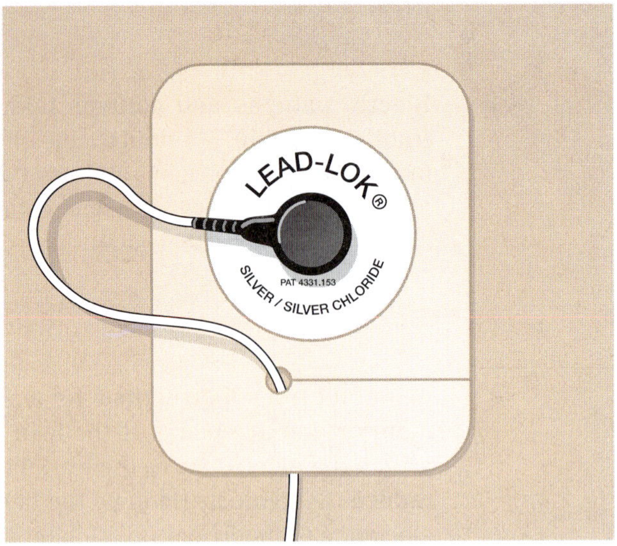

Figure 12-13 Individual stress loops take up slack and prevent tension on the lead wires and electrodes during ambulatory monitoring.

Checkpoint Question (LO 12.6)

1. What kind of problems could the patient encounter during monitoring?

____

____

12.7 Removing an Ambulatory Monitor and Reporting Results

When the patient returns to have the monitor removed, briefly review the completed diary with him or her. Turn off the monitor and detach it from the lead wires, then detach the lead wires and cables from the patient. Remove the tape and electrodes from the patient's chest. Clean the skin where the electrodes had been placed. Record the removal procedure on the patient's chart.

Law & Ethics

Document and Label

Carefully document and label the report, diary, and digital disk with all required information as established by the facility protocol.

Once the monitoring is complete, your next responsibility is to see that the results are evaluated and a report is placed in the medical record. In order for the results of the recording to be evaluated, they must be put in the proper format. Each type and brand of ambulatory monitor has a slightly different procedure for preparing the recording for analysis. In some circumstances, you may need to attach the machine to a scanner or computer. The recording will be viewed on an output device such as an LED or LCD monitor or printer. The computer may provide an analysis as well. A physician, usually a cardiologist, must view the recording and the patient diary in order for a final interpretation to be completed. Computer interpretation and evaluation by a cardiologist may occur within your facility, or the digital disk may be sent to an outside laboratory, known as a reference laboratory, for analysis. If the results are sent to a reference laboratory, they are returned to the patient's physician so that the results can be provided to the patient.

Law & Ethics

Ensure Accurate Results

You are assigned to apply a new type of Holter monitor that has a five-lead system. Because you have never used this type of five-lead system before, you should check the manufacturer's instructions prior to placing the electrodes. Ambulatory monitors can vary, and correct placement of the electrodes is essential for accurate results. If you cannot locate the directions or still do not understand the correct placement, you should consult your supervisor.

Accurate results must be provided for correct interpretation of the ECG tracing. Many factors can affect these results, such as improper lead attachment, incomplete patient diary, and failure of the patient to maintain a normal routine. You can reduce the chances of having to repeat the procedure by ensuring proper lead attachment, patient education, and recording of results. The test may need to be repeated if the results are inconclusive.

When the results are sent to an outside lab, it usually takes 7 to 10 days to get the report. The final report must be placed on the patient's chart for the physician to provide the patient with the results of the test. Abnormal results may indicate any of the following:

- Electrical-conduction defects in the heart's rate and rhythm-controlling system
- Rhythm abnormalities
- Premature atrial or ventricular contractions

Troubleshooting

No Diary

When your patient returns to have his or her monitor removed, you should first ask for the patient diary. If the patient has forgotten to bring the diary, the results of the recording cannot be evaluated.

What do you think you should do if a patient arrives without the diary?

Advise your patient to discuss the results of the ambulatory monitoring with his or her physician. It is important to note that the ambulatory monitor is only part of the diagnostic process. Results of the ambulatory monitoring will correlate the patient's symptoms with changes on the ECG tracing. Additional tests may be required, depending on the patient's condition. Some examples of additional tests that may be needed include the following:

- Echocardiogram
- Coronary angiogram
- CT (computerized tomography) scan
- MRI (magnetic resonance imaging) scan
- PET (positron emission tomography) scan

Checkpoint Question (LO 12.7)

1. What factors can affect the results of ambulatory monitoring?

____

____

Chapter Summary

Learning Outcomes	Summary	Pages
12.1 Identify the types of ambulatory monitors and their functions.	The most common type of ambulatory monitor is the Holter monitor. Telemetry is typically real-time monitoring. Transtelephonic is through a phone, most commonly a wireless phone. Ambulatory monitoring can be either continuous or intermittent. Intermittent records only when the patient is experiencing symptoms and the tracing is shorter. During continuous monitoring the patient uses an event marker or voice activation.	282–284
12.2 Explain why ambulatory monitoring is used in addition to the 12-lead ECG.	Unlike an ECG, which evaluates the heart at one point in time, ambulatory monitoring is used to evaluate the heart during an extended period of time when symptoms or problems could occur.	284–285
12.3 Summarize the common uses and variations of ambulatory monitoring.	Ambulatory monitoring is used to evaluate for dysrhythmias and correlate them to symptoms the patient is experiencing, to evaluate the effectiveness of cardiac medications, and to check the functioning of an artificial pacemaker.	285–290
12.4 Educate the patient about ambulatory monitoring.	The patient undergoing ambulatory monitoring must be educated about the procedure; its reasons; how long it will last and when to return; the equipment, including marking the tracing during symptoms and electrode problems; the diary; and when and how to contact the medical facility.	290–292
12.5 Prepare a patient for application of an ambulatory monitor.	A patient must be prepared physically and emotionally before the ambulatory monitoring procedure. Reducing a patient's fear may help improve cooperation during the procedure.	292–293
12.6 Describe the procedure for applying an ambulatory monitor correctly.	After educating the patient, the equipment must be gathered and prepared, and the electrodes are placed on the patient's chest.	293–296
12.7 Describe the procedure for removing the ambulatory monitor and reporting the results.	Before removing the ambulatory monitor, ask the patient to provide the completed patient diary, then turn off the recording, remove the leads, clean the skin, and report the results. The ambulatory monitor recording must be prepared for review and evaluation. This process is based on the type of equipment used.	296–298

Chapter Review

Ordering

The following is a list of steps for applying the Holter monitor. Number the steps in sequential order from 1 to 13. (LO 12.6)

_______ **1.** Prepare the chest for lead placement.

_______ **2.** Identify the patient.

_______ **3.** Remove the patient's clothes from the waist up, and use a drape for female patients.

_______ **4.** Explain the procedure.

_______ **5.** Record the procedure in the patient's chart.

_______ **6.** Attach the lead wires.

_______ **7.** Record the start time in the patient's diary.

_______ **8.** Start the monitor, and make sure that it is functioning correctly.

_______ **9.** Remove the adhesive backing, and apply the electrodes at the correct sites.

_______ **10.** Place the monitor in its holder, and strap it comfortably to the patient.

_______ **11.** Give the patient the diary, and review the instructions.

_______ **12.** Attach the cable to the monitor.

_______ **13.** Secure the lead wires to the electrodes with tape.

Matching

Match the key terms on the left with their definitions on the right.

_______ **14.** Holter monitor (LO 12.1)

_______ **15.** palpitation (LO 12.2)

_______ **16.** stress ECG (LO 12.1)

_______ **17.** myocardial infarction (LO 12.3)

_______ **18.** syncope (LO 12.2)

_______ **19.** ambulatory monitoring (LO 12.1)

_______ **20.** transtelephonic monitoring (LO 12.3)

_______ **21.** ambulate (LO 12.3)

_______ **22.** antidysrhythmic (LO 12.2)

a. walk

b. medication given to prevent dysrhythmias

c. ECG monitoring performed outside a healthcare facility

d. ambulatory monitor used with patient diary

e. heart attack

f. recording an ECG for an extended period of time while the patient performs daily activities

g. fast, irregular heartbeat sensation felt by the patient

h. exercise electrocardiography

i. fainting

Patient Education

You are assigned to teach Mr. Booth about ambulatory (Holter) monitoring. From the following list, determine which are correct patient instructions for ambulatory monitoring and which are not. Place a *C* beside the correct statements and an *I* beside the incorrect statements. For each of the incorrect (*I*) statements, write the correct instructions for the patient. (LO 12.4)

_______ **23.** You should avoid alcohol and caffeine during ambulatory monitoring.

____

____

_______ **24.** During ambulatory monitoring, you will need to record your activities and any symptoms in your diary.

____

____

_______ **25.** Mr. Booth, you may take a tub bath as long as you do not let the monitor drop into the water.

____

____

_______ **26.** Wear a loose-fitting shirt, preferably one that buttons down the front, and you will be more comfortable during the procedure.

____

____

_______ **27.** Mr. Booth, you should not take your heart medications during the ambulatory monitoring procedure unless instructed to do so by the physician.

____

____

Multiple Choice

Circle the correct answer.

28. Mr. Jones will be attached to a transtelephonic monitor. How long will he have the monitor in place? (LO 12.3)

- **a.** 2 to 4 hours
- **b.** 24 to 48 hours
- **c.** Up to 30 days
- **d.** Only during his hospital stay

29. Ms. Buckwalter is attached to a real-time telemetry monitor. What does this mean? (LO 12.3)

- **a.** She has 12 leads attached to her chest.
- **b.** She must be at an inpatient facility.
- **c.** She is going to send her results over the telephone.
- **d.** She has her ECG tracing being monitored at all times.

30. Mr. Casler is having an ambulatory (Holter) monitor attached and asks you how long it will remain in place. Your answer would be (LO 12.4)
   a. "2 to 4 hours."
   b. "24 to 48 hours."
   c. "Up to 60 days."
   d. "Only during your hospital stay."

31. Your patient Mrs. Jackson asks, "Why am I having this ambulatory monitor attached when I just had an ECG the other day?" What would be your *best* answer? (LO 12.3)
   a. "Ambulatory monitors record your heart activity in a different way than an ECG does."
   b. "Your doctor wants to find out what is happening to your heart during a longer period of time than an ECG can provide."
   c. "It is necessary to monitor your heart while you are walking. That is why it is called ambulatory monitoring."
   d. "I cannot answer that question. You should speak to your doctor."

32. Which of the following is *not* a common use of the ambulatory monitor? (LO 12.3)
   a. To monitor the blood pressure
   b. To monitor the heart during a typical day
   c. To evaluate pacemaker function
   d. To correlate symptoms and heart activity

Holter Diary

At 4:20 p.m. today, Sam McDaniel, a 54-year-old male patient, turned in the Holter monitor diary shown below. He was connected to the monitor yesterday at 8:00 a.m. Looking at his medical record, you see that he takes Plavix 75 mg daily and Lipitor 20 mg daily. Disconnect the monitor and turn it over to the physician.

33. Complete your portion of the diary with the information provided above.

34. Did the patient complete his portion of the diary? If not, what is missing?

35. If the diary was not complete, what should you do?

Sample Diary

A portion of a sample diary is shown below. Remember that the more complete your diary, the more valuable it is for your doctor. If in doubt, write it down. Please print clearly so that your doctor or technician will understand your comments.

TIME	ACTIVITY	SYMPTOM
10:35 am	walked to mailbox	chest felt funny
11:45 pm	Took Plavix and Lipitor	
1:00 pm	walked around block	flutter
6:00 pm	sitting watching TV	
8:00	Bed	feeling tired

Patient Instructions

Carry this diary and a pencil with you at all times and enter your activities, symptoms, and times they occur. Generally you should record:

Time of Day: For every entry in the diary.

Activities: Routine and strenuous exercise, bowel movements, taking medication, or emotional upsets, such as anger.

Symptoms: Chest, neck, arm, or face pain; heart pounding; dizziness; nausea; shortness of breath; or any other—whether or not you feel they are important. If in doubt, write it down.

Important:
1. Do not tamper with the recorder, electrodes, or electrode leads.
2. Do not get the recorder wet.
3. Your recorder is equipped with a digital clock display and an event marker button; activate it when symptoms occur.

Patient Activity Diary

( )hr ( )12 hr ( )24 hr

Patient's Name____________

Patient's Addr.____________

____

Age:_____ Sex:_____

Phone:____________

Medication:____________

____

Date of Recording:____________

Started:__________a.m./p.m.

Connected By:____________

____

Ended:__________a.m./p.m.

Disconnected By:____________

____

Critical Thinking Application *What Should You Do?*

Read the following situations and use critical thinking skills to determine how you would handle each. Write your answer in detail in the space provided.

36. While working in an ambulatory care facility, you are preparing an ambulatory monitor for placement. You are about to insert the batteries when the monitor slips out of your hands. You are by yourself, and no one sees or hears you drop the monitor. What should you do? (LO 12.6)

____

____

37. When a patient returns to have her Holter monitor removed, you check the patient's diary. You notice that many places have been left blank, and the diary does not appear complete. What should you do? (LO 12.7)

____

____

38. Mr. Hernandez, a 67-year-old man with a pacemaker, has just had his Holter monitor applied. You ask Mr. Hernandez to write the first entry into his diary before he leaves. He appears hesitant. You try to encourage him, and he flatly refuses. What should you do? (LO 12.4)

____

____

39. You are applying an ambulatory monitor to Ms. Lin. She states that she will be going into court tomorrow before she returns to have the monitor removed. Should this be a concern to you or Ms. Lin? How would you respond to her statement? Is there a reason why Ms. Lin should or should not go to court, and if so, what is it? (LO 12.7)

____

____

connect® Now that you have completed the material in the chapter text, go to Connect and complete any chapter activities you have not yet done.

PROCEDURES CHECKLIST 12-1

Applying and Removing an Ambulatory (Holter) Monitor

Procedure Steps (*Rationale*)	Practice Yes	Practice No	Practice Yes	Practice No	Performed Yes	Performed No	Mastered Date	Mastered Initials
Preprocedure								
1. Gather supplies and equipment.								
• Prep razor								
• Alcohol								
• Electrodes								
• Gauze pads								
• Skin rasp								
• Tape								
• Holter unit with strap and case								
• Fresh batteries								
• Digital disk (SD card)								
• Pen and patient diary								
2. Review patient instructions per facility policy (to ensure accuracy and prevent problems during the testing procedure).								
• Documentation (diary), activities of daily living (ADLs), when symptoms occur.								
• Medications.								
• Physical restrictions such as new activities (should maintain normal routine), bathing, showers, swimming while wearing the device.								
• How to operate the event marker.								
• How to reapply an electrode if one comes loose or falls off.								
• Must return with the Holter and diary to complete the test.								
• Must wear loose-fitting garments on the upper body to reduce artifact.								
• Provide facility phone number, copy of instructions, and "point of contact" if the patient has questions, problems, or concerns.								
• Provide picture of electrode locations, extra electrodes, and adhesive tape per clinic policy.								

(*Continued*)

Procedure Steps (*Rationale*)	Practice Yes	Practice No	Practice Yes	Practice No	Performed Yes	Performed No	Mastered Date	Mastered Initials
Procedure								
1. Apply the electrodes.								
• Using alcohol pads, gently rub and cleanse the patient's skin to obtain a good skin-to-electrode contact (reduces artifact).								
• Dry each site completely by rubbing the skin with a gauze pad until it is dry.								
• Shave and/or clip any hair in the areas where the electrodes will be attached.								
• Wrap tape with adhesive side facing outward from hand, and pat gently to remove any loose hairs remaining on the patient's skin.								
• Remove the electrodes from their package and snap onto the patient leads. (This prevents pressure on the patient's chest caused by applying leads to electrodes after they are placed on the chest.)								
• Peel the protective backing off the electrodes one at a time as they are placed on the patient.								
2. Place the leads.								
• Place the electrodes in the appropriate position. (Follow the physician's preference or manufacturer's instructions.)								
• Try to center the electrodes over the ribs by gently setting the gelled center against the skin. (A wrinkled electrode or dispersed gel would cause an inaccurate tracing.)								
• If the electrode wrinkles or gel is dispersed, apply a new electrode.								
• Form a stress loop for each electrode and tape the cable, loop, and electrode to the skin.								
• Leave enough slack between the electrode and the stress loop to allow the patient to move without pulling or stressing the electrodes (prevents inaccurate tracing).								
• Verify that all leads are firmly inserted into the monitor.								
3. Prepare the equipment.								
• Insert the digital disk into the recorder.								
• Insert the appropriate number and size of new batteries into the recorder.								

(*Continued*)

Procedure Steps (*Rationale*)	Practice Yes	Practice No	Practice Yes	Practice No	Performed Yes	Performed No	Mastered Date	Mastered Initials
Procedure (*continued*)								
• Once the batteries have been inserted, avoid removing the digital disk. Some disks may become unusable if this is done.								
• Slide and secure the battery cover onto the recorder.								
• An LED may blink as the recorder performs an initialization sequence and self-diagnostics. This will take approximately 20 seconds.								
4. Start the recording.								
• Wait for the green LED to stop flashing and stay lit. This indicates that the recorder is collecting ECG data and functioning properly.								
• Note the start time on the enrollment form and patient's diary.								
• Place the recorder in the pouch and review the instructions with the patient.								
• Have the patient sign the Patient Responsibility Statement on the enrollment form.								
• Complete the paperwork.								
Postprocedure								
1. End the recording.								
• Collect the patient diary—check to ensure that entries were made.								
• Check with the patient to make sure no problems occurred during the recording procedure.								
• Report problems to the licensed practitioner per facility policy.								
• Turn off and disconnect the device per manufacturer's instructions.								
• Disconnect the cable from the ambulatory unit.								
• Remove the recorder from the pouch.								
• Carefully remove the electrodes from the patient. (This prevents irritation and tearing of the skin, especially for patients with paper-thin skin.)								

(*Continued*)

Procedure Steps (*Rationale*)	Practice Yes	Practice No	Practice Yes	Practice No	Performed Yes	Performed No	Mastered Date	Mastered Initials
Postprocedure (*continued*)								
• Clean any residual electrode gel from the patient's skin, and assist the patient as necessary.								
• Remove and discard the batteries.								
• Remove the digital disk from the recorder.								
• Remove excess tape, and clean cables with a nonalcohol adhesive remover.								
• Turn in the recording and diary for analysis per facility policy.								
• Document the completed procedure according to your facility policy.								
• Explain to the patient that results may take 7 to 10 days and when he or she will be notified of the results.								

Comments: ______________________________

____

____

____

____

Signed

Evaluator: ______________________________

Student: ______________________________

Clinical Presentation and Management of the Cardiac Patient 13

Learning Outcomes

13.1 Identify the major coronary arteries, and describe the structure of arteries.

13.2 Describe typical cardiac symptoms and unstable angina.

13.3 Summarize atypical patient types and presentation.

13.4 Compare ST segment elevation and non-ST segment elevation.

13.5 Explain heart failure.

13.6 Identify assessment and immediate treatment needed for the cardiac patient.

13.7 Discuss treatment modalities for the cardiac patient.

Key Terms

acute coronary syndrome (ACS)
angina
angioplasty
anorexia
ascites
atherosclerotic plaque
bolus
cardiac enzymes (cardiac markers or cardiac biomarkers)
cardiogenic shock
circumflex artery
collateral blood vessels
coronary angiography
coronary artery bypass graft (CABG) surgery
electrocardiogram (ECG)
enhanced external counter pulsation (EECP)
fibrinolytic agent
hypercoagulopathy
IV fluid challenge
left anterior descending artery
neuropathy
non-ST segment elevation MI (NSTEMI)
pallor
posterior descending artery
pulmonary edema
rales (crackles)
restenosis
stent
ST segment elevation MI (STEMI)
sudden cardiac arrest
thrombolytic agent
unstable angina (pre-infarction angina)
volume expander

13.1 Coronary Arteries

posterior descending artery One of the primary branches of the right coronary artery providing blood to the posterior wall of the heart.

circumflex artery One of the primary branches of the left coronary artery, which winds around, supplying blood to the lateral wall of the left ventricle.

left anterior descending artery One of the primary branches of the left coronary artery supplying blood to the anterior wall of the left ventricle.

The heart, like all of the other organs in the body, needs nutrition and an oxygen supply in order to function. Recall from the chapter *The Cardiovascular System* that this is accomplished by the coronary arteries (Figure 13-1). The first two branches of the aorta are the left and right coronary arteries. The right coronary artery passes along the atrioventricular sulcus (groove) between the right atrium and the right ventricle. It has two major branches. One is the **posterior descending artery** (posterior interventricular artery), which supplies blood to the walls of both ventricles. The other is the marginal artery, whose branches supply the walls of the right atrium and the right ventricle. One branch of the left coronary artery is the **circumflex artery.** This artery follows the atrioventricular sulcus between the left atrium and left ventricle. Its branches supply blood to the left atrium and left ventricle. Another branch of the left coronary artery is the **left anterior descending artery** (anterior interventricular artery), which supplies blood to both of the ventricles (see Figure 13-1).

The coronary arteries, just like all arteries and veins, have three layers (Figure 13-2). The outermost layer of the artery is the tunica adventitia. This layer is composed of tough fibrous connective tissue whose function is to keep the vessel open. The middle layer, the tunica media, is composed of smooth muscle. Its job is to dilate and constrict to maintain normal blood pressure, thus maintaining homeostasis. When certain medications, such as nitroglycerine, are administered to the chest pain patient, they directly affect this layer of the artery. These medications are discussed later in this chapter.

Figure 13-1 Blood vessels on the surface of the heart. *A.* Anterior view. *B.* Posterior view (next page).

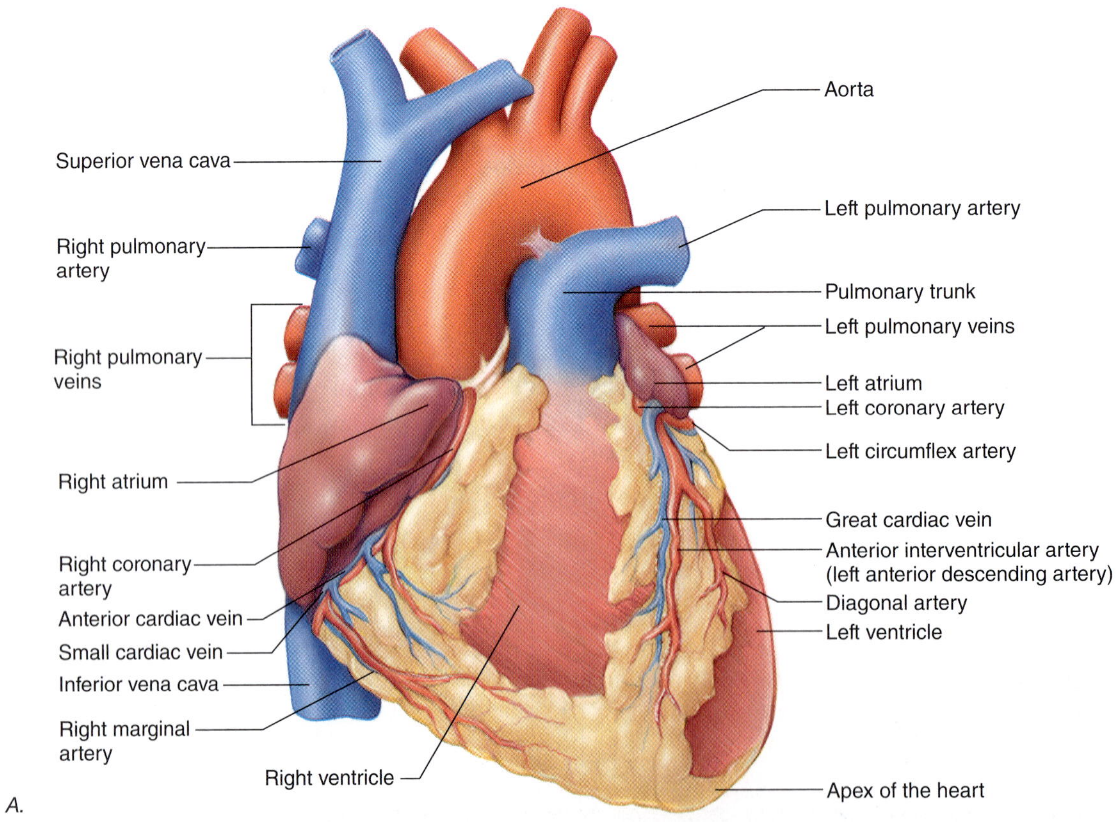

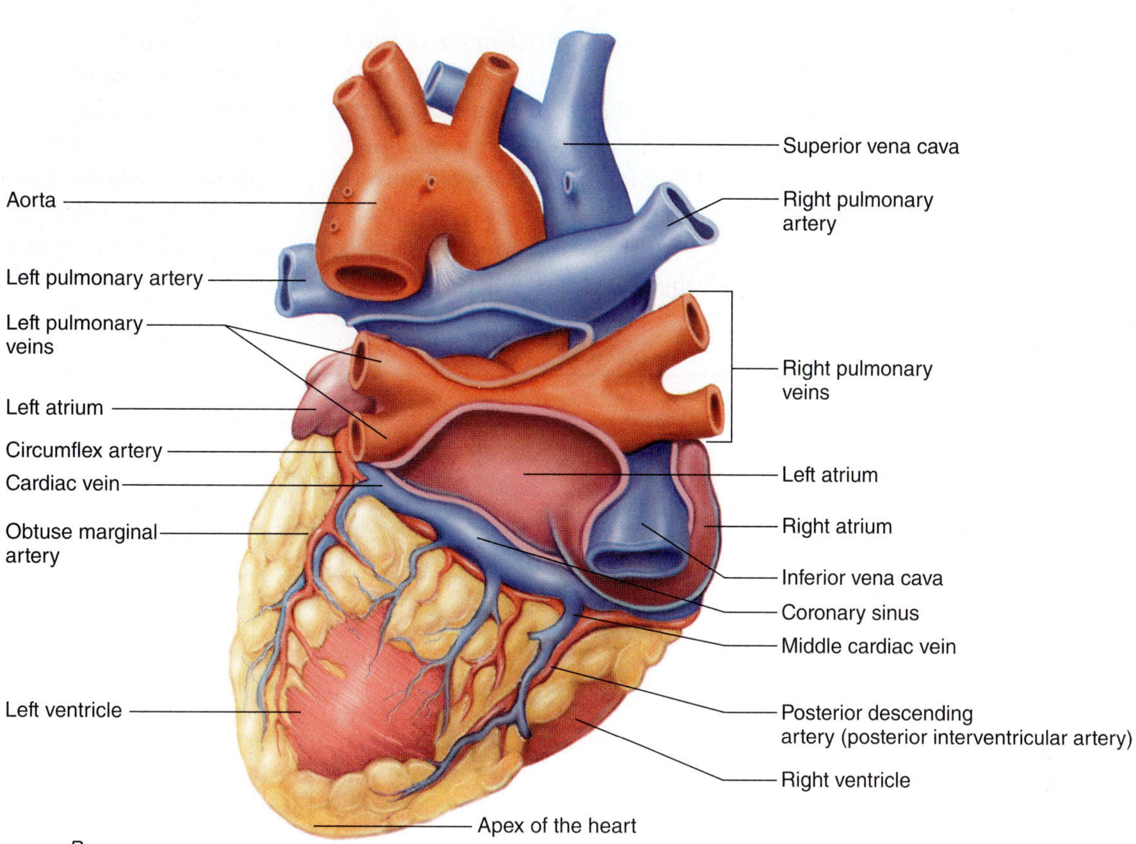

B.

Figure 13-2 Blood vessels have three layers. *A.* The wall of an artery. *B.* The wall of a vein.

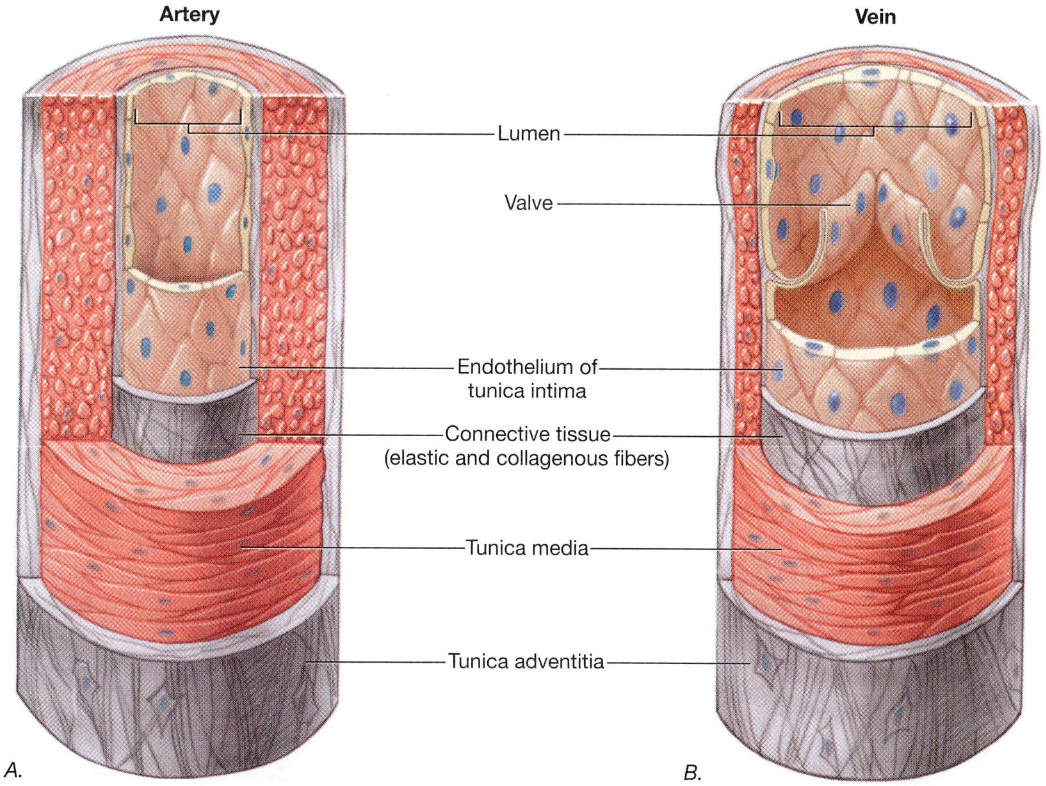

The third and innermost layer is the tunica intima. This is the layer of the artery that comes in direct contact with the blood. It is a single-cell layer of endothelial cells that is normally very smooth. This delicate layer is prone to disruption when atherosclerotic plaque is ruptured and peels away. When this happens, chemicals are released into the bloodstream, where they cause the platelets to stick together, and to the site of injury, forming a clot. The progressive growth of this clot reduces blood flow at the site of injury and causes ischemia distally to this site within the heart.

Checkpoint Question (LO 13.1)

1. Name the three layers of an artery and their functions.

____

____

13.2 Cardiac Symptoms

If normal blood flow through the coronary arteries is interrupted or diminished, a patient may experience symptoms of a heart attack. According to the National Institutes of Health's National Library of Medicine (MedlinePlus), the average person waits three hours before seeking help for symptoms of a heart attack. The National Health and Nutrition Examination of 2006 indicates that over 10,200,000 people in the United States suffer from angina.

Not all chest pain is cardiac in origin. Patients may experience chest pain due to inflammation of the costal cartilage or lungs, gastric or esophageal irritation, gallbladder, or dental pain, to name a few. The difficulty lies in knowing whether or not the patient's symptoms are related to a myocardial infarction (MI). However, it is best *not* to discredit the patient with jaw pain as being a "dental problem" because, the one time you do, your patient actually could be experiencing a heart attack.

angina An oppressive pain or pressure in the chest when the heart muscle does not receive enough oxygen due to partial or complete blockage of a coronary artery.

Chest pain or chest discomfort may present suddenly or gradually. It may stay in one location or may radiate or travel to other locations. It may be described as pressure or pain within the chest. The patient experiences chest pain or pressure when the heart muscle does not receive enough oxygen due to partial or complete blockage of a coronary artery. This discomfort or pain is referred to as **angina.**

Safety & Infection Control

To protect the patient, *consider all chest discomfort or pain as being cardiac in origin until proven otherwise.* It is better to consider discomfort or pain as a cardiac problem and be incorrect than to ignore chest pain or discomfort as a cardiac problem and have it turn out to be an untreated myocardial infarction or other serious cardiac condition. When chest pain is involved, always consider and treat the worse case scenario first.

Anginal symptoms are the heart's way of complaining that it is not receiving enough oxygen. The blockage of coronary arteries can cause ischemia, injury, and even death in the affected areas of the heart muscle. In addition to chest pain or pressure, patients may present with other complaints. The following is a list of complaints that may occur due to blockage of the coronary arteries.

- Shortness of breath
- Sweating
- Chest pain
- Epigastric discomfort (bad indigestion)
- Neck pain
- Cough
- Back pain (between shoulder blades)
- Squeezing sensation
- Dizziness
- Pressure in the chest
- Nausea
- Fullness in the chest
- Tight band around the chest
- Palpitations
- Anxiety
- Sense of impending doom
- Jaw pain
- Arm pain (one or both arms)

It is not likely a patient would present with all the symptoms together, but any of these symptoms could indicate a possible cardiac problem. Frequently the patient describes the pain as "it feels like an elephant is sitting on my chest."

unstable angina (pre-infarction angina) A warning sign that the disease that has been causing angina has worsened. Signs and symptoms are less predictable, last longer, and are more painful than previously experienced.

Unstable Angina

Patients with a known cardiac condition or disease may experience angina. However, **unstable angina** is a signal to these patients that the angina that they have experienced in the past has changed or worsened. It is a warning sign that the cardiac disease has advanced and may indicate acute coronary syndrome (discussed later in this chapter). Unstable angina is a state between angina and myocardial infarction. Patients with unstable angina will experience symptoms at rest or with minimal exertion. Symptoms will become less predictable and will remain longer. Signs of unstable angina that may be confused with myocardial infarction are described in Table 13-1.

Checkpoint Question (LO 13.2)

1. Briefly explain why all chest pain is initially treated as cardiac in origin.

____

____

TABLE 13-1 Signs of Unstable Angina—Chest Pain

Chest Pain	Examples
Change in severity and frequency	Pain is more frequent or severe; pain increases to three or more times a day.
Change in cause	Occurs with less and less exertion; occurs at rest or awakens the patient from sleep.
Change in duration	The symptoms last longer; often greater than 20 minutes.
Change in responsiveness to treatment	Pain is less responsive to nitroglycerin. The patient needs to take more nitroglycerin than previously for the same or less reduction of pain.

13.3 Atypical Patient Presentation

Not all patients experience the same symptoms. It is important to know three groups of patients whose complaints and problems are often atypical (different). These include women, patients with diabetes, and elderly individuals.

Women

Chest pain is identified by doctors as the most important heart attack symptom in both women and men. However, women often present with different complaints. According to the Centers for Disease Control and Prevention, over 40% of women having a heart attack never experienced chest pain. This makes it very important to us as healthcare providers to be aware of other, subtler complaints that this large patient population may have. Cardiac symptoms are less predictable in women than men. Women are more likely than men to experience some of the other common symptoms, particularly shortness of breath, nausea and/or vomiting, and back or jaw pain. Table 13-2 lists common cardiac symptoms and their occurrence in women.

TABLE 13-2 Common Cardiac Symptoms in Women

Common Symptoms	Percentage of Occurrence*
Shortness of breath	58%
Weakness	55%
Unusual fatigue	43%
Cold sweat	39%
Dizziness	39%
Indigestion	39%

*Percentage of women who experience this symptom as a symptom of a cardiac event.

Diabetes

Chronic diabetes or poorly managed diabetes with high blood glucose levels damages nerves and blood vessels. The elevated glucose level leads to an accumulation of fatty deposits called **atherosclerotic plaque.** The blood vessels can accommodate the presence of up to as much as 40% of this plaque. The vessels will expand and reshape or remodel themselves in an effort to maintain normal blood flow. Eventually, however, the vessel can no longer expand. As plaque continues to accumulate, it further reduces blood flow to

atherosclerotic plaque Fatty deposits accumulated due to elevated glucose levels.

the heart muscle. This often leads to complications such as heart disease and stroke. Because of the damage to the blood vessels, a patient with diabetes is twice as likely to experience a heart attack or stroke. Heart attacks in people with diabetes are more serious and more likely to result in death.

Patient with diabetes have similar cardiac symptoms; however, the symptoms experienced by a patient with diabetes may be transient. The most common symptoms include:

- Chest pain or discomfort
- Pain or discomfort in arms, back, jaw, neck, or stomach
- Shortness of breath
- Sweating
- Nausea
- Light-headedness

neuropathy Nerve damage that causes vascular and autonomic nervous system problems, with loss of ability to maintain blood pressure and loss of or impaired sensation. Common cause is chronic diabetes mellitus.

The problem for patients with diabetes is that their symptoms may be mild or absent due to a condition in which the heart rate stays at the same level during exercise, inactivity, stress, or sleep. Additionally, **neuropathy** (nerve damage) caused by diabetes may result in lack of, or impaired perception of, pain during a heart attack.

Women have the additional benefit of protective hormones produced during their childbearing years that help reduce the risk of cardiac problems. However, women with diabetes have an increased risk of heart disease because diabetes cancels out the benefits of these protective hormones.

Elderly Patients

Various studies indicate that approximately 50% of elderly patients with an acute coronary syndrome reported atypical symptoms, including shortness of breath, nausea, profuse sweating, pain in the arms, and fainting. These symptoms are more likely to occur in patients with personal or family history of heart disease. Although classic symptoms of heart disease may be experienced by any patient regardless of age, gender, or medical history, elderly patients are likely to experience milder symptoms. As a result, they are more likely to delay medical treatment. The most common symptoms in elderly patients include:

- Shortness of breath
- Nausea
- Profuse sweating
- Pain in the arms
- Syncope
- Weakness or fatigue

Checkpoint Questions (LO 13.3)

1. Which of the following patient groups present atypically? Select a or b.
   a. Children, African Americans, and men
   b. Patients with diabetes, women, and elderly individuals
2. Why are these groups considered atypical?

____

____

____

artery, whereas sudden cardiac arrest is an electrical event that affects the entire heart. Sudden cardiac arrest is a separate event that can occur during recovery from a heart attack and can cause death if CPR is not initiated promptly.

Checkpoint Question (LO 13.4)

1. List two changes in the cardiac complex that may indicate ischemia.

   a. ______________________________

   b. ______________________________

13.5 Heart Failure

Heart failure occurs when the heart muscle has sustained enough injury that it is unable to perform as an effective pump. This occurs when a lack of blood supply causes the tissue of the heart to die, making it unable to contract. Heart failure differs depending on which side of the heart is affected. Recall from the chapter *The Cardiovascular System* that the left side of the heart receives the blood from the lungs and pumps the blood to the body. The right side of the heart receives the blood from the body and pumps the blood to the lungs. Because each side functions differently, failure is different based on location of the heart muscle damage (Figure 13-4).

The most common cause of pump failure is myocardial infarction. It is important always to remember that the heart is a pump. When the heart is damaged and doesn't work the way it should, the tissues of the body do not receive enough oxygen-carrying blood, and sometimes do not receive any oxygen at all. This is often referred to as **cardiogenic shock.** Cardiogenic shock results in different effects on the systems of the body. For example, when the kidneys are not perfused well enough, urinary output is decreased. The elimination of waste from the body is very important to heart function. When the liver is not perfused well enough, special proteins important to blood clotting are reduced, increasing the patient's risk of bleeding in the event the patient is injured.

cardiogenic shock Inadequate flow of arterial blood, typically as a result of left heart failure.

Left Ventricular Failure

The left ventricle plays perhaps the most important role of the heart in its job of providing oxygenated blood for systemic circulation. When the left pump (ventricle) fails, blood will stall and back up in the lungs, often causing **pulmonary edema.** Respiratory assessment will often reveal noisy, "wet"-sounding lungs, referred to as **rales (crackles).** Additional signs and symptoms of left heart failure include:

- Shortness of breath or trouble breathing
- Fatigue (tiredness)
- Tachycardia
- Confusion
- Shortness of breath
- **Anorexia** (lack of appetite)
- Decreased or absent urine production
- **Pallor** (pale skin)

pulmonary edema Abnormal collection of fluid within the pleural space (lungs) due to congestive heart failure (left ventricle).

rales (crackles) Noisy breath sounds during inhalation caused by retained airway secretions. When caused by pulmonary edema, rales are heard as very short, soft, bubbling or rattling lung sounds.

anorexia Decreased or loss of appetite.

pallor Pale skin.

Figure 13-4 Effects of heart damage on function.

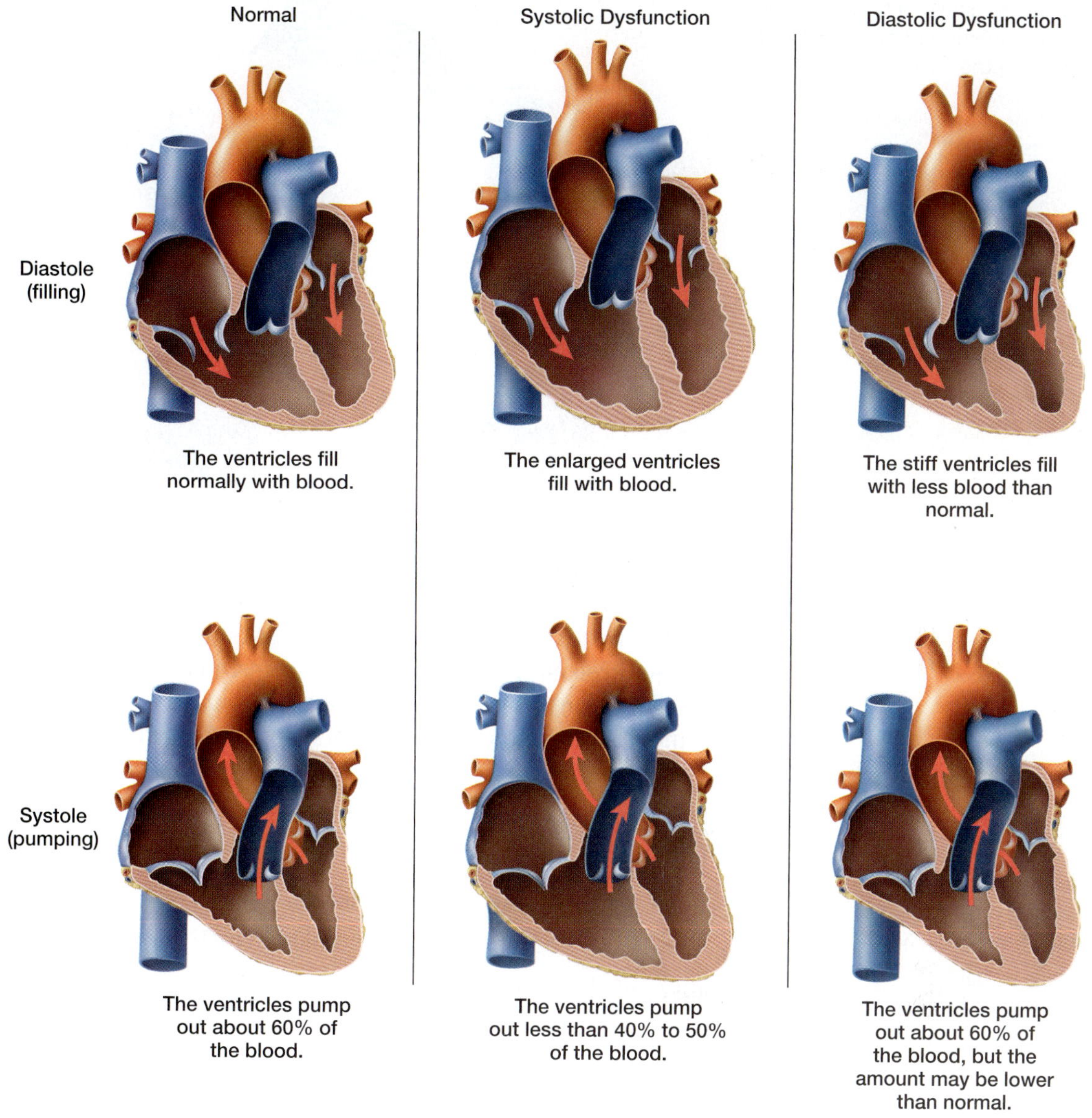

Left heart failure always leads to right heart failure. Common causes of left ventricular failure include, but are not limited to:

- ST-segment elevation myocardial infarction (STEMI)
- Hypertension
- Cardiac dysrhythmias, such as atrial fibrillation

Right Ventricular Failure

Right ventricular failure has a different effect on the body. When the right ventricle fails, less blood is being pumped into the lungs. This in turn reduces the amount of blood reaching the left ventricle. The left heart can only pump out what it receives, and this reduction in cardiac output then affects blood pressure. Hypotension is one of the leading signs of right ventricular failure.

Figure 13-5 Clinical triad. These three symptoms are indicative of right-side heart failure and are considered ominous when they present together.

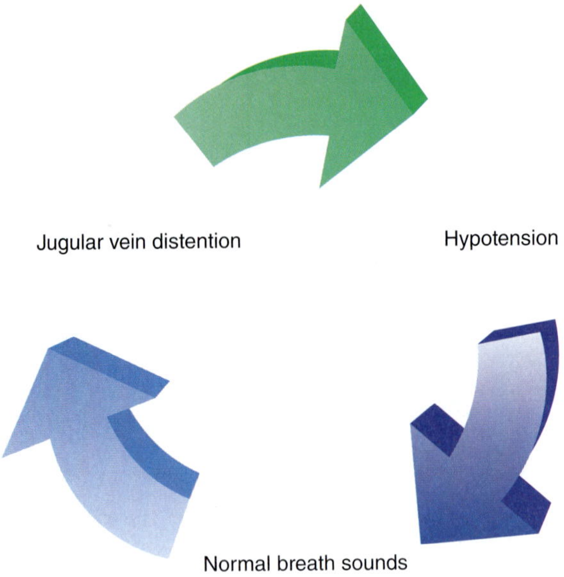

Blood is not backing up in the lungs, so respiratory assessment will demonstrate clear, "normal" breath sounds; however, it *is* still backing up on the venous side. This will frequently cause the patient's jugular veins to distend or "bulge." These three clinical signs are often referred to as the clinical triad (Figure 13-5). They don't always present together, but all three together represent an ominous sign. Signs and symptoms of right heart failure include:

- Hypotension
- Jugular vein distention
- Clear lung sounds
- Swelling in the ankles, feet, legs, abdomen (pitting edema)
- **Ascites** (fluid collecting in the abdominal cavity)

ascites Abnormal collection of serous fluid within the abdomen (peritoneal cavity). This may occur secondary to congestive heart failure.

Common causes of right ventricular failure include, but are not limited to:

- Left-sided heart failure (most common)
- Coronary artery disease
- Chronic lung disease
- Extensive right ventricular infarction

Checkpoint Question (LO 13.5)

1. Explain what can occur from left ventricular heart failure.

____

____

13.6 Cardiac Patient Assessment and Immediate Treatment

Cardiac patients may present with a number of different physical complaints and a different duration of symptoms. It is important to approach all cardiac patients the same way. Two types of mnemonics (memory devices) can be used when assessing the patient: O-P-Q-R-S-T and S-A-M-P-L-E. The

O-P-Q-R-S-T mnemonic device is used to evaluate pain, and the S-A-M-P-L-E mnemonic device gathers more information. No matter what method of questioning or evaluation is used, the information must be efficiently gathered, recorded, and/or reported to the physician or treating practitioner.

O-P-Q-R-S-T

The O-P-Q-R-S-T mnemonic will help you evaluate the pain or discomfort a patient is experiencing. Each letter of this memory device corresponds with a specific question related to the patient's pain level. This creates the logical flow for patient questioning and information gathering that is necessary for the most prompt medical care (Figure 13-6).

O—*Onset:* What were you doing when it started? Did it occur suddenly or gradually?

P—*Provoke:* What provokes (causes) the pain or makes it better or worse?

Q—*Quality:* Can you describe what the pain feels like? Is it sharp, dull, aching, and so on?

R—*Radiation:* Does the pain stay in one location or travel in a particular direction? Can you touch a spot that hurts the most?

S—*Severity:* Rate your pain on a scale of 0 to 10, with 0 = no pain and 10 = most pain ever experienced. What number was it when it started? What number is it now? If the patient cannot understand this scale or does not speak English, use a visual pain scale like the one shown in Figure 13-7.

T—*Time:* How long has it been going on?

S-A-M-P-L-E

S-A-M-P-L-E is another mnemonic tool used when evaluating patients. O-P-Q-R-S-T is specific to the pain or discomfort level, while the S-A-M-P-L-E memory tool includes additional information gathering (Figure 13-8).

S—*Signs and symptoms:* Signs are things you can actually see, feel, or measure, such as pallor (pale skin), cyanosis (blue tint) to skin or other body parts such as lips or nail beds, or vital signs. Symptoms are patient complaints such as pain, tingling, or pressure. Note that the O-P-Q-R-S-T actually gathers information about pain, which is one of the most important symptoms to be evaluated, so O-P-Q-R-S-T is actually part of the first step in the S-A-M-P-L-E mnemonic.

Figure 13-6 Patient pain assessment using a mnemonic (memory device): O-P-Q-R-S-T.

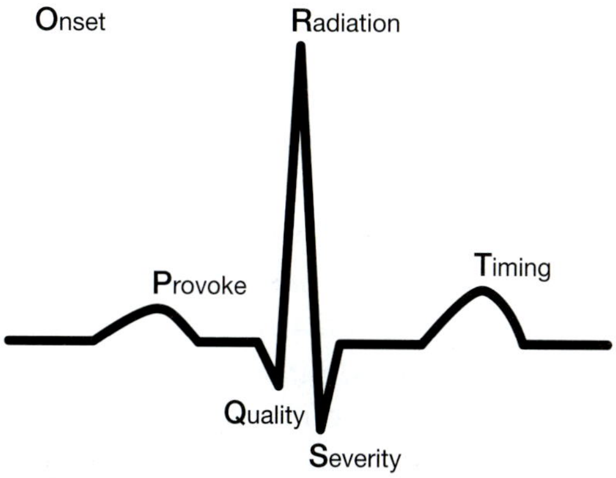

Figure 13-7 When evaluating the severity of pain that a patient is experiencing, a pain scale can be used. This is especially helpful for patients with language, educational, or other understanding barriers.

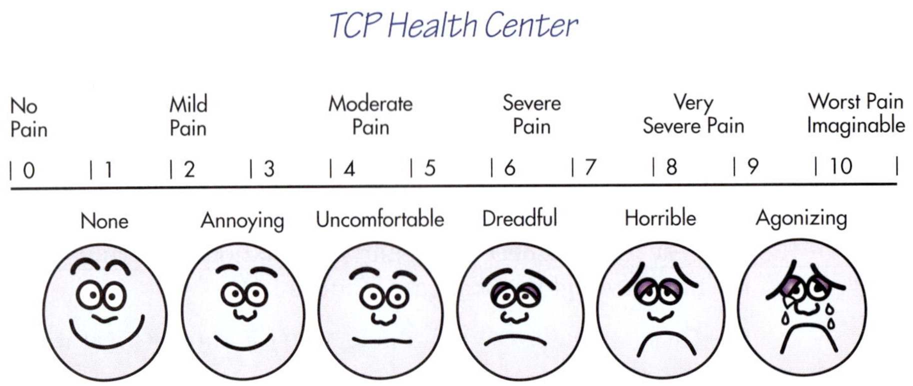

Figure 13-8 Patient assessment using a mnemonic (memory device): S-A-M-P-L-E.

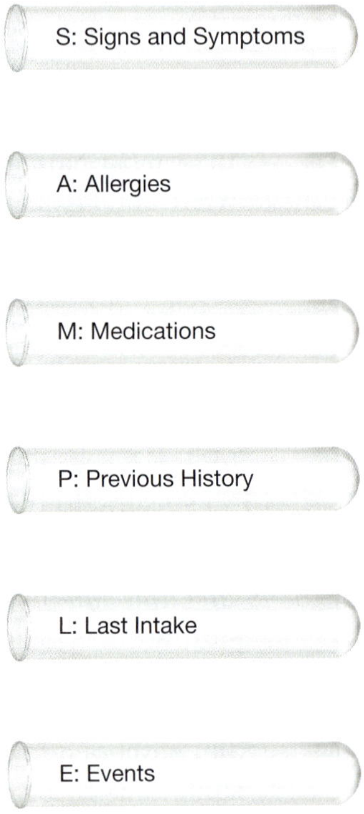

A—*Allergies:* Record any known allergies and, for inpatients (patients admitted to a hospital), place a wrist band identifying the allergy on an arm. If there are no allergies, be sure to document this so it is known that the question has been asked.

M—*Medications:* Record all prescription, over-the-counter, and herbal medications.

P—*Previous history:* Record any pertinent information related to the patient's cardiac health or previous cardiac events.

L—*Last intake:* This would include food or liquids, when they were eaten, and how much.

E—*Events:* Record anything that led up to the problem.

Safety & Infection Control

With a cardiac patient, you should gather and record information as quickly and clearly as possible to report to the physician or treating practitioner. It is not your responsibility to diagnose the patient. Remember that time is muscle—the patient's heart muscle!

Immediate Care

When providing care to chest pain patients, it is necessary that medical care be delivered immediately and effectively. Communication within the team creates success. This is a very busy time, so precise and complete communication is essential. Each member of the healthcare team typically will be assigned to perform very specific tasks.

Using the ACC/AHA guidelines, the following is a list of tasks to be performed within 10 minutes of the patient's arrival:

1. Assess pain level: quality, duration, location, radiation. Use the O-P-Q-R-S-T technique.
2. Check vital signs, including pulse oximetry (Figure 13-9), which measures the oxygen saturation (SpO_2) of the blood.
    - Pulse reporting is more than just the number. It is important to report regularity and strength of the pulse. It will be important to report your observations to the physician.
    - Is the pulse thready (weak), full (normal), or bounding?
    - Are the respirations regular or in a pattern? Does it appear as though the patient is struggling to breathe? Is the patient breathing through his or her mouth, or is tissue around the neck or upper chest pulling back with each respiration (tracheal tugging)?

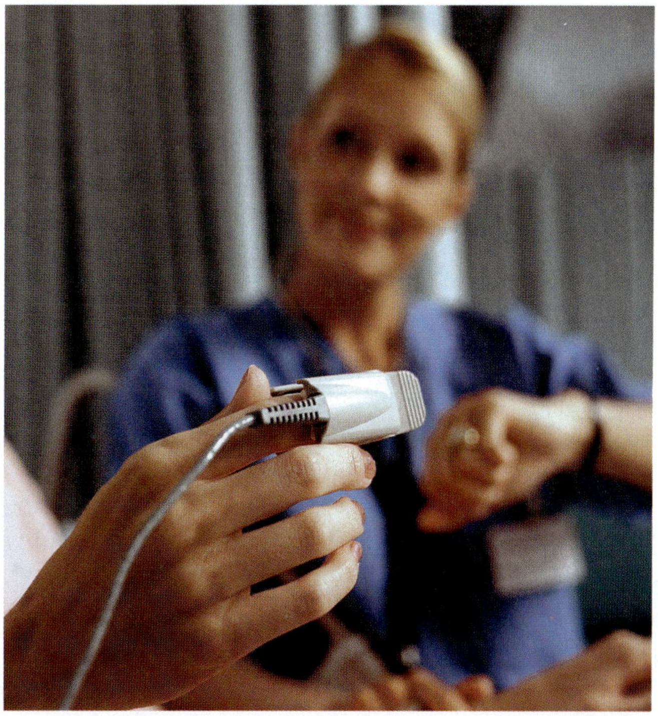

Figure 13-9 Pulse oximetry. A small device that uses red and infrared light passing from one side of the finger to the other to measure the SpO_2.

3. Start oxygen at 4 liters/min by nasal cannula (or per local protocol).
4. Obtain 12-lead ECG immediately and with each set of vital signs.
5. Notify physician or treating practitioner of patient with chest pain.
6. Physician or treating practitioner interprets ECG.

Once the initial tasks have been performed, the physician or treating practitioner will direct further care based on clinical impression or index of suspicion. Further treatment may include the following orders.

1. Determine cardiac rhythm on monitor.
2. Start an intravenous line or saline lock. This must be done before medications such as nitroglycerin or morphine are administered.
3. Obtain a blood specimen. It is common for the blood to be drawn by the person starting the IV. This is done to save time and to avoid the need for an additional needle stick.
4. Order laboratory tests, including CBC, electrolytes, PT/PTT or PT/INR, lipid panel, and **cardiac enzymes (cardiac markers or cardiac biomarkers)** such as troponin and CK-MB. Blood tests can help the doctor determine if there is evidence of heart tissue death (infarction or necrosis). When cardiac myocytes (muscle cells) die, intracellular chemicals are released into the bloodstream. Increased levels of these chemicals are indicators or markers for MI. This is very useful in cases when a patient is having or recently has had an MI and the usual changes are not seen on an ECG.
5. Aspirin is typically administered; the doctor will order either a 325-mg tablet or two to four 81-mg chewable baby aspirin tablets if no aspirin has been taken in the past 3 hours.
6. Nitroglycerin (0.3 or 0.4 mg under the tongue [SL]) is administered as long as systolic blood pressure (BP) is greater than 100 mmHg. A tablet or spray is used.
   - A systolic BP of less than 100 mmHg is an indicator of hypotension. It is especially important that hypotensive MI patients have an intravenous line or saline lock in place before nitroglycerin or morphine is administered. The hypotensive MI patient will still need these medications, but the doctor will order an **IV fluid challenge** or **bolus** of between 250 and 500 milliliters (mL) of fluid administered as a **volume expander.** This is done in an effort to raise the patient's systolic blood pressure to a safe level in anticipation of the pressure drop that occurs with the administration of drugs such as nitroglycerin. If this is not done, the patient's blood pressure may drop to the point of hypoperfusion (low blood circulation), further complicating ischemia, injury, and infarction. The hypotensive MI patient will require frequent reassessment as these drugs are often administered several times in an effort to reestablish blood flow within the heart and to achieve proper pain management.
7. Repeat nitroglycerin administration for two more doses, five minutes apart, if chest pain persists and as long as systolic pressure remains over 100 mmHg.
8. Monitor vital signs every 15 minutes.
9. Start morphine IV as ordered, if chest pain is not relieved by nitroglycerin and systolic pressure is above 100 mmHg.

cardiac enzymes (cardiac markers or cardiac biomarkers) Chemicals found in the bloodstream that are indicators of myocardial cell death (infarction). Common examples include troponin, CK-MB, and myoglobin.

IV fluid challenge Administration of IV fluid (such as 0.9% NaCl) to offset the effect of administered medication or to treat for hypovolemia. Often referred to as a fluid resuscitation.

bolus A concentrated amount of medication or fluid to be administered over a prescribed short period of time.

volume expander IV solution administered to fill fluid volume or replace the space that blood normally takes up. In the context of this book, volume expanders are inert fluids, specifically 0.9% NaCl. It is given to increase blood volume in the hypotensive or potentially hypotensive patient in an effort to maintain homeostasis.

10. Beta blocker medications are given per the protocol of the facility. (See the appendix *Cardiovascular Medications* for more information about beta blockers and other cardiovascular medications.)
11. Other tasks may include contacting radiology for a portable upright chest x-ray and cardiopulmonary or laboratory for a blood gas analysis.

Law & Ethics

If there is a possibility that the patient will be undergoing an invasive procedure such as a cardiac catheterization or operation, an operative permit or consent must be signed before any narcotic is administered. Informed consent is violated if the patient is chemically impaired from a narcotic when signing this document.

Additional Cardiac Tests

Additional tests are used to evaluate the heart and its function. These include the following:

coronary angiography
An x-ray visualization of the coronary vessels after a radiopaque dye is injected into the patient.

Coronary angiography. This is usually done in the cath (short for catheter) lab. A radiopaque dye is injected into the patient to assist with visualizing the heart structures and especially the coronary arteries (Figure 13-10).

Figure 13-10 During a coronary angiography, radiopaque dye is injected into the patient to assist with visualizing the heart structures, and especially the coronary arteries.

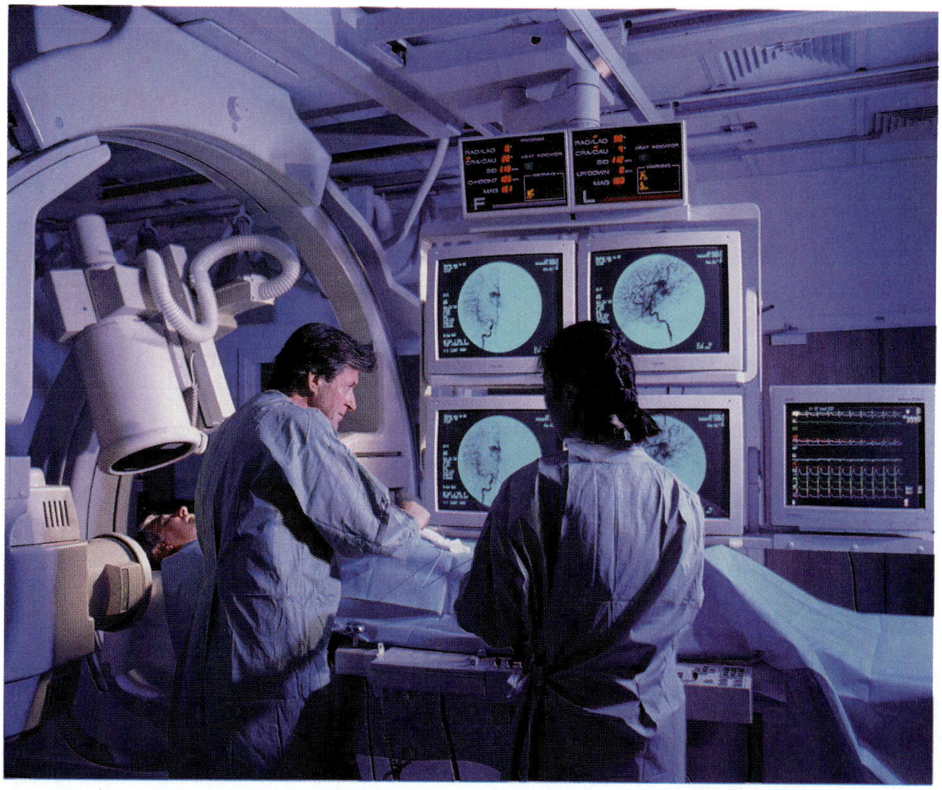

electrocardiogram (ECG) A tracing of the heart's electrical activity recorded by an electrocardiograph.

Electrocardiogram (ECG). Serial or repeated ECGs are performed at regular intervals over several hours to observe for subtle changes in the cardiac complexes.

Checkpoint Questions (LO 13.6)

1. List and describe the two common memory devices used in assessment of the cardiac patient.

   a. ______________________________

   b. ______________________________

2. Why are tools like these important in the care and management of the chest pain patient?

   ____

   ____

13.7 Treatment Modalities for the Cardiac Patient

Life-threatening irregular heartbeats, or dysrythmias, are the leading cause of death in the first few hours of a heart attack. Dysrythmias may be treated with medications or electrical cardioversion (defibrillation). In many instances it is necessary to perform other procedures as well. The following are common examples of interventional procedures. Not every patient is a good candidate for each procedure. Some patients are not strong enough, the occluded coronary vessel may not be accessible enough, or there may not be a facility with the capabilities to perform the intervention nearby.

Thrombolytic or Fibrinolytic Therapy (Clot Busters)

Thrombolytic or fibrinolytic therapy has been an important addition to the world of emergency cardiovascular care. Known as clot busters, these medications are used to prevent or break down clots that cause blocked coronary vessels. In order to understand this type of therapy, you must first understand how clots are formed. The three main components of a blood clot are platelets, thrombin, and fibrin. During thrombus formation, activated platelets convert circulating prothrombin to the active clotting factor thrombin. Fibrinogen is converted to fibrin by the newly activated thrombin. Fibrin then forms a matrix to which the platelets can adhere.

thrombolytic agent Medication administered intravenously that possesses the ability to break down a clot.

fibrinolytic agent Medication administered to break down the fibrin in a blood clot, essentially dissolving it.

Thrombolytic agents work by converting plasminogen to the natural fibrinolytic agent plasmin. Plasmin lyses clots by breaking down the fibrin contained in a clot. **Fibrinolytic agents** work by breaking down the fibrin in the clot, causing lysis (destruction) of the clot. The small remaining fragments of this clot are metabolized by the liver and kidneys and eliminated from the body.

These agents are especially beneficial in regions of the country where a cath lab or cardiovascular operating room is not immediately available. The sooner the symptomatic cardiac patient receives this drug, the better the chances of survival. It is often referred to as door-to-drug or door-to-needle time. Thrombolytics or fibrinolytics can be given in the prehospital setting to further reduce the time to treatment. The goal is a door-to-drug or door-to-needle time of less than 30 minutes. Every effort must be made to expedite the intervention.

Thrombolytic or fibrinolytic therapy is not appropriate in cases of:

- Brain bleeding (intracranial hemorrhage)
- Stroke within the past three months (or possibly longer)
- Head trauma within the past three months
- Bleeding disorders
- Bleeding ulcers
- Pregnancy
- Uncontrolled high blood pressure
- Recent trauma or surgery

Thrombolytics are given intravenously. They will dissolve formed clots anywhere in the body, so it is important to realize the systemic (entire body) impact. The patient is at risk for hemorrhage from other locations of recent injury or even at the IV puncture site itself.

Angioplasty and Stents

angioplasty A minimally invasive procedure performed to open narrowed or blocked blood vessels.

Angioplasty is a minimally invasive procedure performed to open narrowed or blocked blood vessels. When angioplasty is performed specifically on coronary vessels, it is referred to as *percutaneous coronary intervention (PCI)* or *percutaneous transluminal coronary angioplasty (PTCA)*. It should be performed within 90 minutes of the patient's arrival at the hospital and no more than 12 hours after a heart attack.

In this procedure, dye is injected for fluoroscopic examination of the arteries to determine the specific location of a narrowed or occluded artery. Once the location has been determined, a catheter with a balloon is inserted, and the balloon is placed at the location of the obstruction and inflated. The balloon outwardly compresses the plaque to reestablish blood flow to the region of tissue distal to the occlusion.

restenosis The return of a blood vessel to a blocked state.

stent A matrix of crisscrossed metal that forms a small tube to help keep an artery open after angioplasty.

Angioplasty alone has a chance of **restenosis,** or returning to the blocked state. For severe blockages, restenosis may occur in up to 60% of cases within six months after the angioplasty is performed. Therefore, a coronary artery **stent** is typically inserted at the time the angioplasty is performed (Figure 13-11). The stent is a matrix of crisscrossed metal that forms a small tube. The stent helps hold the artery open after the angioplasty. Some stents have medication in them (drug-eluting stent) that also helps prevent restenosis.

Coronary Artery Bypass Graft (CABG) Surgery

Coronary angiography is performed for diagnostic purposes. When this test is performed, sometimes it reveals extensive coronary artery disease or disease in the left main coronary artery. Disease of the left main coronary artery is a very dangerous circumstance requiring immediate intervention. Occlusion of the proximal left main coronary artery leads to cardiogenic shock and sudden death and is often referred to as the "widow maker." Occlusion of this vessel will lead to death of the septum and the anterior and lateral walls of the left ventricle, with subsequent left pump failure and death.

Figure 13-11 Coronary angioplasty with stent.

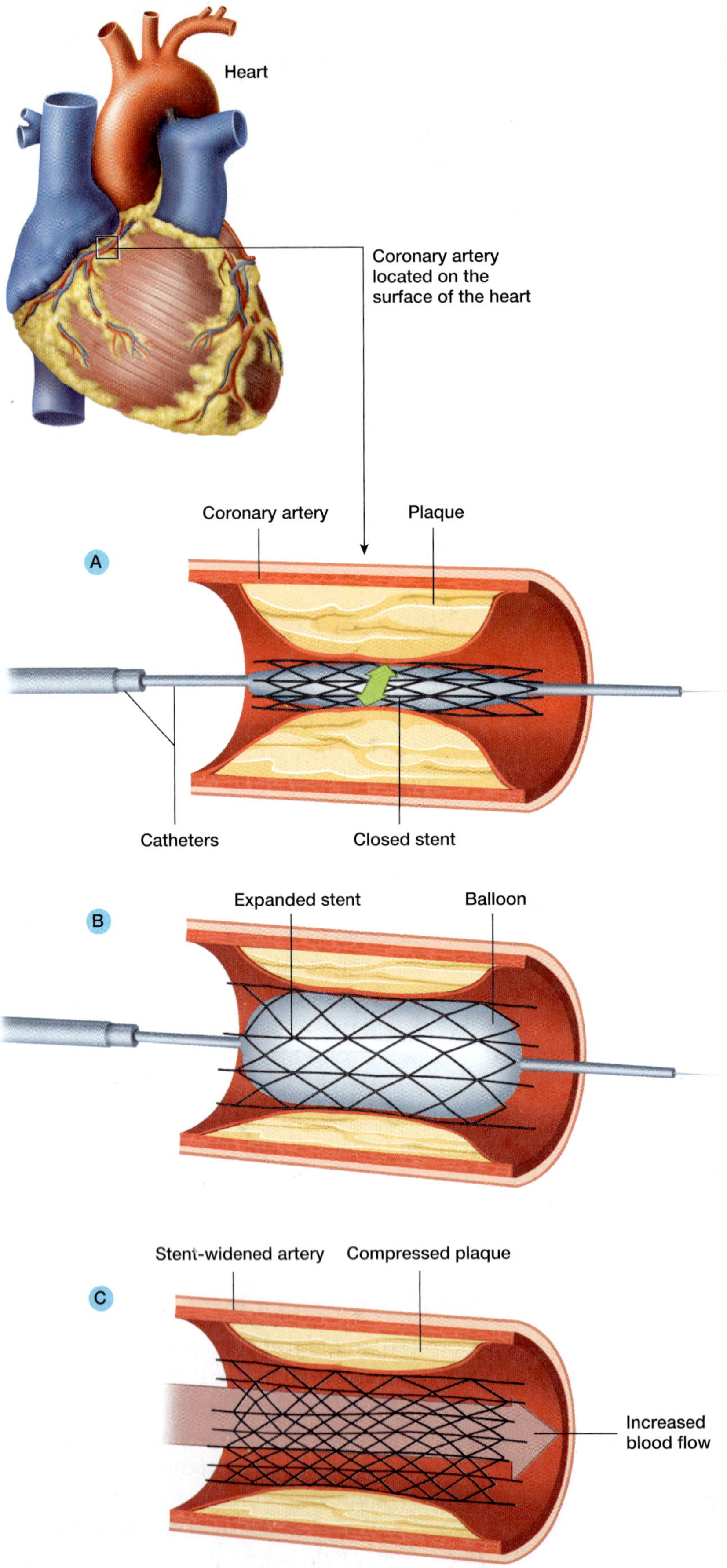

coronary artery bypass graft (CABG) surgery Surgical intervention performed by taking a grafted or transplanted blood vessel and attaching it to the heart at a point beyond an occluded coronary artery to reestablish blood flow.

The main coronary arteries are repaired using a procedure called **coronary artery bypass graft (CABG) surgery.** This surgical procedure is performed while the patient is under anesthesia and placed on a heart–lung machine. The surgeon will either graft the internal mammary artery directly to the heart just past the occlusion to reestablish blood flow or obtain grafts from the greater saphenous vein in the leg. Typically the surgeon will connect the vein graft to the ascending aorta and attach it to a point on the heart just distal to an occluded vessel. Whichever vessel is used, the intent is to reestablish blood flow to ischemic regions of the heart due to blood vessel disease (Figure 13-12).

Coumadin Clinic

hypercoagulopathy An increased ability of the blood to form clots.

Coumadin clinics provide an essential service to patients taking the oral anticoagulant Coumadin. Patients are prescribed this drug due to either a heart rhythm disturbance such as atrial fibrillation or a problem with **hypercoagulopathy.** In either case, the drug is used to reduce the clot formation in the blood.

The Coumadin works by decreasing the activity of vitamin K, so while taking Coumadin the patient needs to keep his or her vitamin K blood level consistent. A sudden increase in vitamin K will decrease the effect of Coumadin. Once this therapy is initiated, the patient is placed on a specific diet that restricts foods that will affect the clotting of the blood. Patients must limit the intake of foods that are high or moderately high in vitamin K, such as spinach, kale, broccoli, turnips, romaine lettuce, and collard greens.

Patients must take the Coumadin at the same time each day and have their bleeding times checked on a regular basis at a Coumadin clinic. This helps ensure that the dose of Coumadin remains within the therapeutic range. These patients are carefully monitored to prevent excessive bleeding or the formation of an embolus.

enhanced external counter pulsation (EECP) Treatment for chronic angina patients who do not have other options due to health status. This procedure is performed five days a week for several weeks, with the intent of developing collateral blood vessels—essentially creating a "natural" bypass around narrowed or blocked arteries.

Enhanced External Counter Pulsation (EECP) Therapy

External counter pulsation therapy may be performed on patients with recurrent angina or, more recently, on heart failure patients who are typically not strong enough to withstand major surgery such as heart catheterization or CABG. **Enhanced external counter pulsation (EECP)** is a safe, noninva-

Figure 13-12 Placement of vessels for coronary artery bypass graft (CABG) surgery.

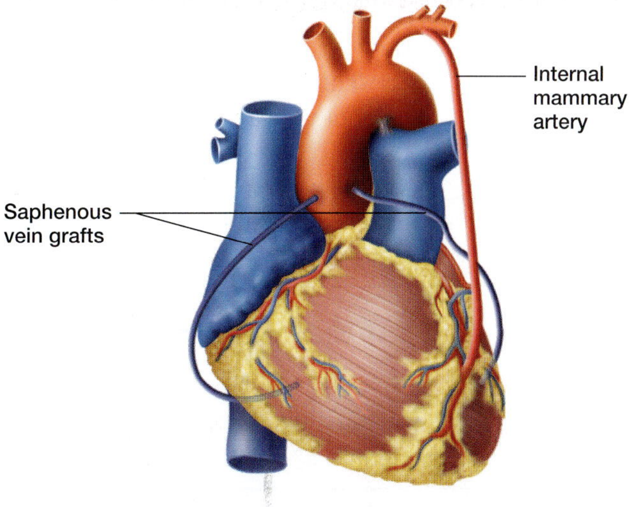

Figure 13-13 Enhanced external counter pulsation (EECP) therapy. Vasomedical™ Lumenair System

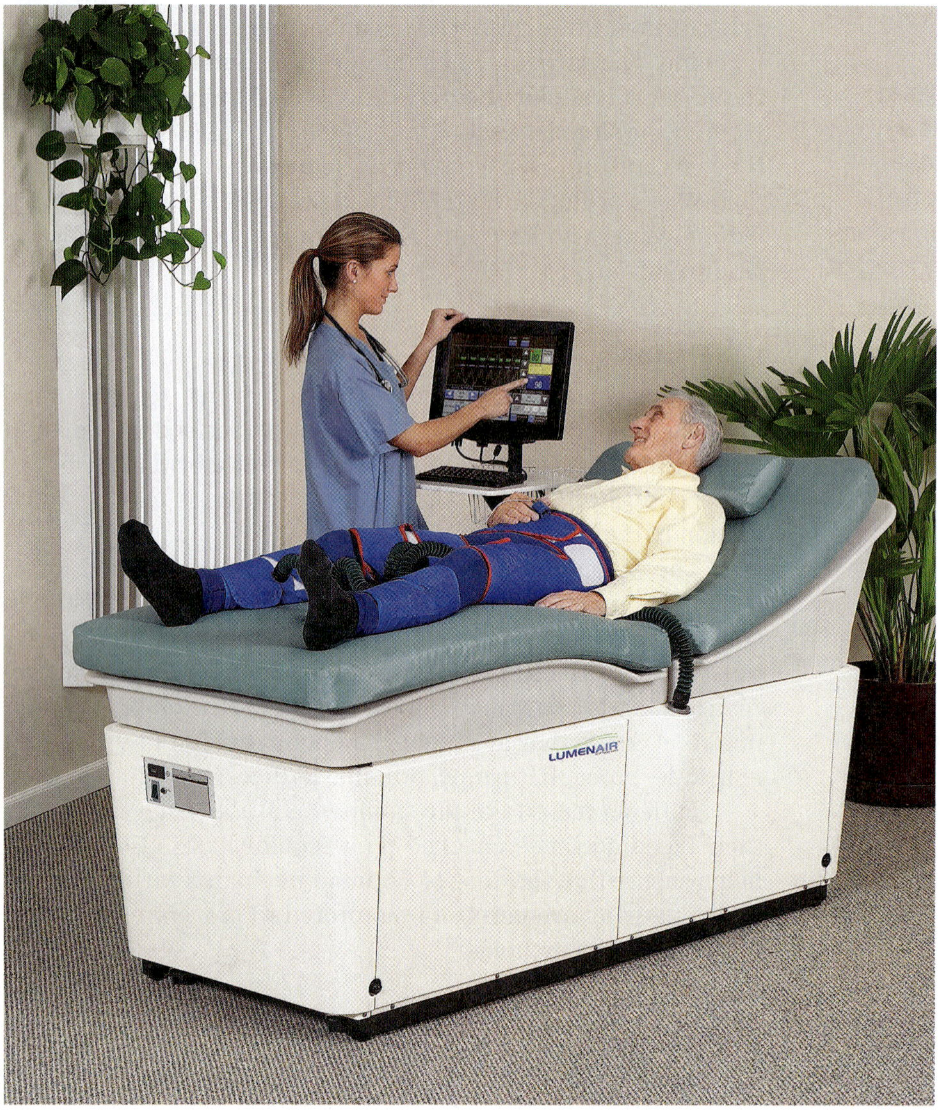

sive, well-tolerated, and clinically effective outpatient physical therapy treatment. During the treatment, the patient lies on a comfortable treatment table with large blood pressure-like cuffs wrapped around his or her legs and buttocks (Figure 13-13). The cuffs are designed to systematically inflate and deflate in coordination with the contraction and relaxation phases of the heart. The idea behind it is to increase the intravascular pressure in an effort to promote the growth of new **collateral blood vessels** and in essence create a "natural" bypass to bridge areas of the heart where occlusions or narrowing of blood vessels have occurred. Each EECP treatment generally lasts one hour per day and is performed five days per week for a total of seven weeks.

collateral blood vessels Side-by-side, as in small vessels providing additional blood flow to a region of tissue.

Checkpoint Question (LO 13.7)

1. Why are stents usually inserted during coronary angioplasty?

____

____

Chapter Summary

Learning Outcomes	Summary	Pages
13.1 Identify the major coronary arteries, and describe the structure of arteries.	The right coronary artery main branches include the posterior descending artery and marginal artery. The left coronary artery main branches are the circumflex and the left anterior descending artery. The coronary artery walls include three layers of tissue: tunica adventitia, tunica media, and tunica intima.	308–310
13.2 Describe typical cardiac symptoms and unstable angina.	Not all chest pain is cardiac in origin; however, all chest discomfort or pain is considered cardiac until proven otherwise. Chest pain may present gradually or quickly, stay in one location, or radiate to other locations. Anginal symptoms are the heart's way of telling us it is not receiving enough oxygen. Unstable angina is a signal to a patient that his or her angina has changed or gotten worse. Signs of unstable angina may be confused with an MI.	310–312
13.3 Summarize atypical patient types and presentation.	Not every patient with MI presents with the same complaints. Women, patients with diabetes, and elderly people are three groups who present atypically.	312–313
13.4 Compare ST segment elevation and non-ST segment elevation.	*Acute coronary syndrome* is a broad term that refers to patients presenting with unstable angina, ST segment elevation MI (STEMI), or non-ST segment elevation MI (NSTEMI). STEMI refers to the classic MI, which occurs 75%–80% of the time. NSTEMI patients don't present with the classic signs and symptoms and represent 20%–25% of cases. NSTEMI patients may be asymptomatic, so the healthcare team must be alert to this type of patient.	314–316
13.5 Explain heart failure.	Heart failure occurs when the heart muscle has sustained enough injury that it is unable to function as an effective pump. The most common cause of heart failure is MI. Left and right ventricular failure have different effects on the body.	316–318
13.6 Identify assessment and immediate treatment for the cardiac patient.	O-P-Q-R-S-T and S-A-M-P-L-E are common mnemonics, or memory tools, used to ensure a consistent approach to information gathering when interviewing cardiac patients. When providing care to the cardiac patient, it is necessary that medical care be delivered immediately and effectively. Communication within the team creates success.	318–324
13.7 Discuss treatment modalities for the cardiac patient.	Additional tests are often used to evaluate the heart and its function. Interventional procedures may be performed for patients in certain circumstances and may include fibrinolytic therapy, angioplasty with stenting of vessels, and CABG surgery. Other types of treatment are prescribed for cardiac patients, such as Coumadin therapy and EECP, depending on the specific diagnosis or patient's health state. When working with a cardiac patient, if there is a chance the patient will be having an invasive procedure, ensure that the consent is signed before the patient receives narcotics.	324–328

Chapter Review

True / False

Read each statement and determine if it is true or false. Circle the T or F. For false (F) statements, correct them on the lines provided.

T **F** **1.** All chest pain is cardiac in origin. (LO 13.2)

____

T **F** **2.** Angina is the heart's way of complaining it needs more oxygen. (LO 13.2)

____

T **F** **3.** All acute myocardial infarctions present with ST segment elevation. (LO 13.4)

____

T **F** **4.** The "A" in S-A-M-P-L-E refers to ascites. (LO 13.6)

____

T **F** **5.** Patients must sign a consent for procedures before receiving narcotics. (LO 13.5)

____

T **F** **6.** Fibrinolytic agents may be used on any patient. (LO 13.7)

____

T **F** **7.** Beta blockers decrease heart rate and blood pressure. (LO 13.6)

____

T **F** **8.** The circumflex artery supplies blood to the right atrium and ventricle. (LO 13.1)

____

Multiple Choice

Circle the correct answer.

9. What is the name of the innermost layer of an artery? (LO 13.1)
- **a.** Tunica adventitia
- **b.** Tunica media
- **c.** Tunica os
- **d.** Tunica intima

10. Which major coronary artery and vessel supplies blood to both ventricles? (LO 13.1)
- **a.** Circumflex artery
- **b.** Left anterior descending artery
- **c.** Right descending artery
- **d.** Right main and marginal arteries

11. Which of the following complaints may be cardiac in origin? (LO 13.2)
   a. Dental pain
   b. Nausea
   c. Indigestion
   d. All of the answers are correct

12. Symptoms of unstable angina include which of the following? (LO 13.2)
   a. Chest pain that lasts greater than 20 minutes
   b. More frequent or severe chest pain
   c. Chest pain that occurs with less exertion
   d. All of the answers are correct

13. Which three groups of patients often present with atypical symptoms of MI? (LO 13.3)
   a. Women, infants, and children
   b. Women, elderly patients, and patients with diabetes
   c. Men, women, and children with diabetes
   d. All of the answers are correct

14. Due to damage to blood vessels, patients with diabetes are __________ as likely as a nondiabetic individual to experience a stroke or heart attack. (LO 13.3)
   a. 10 times
   b. 5 times
   c. twice
   d. not

15. Which of the following are included when referring to acute coronary syndrome? (LO 13.3)
   a. STEMI, NSTEMI, and unstable angina
   b. STEMI, NSTEMI, and stable angina
   c. STEMI, NSTEMI, and diabetes
   d. STEMI, NSTEMI, and CVA

16. What percentage of patients may present with STEMI? (LO 13.4)
   a. 20%–25%
   b. 40%–45%
   c. 75%–80%
   d. 100%

17. What percentage of patients may present with NSTEMI? (LO 13.4)
   a. 20%–25%
   b. 40%–45%
   c. 75%–80%
   d. 100%

18. Heart failure is simply defined as __________. (LO 13.5)
   a. pulmonary edema
   b. hyperlipidemia
   c. pulmonary failure
   d. pump failure

19. Which type of heart failure causes fluid to back up in the lungs, causing pulmonary edema? (LO 13.5)
   a. Right atrial
   b. Right ventricular
   c. Left atrial
   d. Left ventricular

20. Mnemonic devices are commonly used in medicine to __________. (LO 13.6)
   a. create a complex tool for specialists only
   b. decrease communication and efficiency of patient care
   c. increase the amount of time before the patient receives care
   d. increase efficiency and present a more logical flow to patient care

21. What does the "S" in S-A-M-P-L-E refer to? (LO 13.6)
   a. Signs and symptoms
   b. Signs of distress
   c. Pain scale
   d. All of the answers are correct

22. How are O-P-Q-R-S-T and S-A-M-P-L-E related?
   a. They are acronyms that determine the patient's vital signs.
   b. The "O" in O-P-Q-R-S-T is one step of S-A-M-P-L-E.
   c. The O-P-Q-R-S-T is an assessment of pain, which is done in the "S" of S-A-M-P-L-E.
   d. They are both acronyms used for identifying pain and other signs and symptoms.

23. Nitroglycerin causes blood vessels to __________ and blood pressure to __________. (LO 13.6)
   a. constrict, increase
   b. relax, increase
   c. constrict, decrease
   d. relax, decrease

24. Which procedure allows visualization of the coronary arteries and placement of a stent? (LO 13.7)
   a. Coronary artery bypass
   b. Echocardiography
   c. Cardiac catheterization
   d. Enhanced external counter pulsation

25. Coumadin is used to __________. (LO 13.7)
   a. increase heart rate
   b. increase clot formation in blood
   c. decrease heart rate
   d. decrease clot formation in blood

Fill in the Blank

26. List at least five things that must be done when caring for a cardiac patient within the first 10 minutes of his or her arrival. (LO 13.6)

__________ __________

__________ __________

__________ __________

27. List five blood tests that the doctor might order when caring for a chest pain patient. (LO 13.6)

__________ __________

__________ __________

__________ __________

28. Occlusion of the proximal left coronary artery is often referred to as the ______________________ ______________. (LO 13.7)

29. Name two vessels that are commonly used in CABG surgery. (LO 13.7)

______________________________ ______________________________

Critical Thinking Application *What Should You Do?*

30. A 68-year-old male is complaining of substernal chest pressure. The pressure is radiating to his left shoulder. This patient has no history of heart disease, diabetes, hypertension, or stroke. His father died from a heart attack at the age of 62. This patient is moderately anxious. He is not obese, and his vital signs are within normal limits except for a blood pressure (BP) of 90/48. (LO 13.2, 13.6)

   a. Is this patient at risk?

   b. Why would this patient be anxious?

   c. What are the tasks that must be performed within the first 10 minutes of arrival?

   d. Why are these tasks performed within the first 10 minutes?

   e. What do you think this patient is experiencing?

connect® Now that you have completed the material in the chapter text, go to Connect and complete any chapter activities you have not yet done.

14 Basic 12-Lead ECG Interpretation

Learning Outcomes

14.1 Discuss the anatomical views represented on a 12-lead ECG and the coronary artery that commonly supplies that region of tissue.

14.2 Identify common morphologic changes associated with ischemia, injury, and infarction.

14.3 Define axis deviation and the steps utilized to determine the presence of axis deviation.

14.4 Differentiate between left and right bundle branch blocks and how they relate to the 12-lead ECG.

14.5 Describe left ventricular hypertrophy (LVH) and the steps to determine the presence of LVH.

Key Terms

anatomically contiguous lead
axis deviation
hypertrophy
myocardial infarction (MI; heart attack)
myocardial injury
myocardial ischemia
pathologic Q wave
physiologic Q wave
QS complex

14.1 The Views of a Standard 12-Lead ECG and Major Vessels

The chapter *The Electrocardiograph* discussed how the 12-lead ECG produces 12 different tracings of the heart. This chapter explains what a standard 12-lead is specifically looking at—essentially what each lead sees.

Think of each lead as a photograph, like taking a picture of a car. If you stand in front of the car and take the picture, you get the front view of the car. If you stand behind the same car and take a picture, you get a different view—the back view—of the same car.

A standard 12-lead ECG focuses directly on the left ventricle but considers the heart from slightly different angles (Table 14-1 and Figure 14-1). Each lead shows the electrical activity occurring in specific regions of the heart. In the presence of ischemia, injury, or infarction due to partial or complete blockage of coronary arteries, changes to the cardiac complex may occur that would often be indicative of these problems. Consider Figures 14-2 to 14-7. Each figure identifies the area of the heart involved and the lead tracing affected by the involvement.

TABLE 14-1 **Standard 12-Lead Views**

Leads	Portion of Heart Viewed	Coronary Artery and Branch
II, III, aVF	Inferior wall of left ventricle	Right coronary—Marginal branch
V1 & V2	Septal wall	Left coronary—Septal branch
V3 & V4	Anterior wall of left ventricle	Left coronary—Left anterior descending branch
I, aVL, V5, & V6	Lateral wall of left ventricle	Left coronary—Left circumflex branch

Figure 14-1 Typically, a 12-Lead ECG focuses on the left ventricle but considers the heart from slightly different angles.

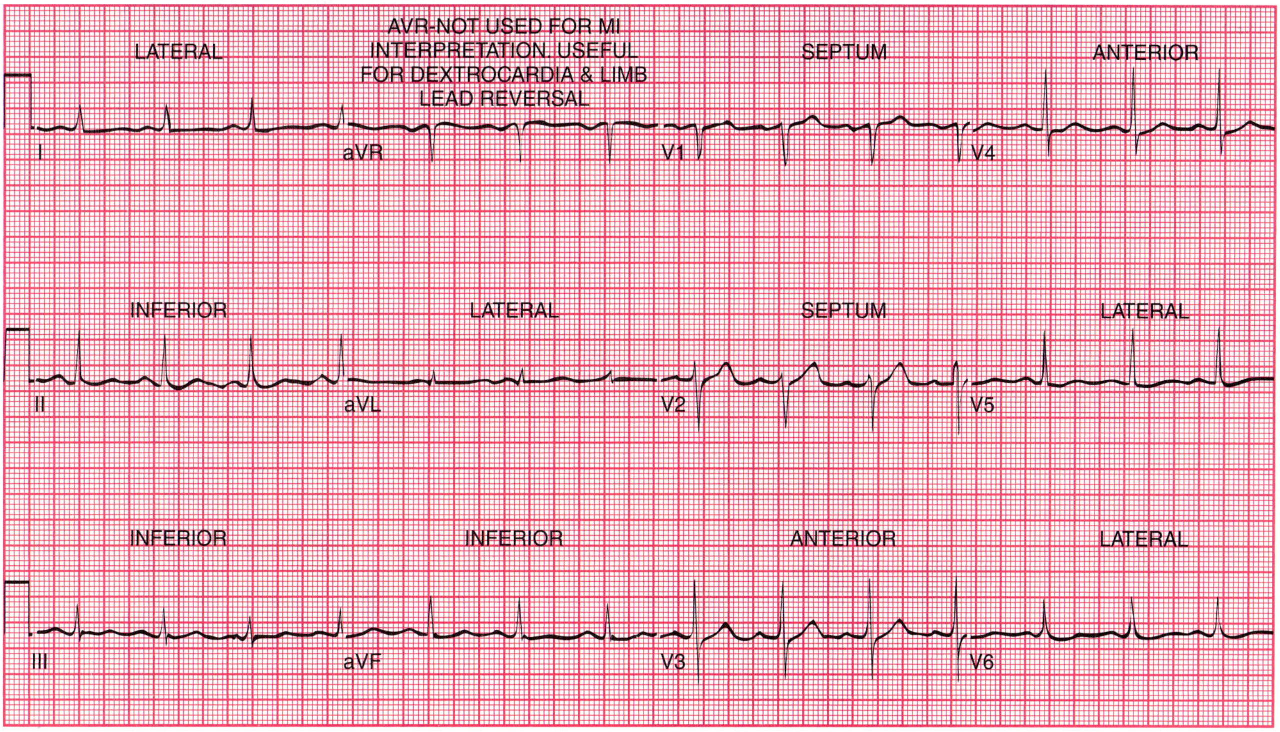

Checkpoint Question (LO 14.1)

1. Why do you think a doctor may order a right-side or posterior 12-lead ECG?

____

____

Figure 14-2 Coronary circulation as it relates to specific portions of the myocardium.

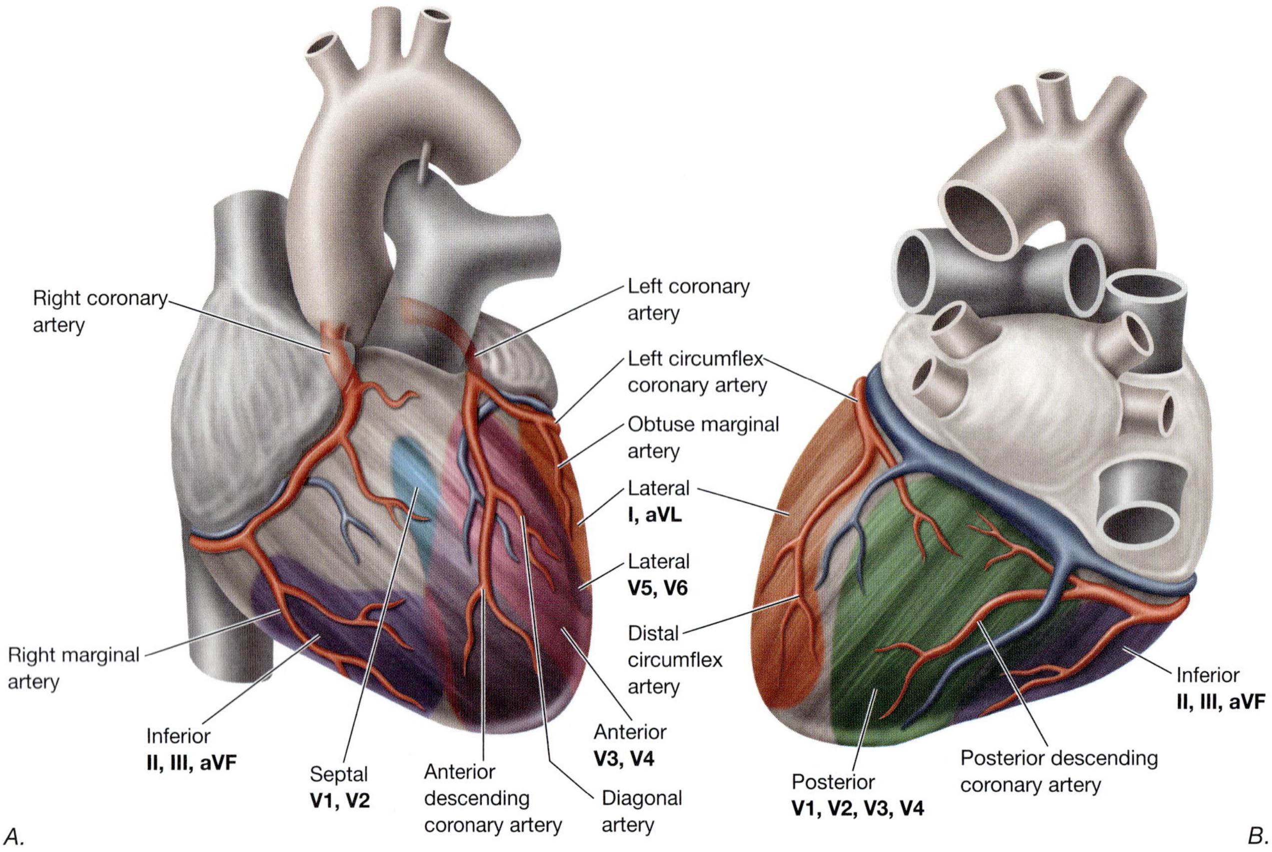

Figure 14-3 Inferior infarction. *A.* Anterior view. *B.* Posterior view.

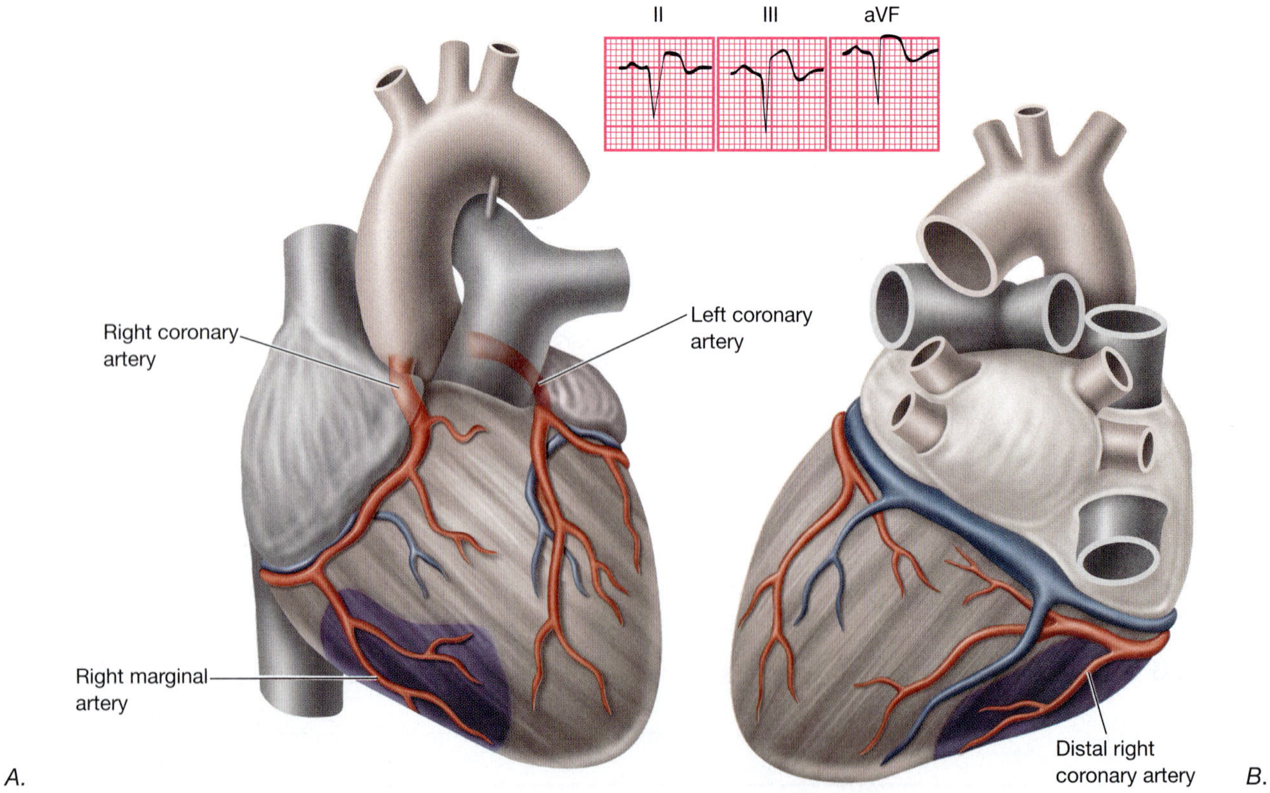

Figure 14-4 Lateral infarction. *A.* Anterior view. *B.* Posterior view.

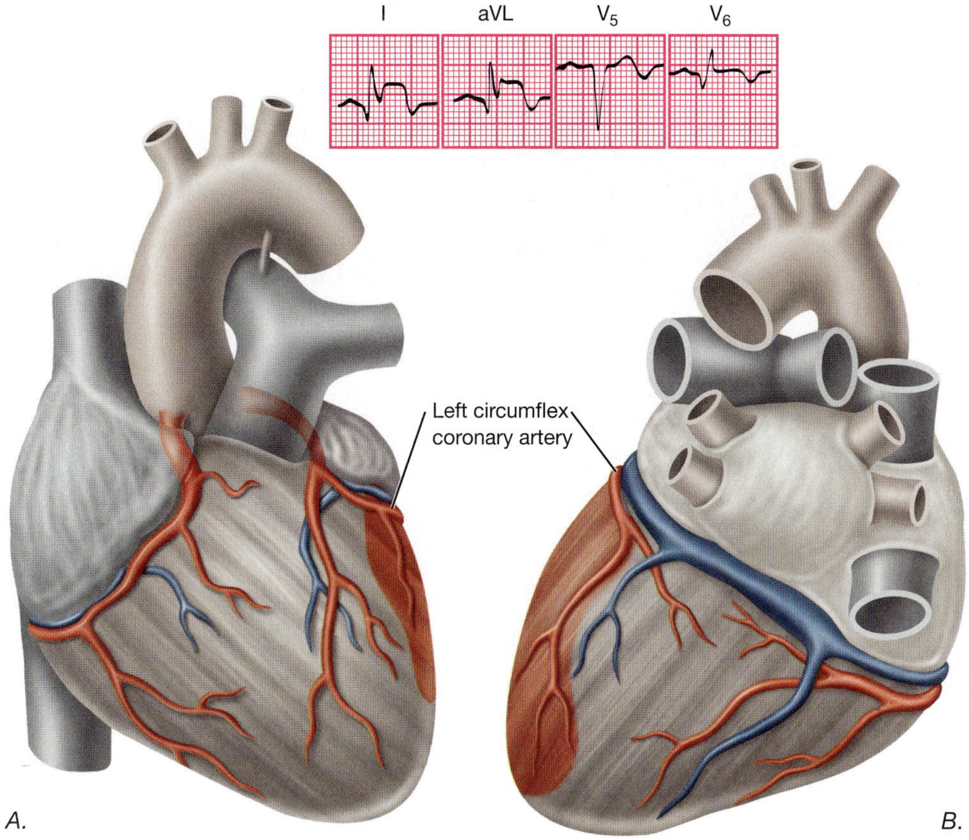

Figure 14-5 Septal infarction.

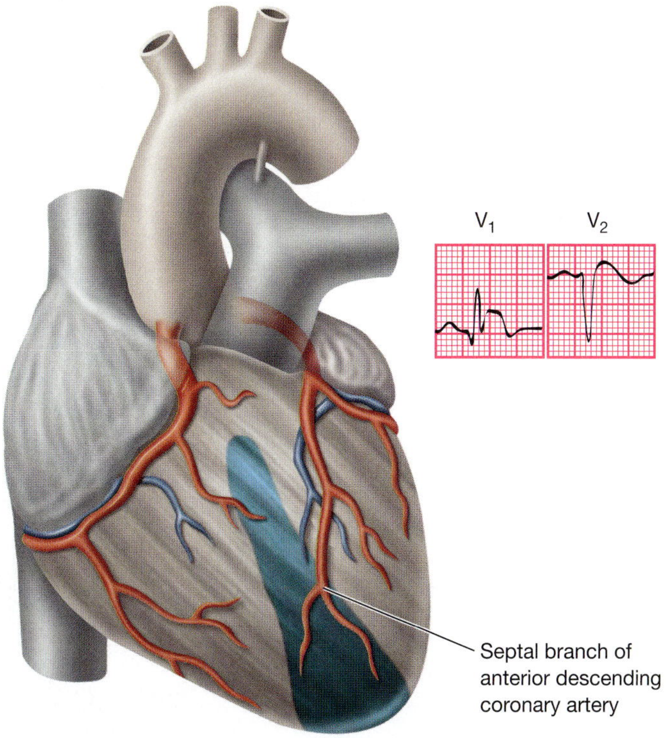

Figure 14-6 Anterior infarction.

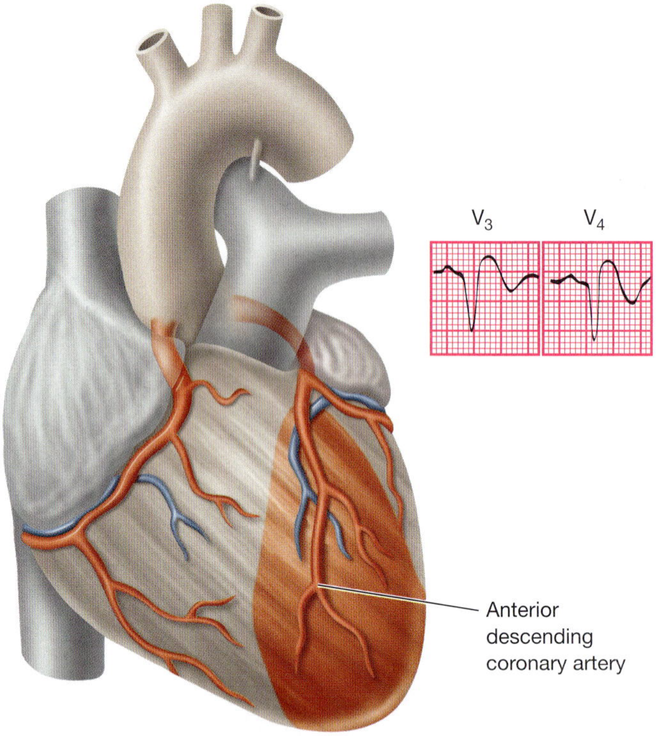

Figure 14-7 Posterior infarction. A posterior wall infarction may result from occlusion of the posterior descending artery, which is formed by the right coronary artery in 90% of the population. Much less frequently, occlusion of the distal portion of the left circumflex artery (10% of the population) may also cause a posterior wall MI.

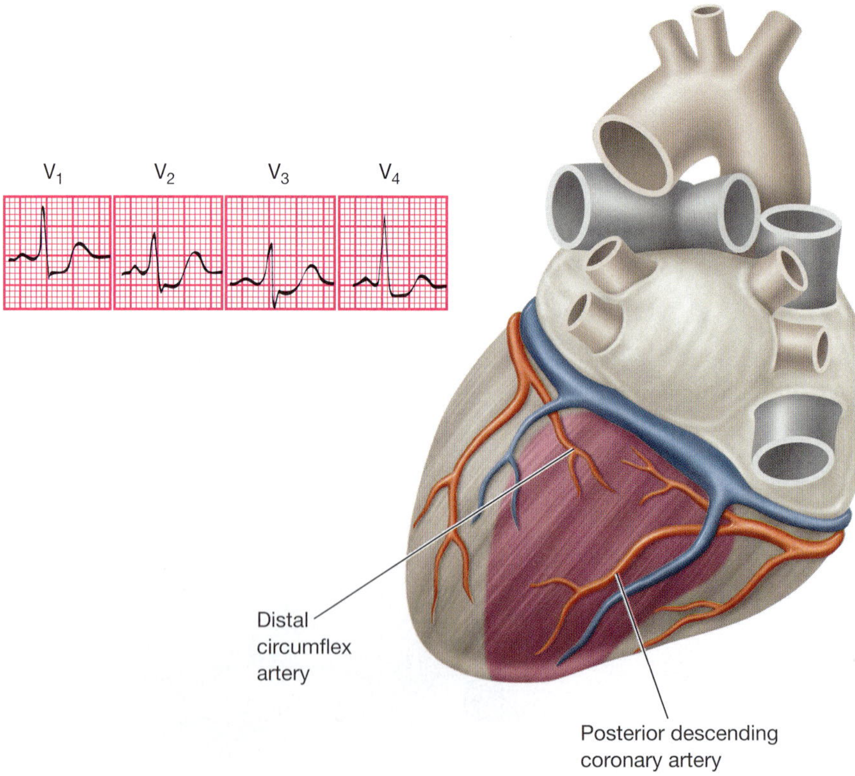

14.2 Ischemia, Injury, and Infarction

When learning how to interpret a rhythm strip, a specific five-step process is followed regardless of how complicated the dysrhythmia may be. In this chapter you will still use the five steps, but you will add two more steps to the process. Presented here are the basics for you to build your skill and competence quickly.

It is important that you get into the habit of analyzing the 12-lead ECG the same way each time. Begin with the five-step process. Recall from the chapter *Rhythm Strip Interpretation and Sinus Rhythms:*

Step 1: Determine the ECG rhythm or regularity.

Step 2: Determine the atrial and ventricular rate.

Step 3: Identify the P wave morphology.

Step 4: Measure the PR interval.

Step 5: Measure the QRS duration and analyze the morphology.

After following the first five steps, view the leads in groups, looking at the same part of the heart and reading from left to right. Focus on ischemia, injury, and infarction; these often cause morphologic changes to the cardiac complexes. Ischemia and injury often cause a delay in repolarization. This delay is represented by ST segment depression or elevation (Figure 14-8). Recall that the ST segment is normally in line with the isoelectric line or baseline.

Think of ischemia, injury, and infarction as a dangerous continuum of worsening cardiac conditions when blood flow to the myocardium is decreased or interrupted for even a few minutes. When seen in two or more anatomically contiguous leads, ST segment depression of 1 mm or more is

Figure 14-8 12-lead ECG with ST deviation.

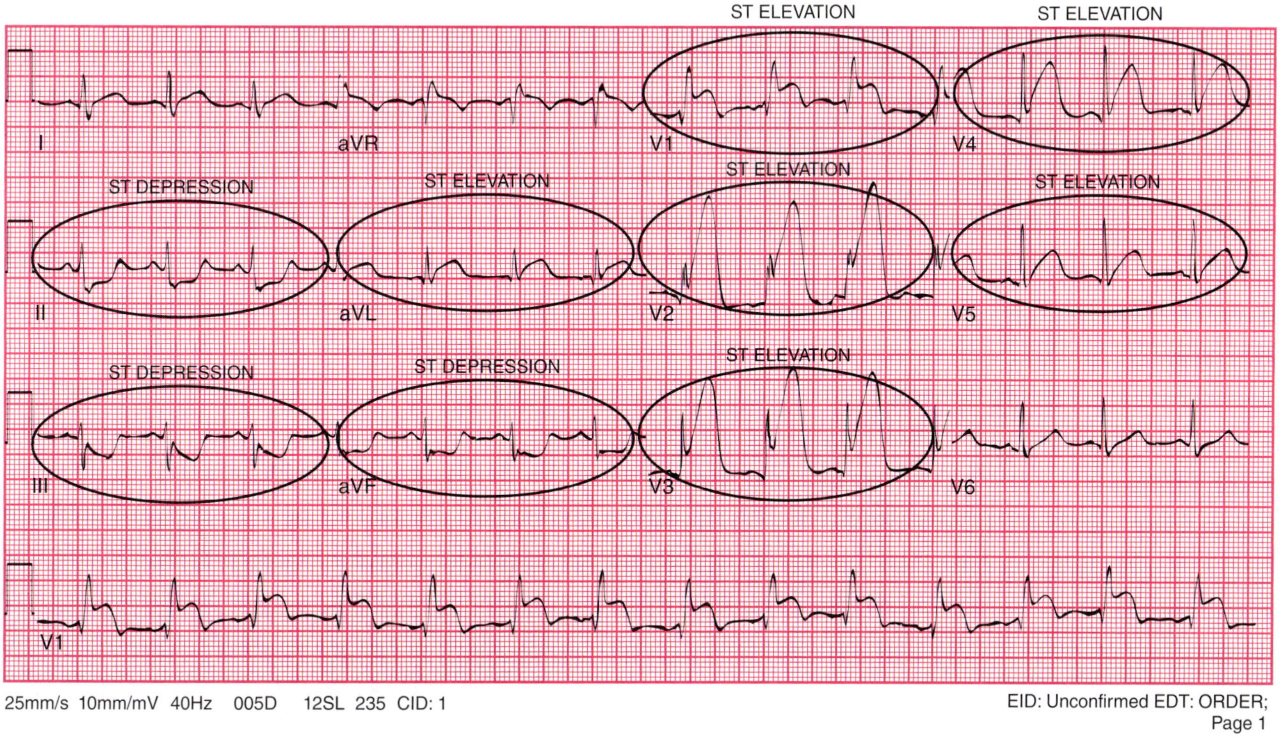

myocardial ischemia A reduction or interruption in blood flow and oxygen to the myocardium for a short period of time.

anatomically contiguous lead Two or more leads looking at the same part of the heart, or numerically consecutive chest leads.

indicative of **myocardial ischemia.** An **anatomically contiguous lead** is defined as two or more leads "looking" at the same part of the heart, or numerically consecutive chest leads. For example, leads II and III look at the inferior wall of the left ventricle, and V3 and V4 are numerically consecutive chest leads that look at the anterior wall of the left ventricle. Examples of anatomically contiguous leads include:

- II, III, aVF
- I, aVL
- V1, V2, V3, V4, V5, V6 (Figure 14-9)

When analyzing the ST segment, it is important to compare the PR segment, ST segment, and TP segment. This will provide you with information about the segments before and after the ST segment. This step is critical for the purpose of analysis. Taking a straight-edge or cardiac ruler and lining up the segments will assist in identifying any deviation of the ST segment from the isoelectric line.

Another indicator of ischemia is T wave inversion. T waves are normally a positively deflected waveform. In some cases of ischemia, the T wave becomes negatively deflected, or inverted. T wave inversion may be seen by itself, as shown in Figure 14-10, but most often T wave inversion is seen with concurrent ST segment elevation (Figure 14-11).

Myocardial ischemia occurs when there is a reduction or interruption in blood flow and oxygen to the myocardium for just a short period. If this reduction or interruption of blood flow persists for more than a few minutes, the affected myocardium enters a more serious state referred to as **myocardial injury.** ST segment elevation is morphologic evidence of acute injury pattern. ST segment elevation of 1 mm or more that is seen in two or more anatomically contiguous leads is indicative of myocardial injury. ST segment elevation may be accompanied by T wave inversion.

myocardial injury Injury to the cardiac muscle caused by prolonged reduction or interruption of blood flow.

Figure 14-9 Anatomically contiguous leads are two leads that are numerically consecutive or look at the same part of the heart. For example, leads V3 and V4 are numerically consecutive and look at the anterior wall of the left ventricle.

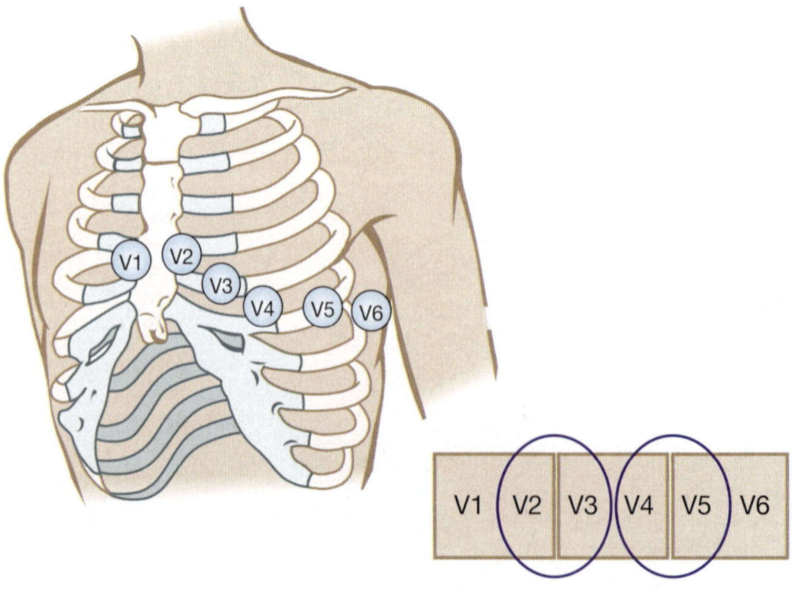

Figure 14-10 T wave inversion.

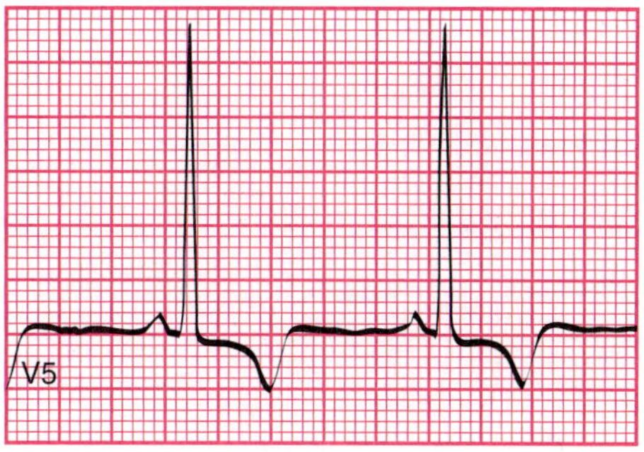

Figure 14-11 T wave inversion with ST elevation.

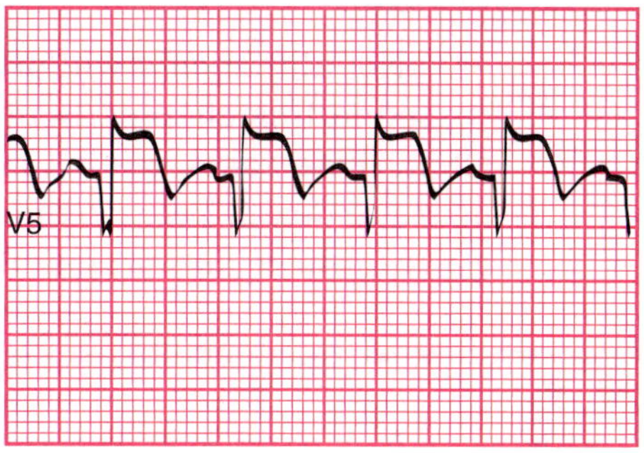

When ST segment elevation is seen on a 12-lead ECG, it is referred to as *myocardial injury, acute injury pattern*, or *acute MI (AMI). When you see ST elevation, it means the problem is happening right now, and the tissue is* ***not*** *dead yet!* It is in that state between ischemic and dead—"stunned" would be a good way to describe it. Unless immediate and effective intervention is established, the tissue soon will begin to die.

Evidence of tissue death (infarction) is often seen as a change in the width and/or depth of the Q wave. A normal or **physiologic Q wave** (Figure 14-12*A*) is defined as one in which the width measures less than 0.04 second and the depth measures less than one-third of the height of the R wave in that lead.

physiologic Q wave A normal Q wave, measuring less than 0.04 second in duration and less than 1/3 the height of the R wave in that lead.

pathologic Q wave A Q wave that measures 0.04 second or wider in duration and/or is 1/3 or more the height of the R wave in that lead.

myocardial infarction (MI; heart attack) Damage to the heart muscle caused by lack of oxygen due to a blockage of one or more of the coronary arteries.

The change in the shape of the Q wave as a result of tissue death (infarction) is called a *pathologic Q wave.* A **pathologic Q wave** (Figure 14-12*B*) is defined as measuring 0.04 second in duration and/or greater than or equal to one-third the height of the R wave in that lead tracing. This indicates tissue death. Pathologic Q waves seen in two or more anatomically contiguous leads indicate that some of the tissue in that part of the heart is now dead (**myocardial infarction**). Note, however, that an absence of Q waves does not eliminate the possibility of myocardial infarction.

(infarcted = tissue necrosis = tissue death)

Many factors combine to determine how dangerous the infarction will be and the potential for recovery. Factors include the involved coronary artery or arteries, location and extent of the infarction, vital structures involved, and time, just to name a few.

When viewing a 12-lead ECG, you should look for the changes (ST depression, ST elevation, T wave inversion, and pathologic Q wave as just described). However, it is most important to know that these changes must be seen in at least two anatomically contiguous leads in order to qualify as indicators of ischemia, injury, or infarction.

Figure 14-12 Q waves. *A.* Physiologic Q wave. *B.* Pathologic Q wave.

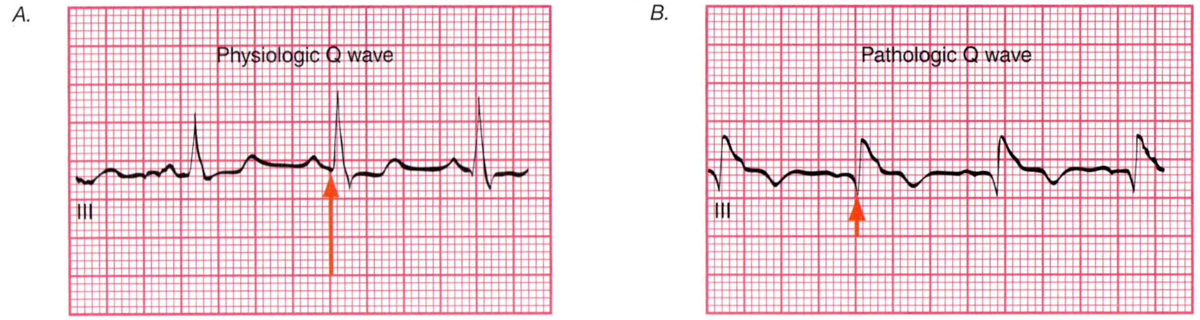

Not all patients will present with the classic morphologic changes discussed in this chapter. Some patients will not present with any changes at all. In these cases, testing is necessary to determine the presence of muscle injury or death. Refer to the chapter *Clinical Presentation and Management of the Cardiac Patient* for more information about these tests.

Safety & Infection Control

ST Segment Elevation

Not every instance of ST segment elevation is indicative of myocardial injury. Time, experience, and further training will help you learn what those instances are. The bottom line is the safety of the patient. ST segment elevation of any kind must *always* be reported.

Checkpoint Questions (LO 14.2)

1. Consider wandering baseline. Why is it important to eliminate this type of artifact from a 12-lead tracing?

____

____

2. Define myocardial ischemia.

____

____

3. What morphologic change provides evidence of myocardial injury?

____

____

4. Describe anatomically contiguous leads.

____

____

5. What is a pathologic Q wave?

____

____

14.3 Electrical Axis

axis deviation Changes that occur on a 12-lead ECG due to the orientation or position of the heart within the chest.

hypertrophy Abnormal thickening of the ventricular wall due to chronic pressure overload; often caused by hypertension.

Electrical **axis deviation** refers to the changes that occur on the 12-lead ECG as a result of the position of the heart within the patient's chest. When the heart is not in its normal location, the deflection of the QRS complex will reflect this abnormality. If you imagine a circle divided into four large, equal quadrants superimposed over a person's chest, the patient's heart would normally be located in the lower left quadrant (Figure 14-13).

Several things may cause the heart to become displaced from its normal location. Displacement of the heart is often seen in conditions such as pregnancy, birth defects, and left ventricular hypertrophy. During pregnancy, the large third-trimester fetus temporarily displaces the heart toward the upper left quadrant. In the case of pregnancy, once the baby is delivered, the heart typically returns to the normal location. With congenital defects, the heart may be permanently displaced. Left ventricular **hypertrophy** is abnormal thickening of the ventricular wall due to chronic pressure overload. Over time the heart may become displaced toward the upper left quadrant.

Axis deviation may be to either the left or right. Left axis deviation is the most common. Other types of deviation are less common but do occur. Table 14-2 provides examples.

Axis deviation changes the direction of ventricular depolarization. A simple way to determine the presence of axis deviation is to refer to leads I and aVF. When "normal," both of these leads have a predominantly positive QRS complex. If either or both of these leads have a prominently negative ventricular depolarization, the electrical axis is considered abnormal. Focus

Figure 14-13 Quadrants used to identify axis deviation.

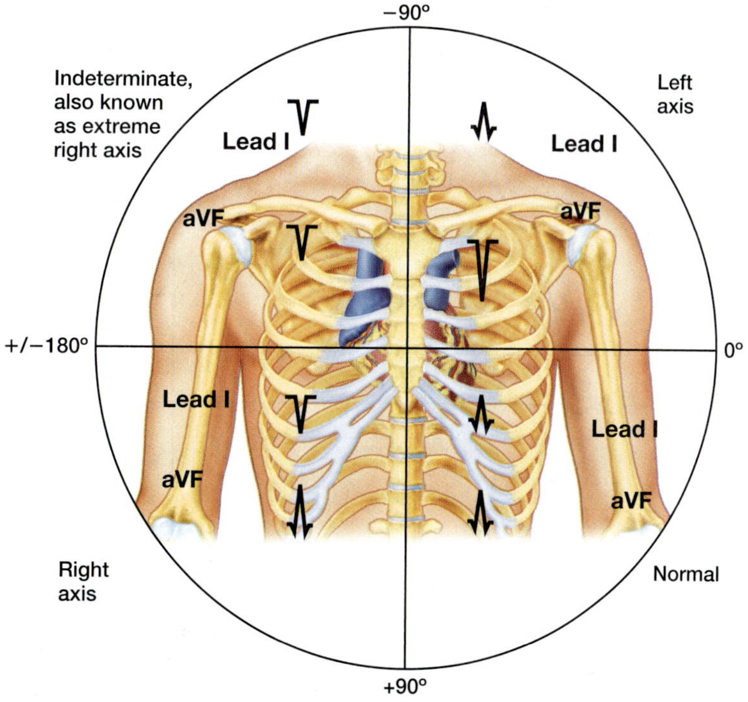

TABLE 14-2 Causes of Axis Deviation

Deviation	Possible Cause
Left axis deviation (most common)	Left ventricular hypertrophy Pregnancy Obesity Emphysema Hyperkalemia
Right axis deviation	Right ventricular hypertrophy Anterolateral wall MI *Note:* Right axis deviation is considered normal in children and tall, thin adults.
Extreme right axis deviation (referred to as indeterminate, NW territory, or No Man's Land)	Situs transversus or dextrocardia (the heart is on the right side of the chest) Pacemaker rhythms COPD patients Hyperkalemia *Note:* Extreme right axis deviation may also indicate lead reversal.

on the QRS complex when referring to leads I and aVF. Review Figure 14-14 and use these steps.

Step One: If lead I is positive and aVF is also positive, the axis is said to be "normal."

Step Two: If lead I is positive and aVF is negative, the patient has left axis deviation.

Step Three: If lead I is negative and aVF is positive, the patient has right axis deviation.

Step Four: If lead I is negative and aVF is also negative, the patient has extreme right axis deviation (also referred to as indeterminate).

Figure 14-14 Axis deviation.

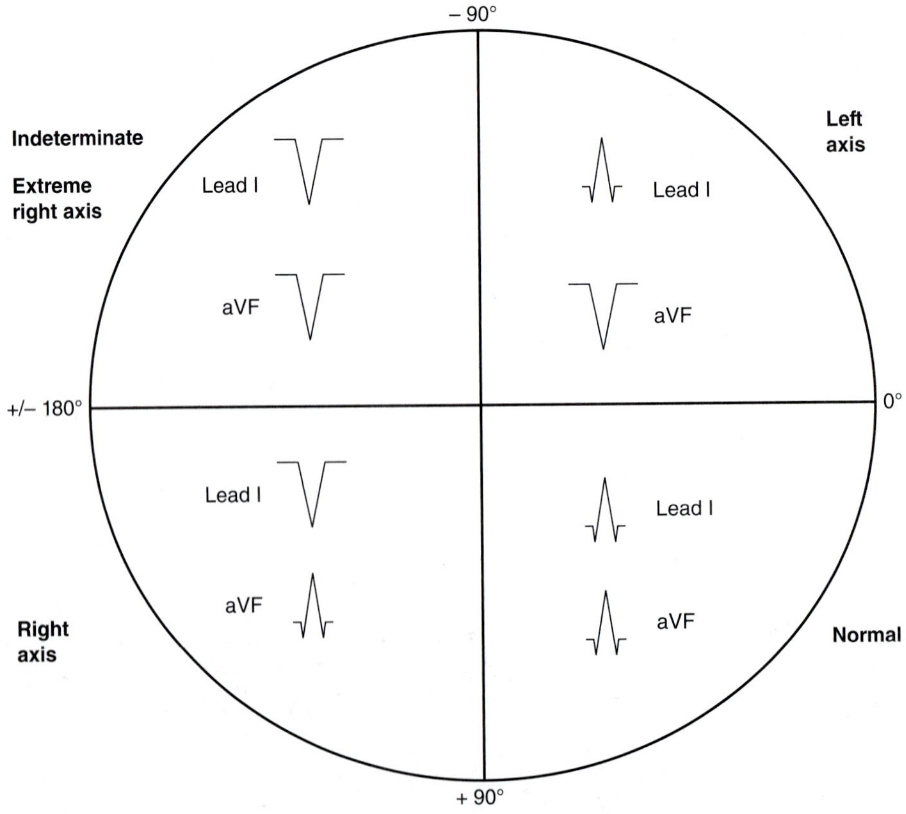

Checkpoint Questions (LO 14.3)

1. What are the two leads we refer to when determining the presence of axis deviation?

____

____

2. When determining the electrical axis, on which portion of the cardiac complex should attention be focused?

____

____

3. Use the two views below from the 12-lead ECG tracing to determine the electrical axis.

____

____

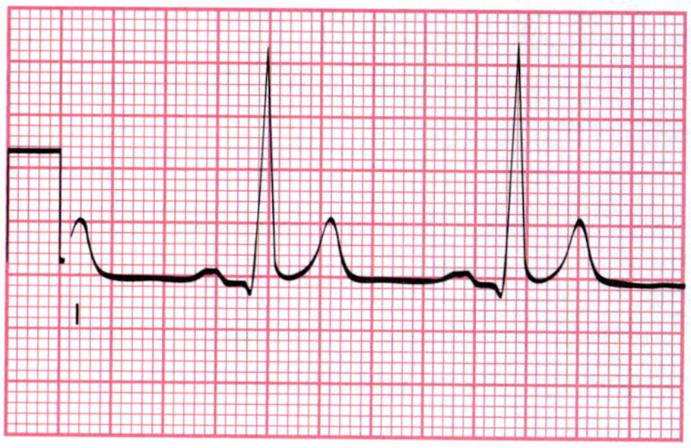

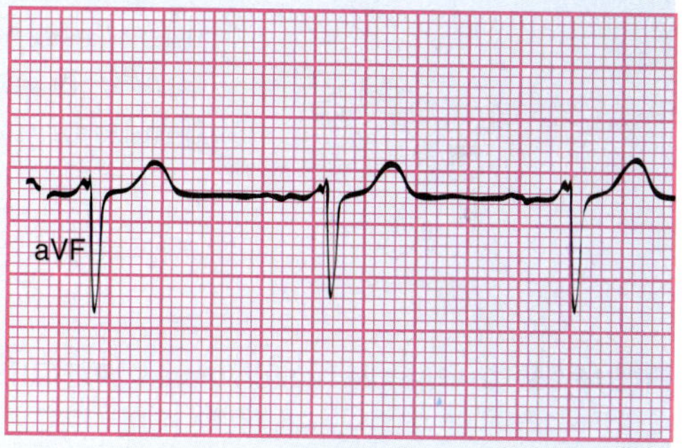

14.4 Bundle Branch Block

As you should know, bundle branch blocks occur when one or both of the ventricular pathways are damaged or delayed due to congenital defects, cardiac disease, drugs, or other conditions (including MI). It is important to realize that bundle branch block alone is typically not considered life threatening. Many people are born with BBB every day and do not even know they have it until much later in life. What *can* can be life threatening is the cause of the BBB, such as myocardial infarction. The development of BBB during MI is cause for significant concern. When an area of one of the bundle branches is damaged, electrical current cannot travel through that tissue to reach the myocardial tissue in its usual fashion. Current travels down the good bundle and activates the myocardial tissue in that corresponding ventricle only. The other ventricle must then receive the impulse as current travels from one cell to the next until the entire myocardial contraction occurs. The cell will not contract until the next cell delivers the energy. Current traveling via the abnormal pathways takes longer to achieve the full ventricular contraction. The increased length of time is reflected in a wider than normal QRS duration (0.12 second or greater). Remember that the QRS duration is a measurement of how long it takes for current to travel through ventricular myocardial tissue.

Characteristics of the right and left bundle branch blocks will be similar over monitoring leads I, II, and III. Specific characteristics of the right or left bundle branch will be present when monitoring with leads V1 to V6. Although bundle branch block is seen in the precordial leads, to distinguish RBBB from LBBB, lead V1 is referenced (Figure 14-15). If the QRS is positively deflected, it is RBBB. RBBB often has a classic RSR pattern in V1 and is often referred to as "bunny ears" or "bunny branch block." If the QRS is negative or a QS complex is present, it is an LBBB. A **QS complex** is a deep Q/S wave with no preceding R wave.

QS complex A deep Q/S wave with no preceding R wave. Can indicate a left bundle branch block.

When analyzing V1 to determine the presence of bundle branch block, look for the following:

1. Evidence of atrial activity (P wave). Remember, the problem is within the ventricles, so we must see a P wave to tell us that the electrical activity was initiated above the ventricles.
2. QRS complex that measures 0.12 second or more in duration.

The question now becomes "which direction is the QRS going and how do you determine this?" Starting at the J point of the QRS, move backward into the ventricular depolarization. If it is going down (negative), it is a left bundle branch block (Figure 14-16*A*). If it is going up (positive), it is a right bundle branch block (Figure 14-16*B*).

Figure 14-15 Bundle branch blocks. *A.* RBBB. Note that the QRS is positively deflected. *B.* LBBB. Note that either the QRS is negative or a QS complex is present.

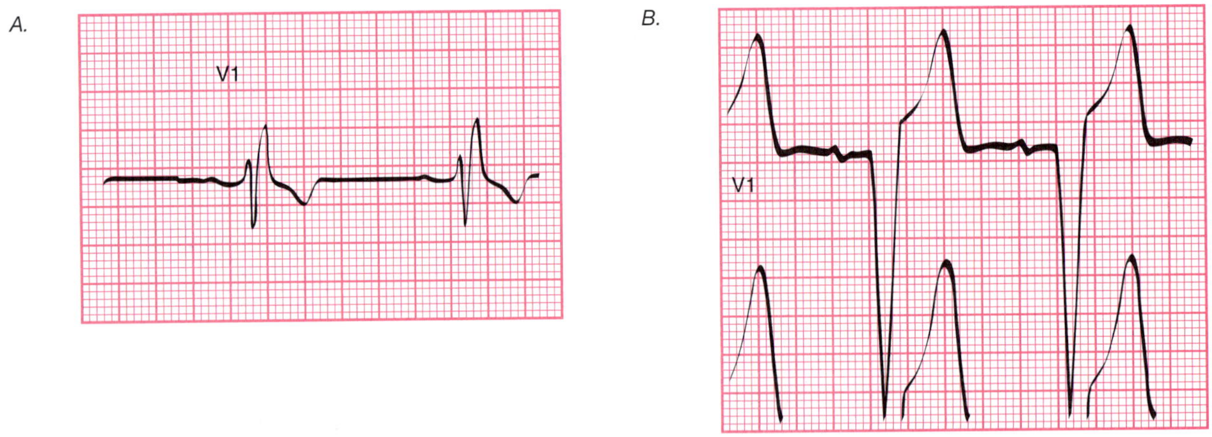

Figure 14-16 Bundle branch blocks. *A.* Left bundle branch block (LBBB). *B.* Right bundle branch block (RBBB). Note the arrow direction in A and B.

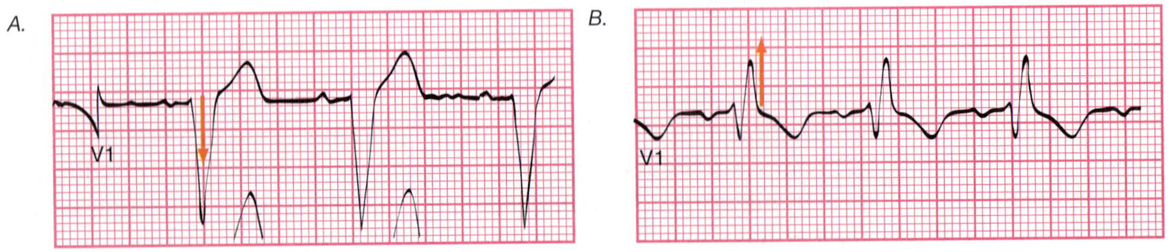

Checkpoint Questions (LO 14.4)

1. Review the following tracings, identify the type of BBB, and then explain how you determined your answers.

   a. ______________________________

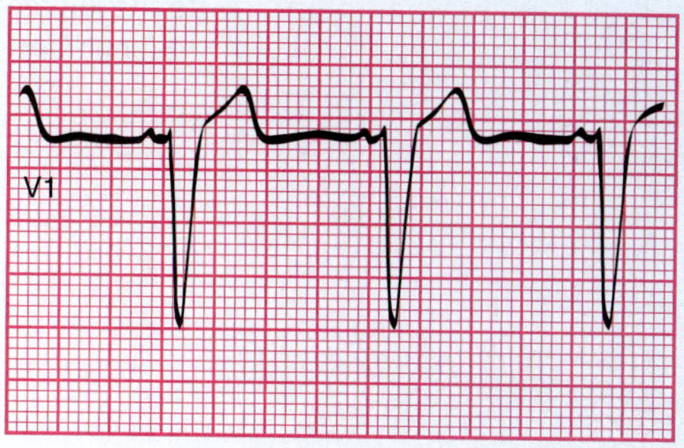

   b. ______________________________

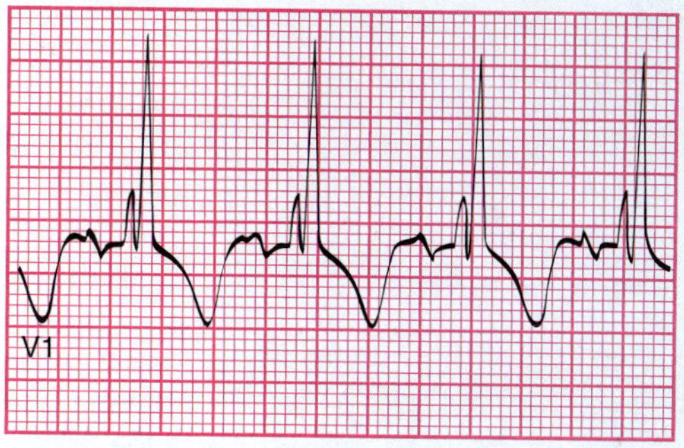

14.5 Left Ventricular Hypertrophy

As discussed earlier, left ventricular hypertrophy (LVH) is the thickening of the ventricular wall due to chronic pressure overload. The effort the heart must exert in order to maintain normal cardiac output is increased due to increased peripheral vascular resistance. This is the same process that would occur if you went to the gym every day and lifted weights: Over time, your muscles would become thicker. As the wall thickens, the depth and height of the ventricular depolarization will increase. More muscle equals more electricity, which is shown as greater amplitude of the QRS complex. This means taller and deeper ventricular depolarization waves will be seen.

When determining the presence of left ventricular hypertrophy, follow these steps (Figure 14-17).

1. Refer to V1 and V2. Select and measure the deeper of the two views. Measure from the isoelectric line down to the tip of the deepest QS complex, count the millimeters, and write down this number.
2. Refer to V5 and V6. Select and measure the taller of the two views. Measure from the isoelectric line to the tip of the tallest R wave, then count the number of millimeters and write it down.
3. Add the two numbers together. If they add up to 35 or more millimeters, clinically you would suspect left ventricular hypertrophy.

Figure 14-17 Assessing for the presence of left ventricular hypertrophy.

A.

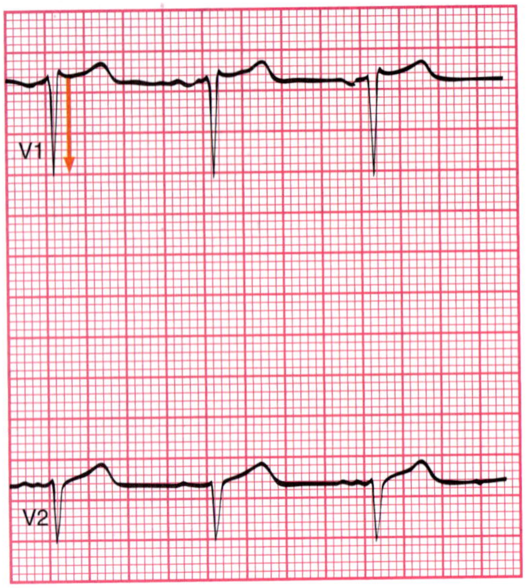

Step 1: Analyze V1 and V2. Measure from the isoelectric line down to the tip of the deepest QS complex. The image to the left measures 12 mm. Write down that number. — 12 mm

B.

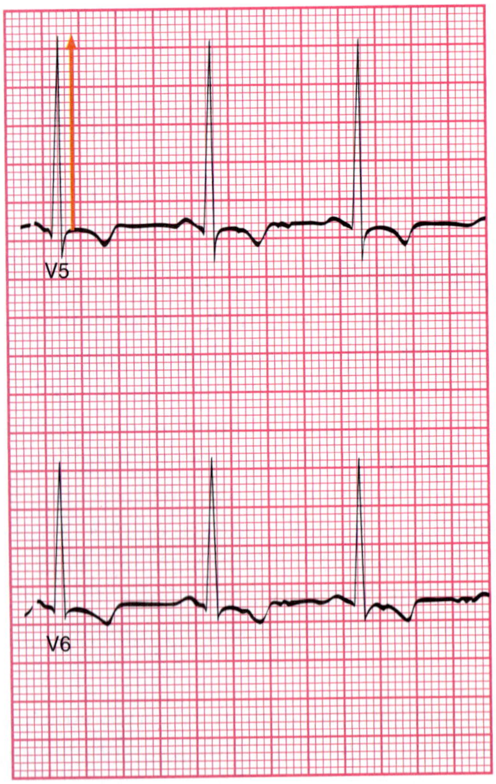

Step 2: Analyze V5 and V6. Measure from the isoelectric line up to the tip of the tallest R wave. The image to the left measures 24 mm. Write down that number. — 24 mm

Step 3: Combine the deepest QS complex measurement with the tallest R wave measurement. If the numbers measure 35 mm or greater when combined, clinically you must suspect left ventricular hypertrophy. — 12 + 24 = 36 mm

Checkpoint Question (LO 14.5)

1. Review the following tracing. Do you suspect left ventricular hypertrophy? Explain how you determined your answer.

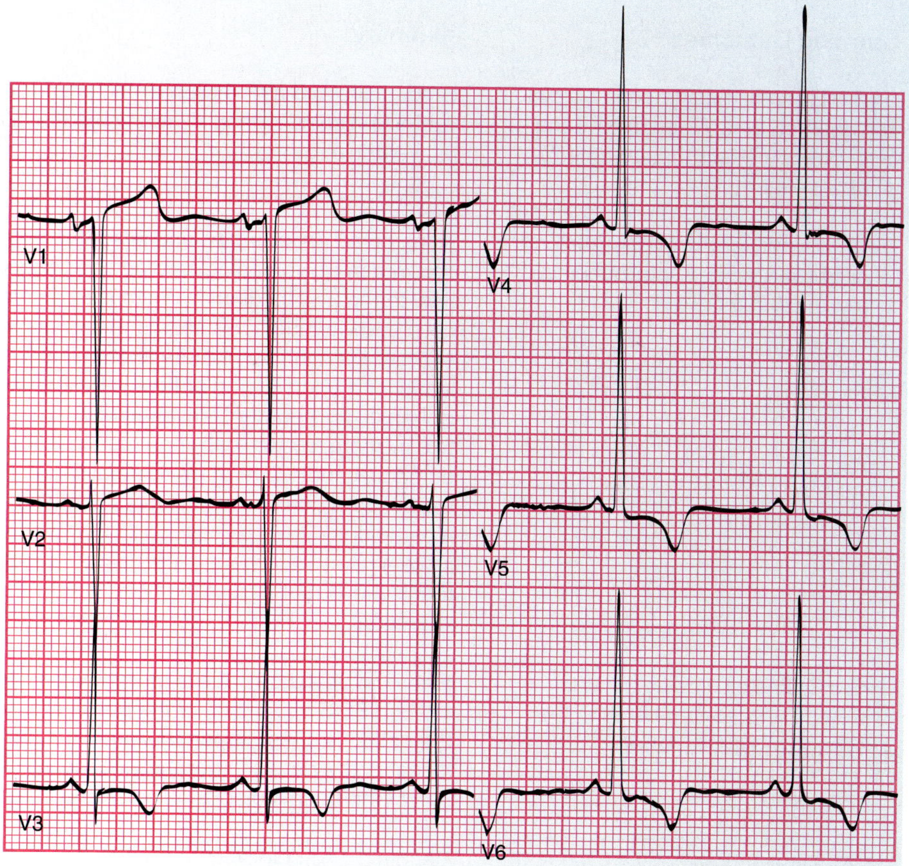

____

____

Chapter Summary

Learning Outcomes	Summary	Pages
14.1 Discuss the anatomical views represented on a 12-lead ECG and the coronary artery that commonly supplies that region of tissue.	Leads II, III, and aVF represent the inferior wall of the left ventricle. Leads V1 and V2 represent the lateral wall of the left ventricle.	334–338
14.2 Identify common morphologic changes associated with ischemia, injury, and infarction.	Think of ischemia, injury, and infarction as a dangerous continuum of worsening cardiac condition when blood flow to the myocardium is decreased or interrupted for even a few minutes. ST segment depression of 1 mm or more seen in two or more anatomically contiguous leads for a short period of time is indicative of myocardial ischemia. ST segment elevation of 1 mm or more seen in two or more anatomically contiguous leads for a longer duration is indicative of myocardial injury. The change in the shape of the Q wave as a result of tissue death is called a pathologic Q wave. Pathologic Q waves seen in two or more anatomically contiguous leads indicate that some of the tissue in that part of the heart is now dead (myocardial infarction).	339–342
14.3 Define axis deviation and the steps utilized to determine the presence of axis deviation.	Electrical deviation causes morphologic changes within the 12-lead ECG as a result of the position of the heart within the patient's chest. When the heart is not in its normal location, the deflection of the QRS complex changes to reflect the heart's displacement in the chest.	343–345
14.4 Differentiate between left and right bundle branch blocks and how they relate to the 12-lead ECG.	Bundle branch blocks occur when one or both of the ventricular pathways are damaged or delayed due to congenital defects, cardiac disease, drugs, or other conditions. The electrical current will not be able to travel through that tissue to reach the myocardial tissue in its usual fashion. The increased length of time is reflected in a wider than normal QRS duration (0.12 second or greater). Refer to lead V1 to differentiate between right and left BBB. • LBBB presents with a P wave and a QS complex measuring 0.12 second or more. • RBBB presents with a P wave and an R wave that often has two points, or "bunny ears." It also measures 0.12 second or more in duration.	345–347
14.5 Describe left ventricular hypertrophy (LVH) and the steps to determine the presence of LVH.	Left ventricular hypertrophy is an abnormal thickening of the ventricular wall due to pumping against increased vascular resistance over a period of time. As the wall thickens, the depth and height of the ventricular depolarization will increase. More muscle equals more electricity and thereby greater amplitude of the QRS complex. This means taller and deeper ventricular depolarizations will be seen.	347–349

Chapter Review

Matching

Match the terms on the left with their definitions on the right.

_______ **1.** axis deviation (LO 14.3)

_______ **2.** contiguous leads (LO 14.3)

_______ **3.** hypertrophy (LO 14.5)

_______ **4.** myocardial infarction (LO 14.2)

_______ **5.** myocardial injury (LO 14.2)

_______ **6.** myocardial ischemia (LO 14.2)

_______ **7.** pathologic Q wave (LO 14.3)

_______ **8.** physiologic Q wave (LO 14.3)

_______ **9.** right marginal branch (LO 14.1)

a. abnormal thickening

b. reduction or interruption in blood flow and oxygen to the myocardium

c. measuring 0.04 second and/or greater than or equal to one-third the height of the R wave

d. supplies blood to both surfaces of the right ventricle

e. tissue death in the heart muscle

f. measures less than 0.04 second, and the depth measures less than one-third of the height of the R wave

g. ST segment elevation of 1 mm or more seen in two or more anatomically contiguous leads over a prolonged period

h. ECG changes due to the position of the heart

i. looks at the same part of the heart or numerically consecutive leads

Multiple Choice

Circle the correct answer.

10. Which leads look at the lateral wall of the left ventricle? (LO 14.1)

a. II, III, and aVF

b. V1 and V2

c. V3 and V4

d. I, aVL, V5, and V6

11. Which leads look at the septal wall of the left ventricle? (LO 14.1)

a. II, III, and aVF

b. V1 and V2

c. V3 and V4

d. I, aVL, V5, and V6

12. Which leads look at the inferior wall of the left ventricle? (LO 14.1)
 a. II, III, and aVF
 b. V1 and V2
 c. V3 and V4
 d. I, aVL, V5, and V6

13. Which leads look at the anterior wall of the left ventricle? (LO 14.1)
 a. II, III, and aVF
 b. V1 and V2
 c. V3 and V4
 d. I, aVL, V5, and V6

14. Which major coronary artery and vessel supply the inferior wall of the left ventricle? (LO 14.1)
 a. Left main and circumflex artery
 b. Left main and left anterior descending
 c. Left main and septal
 d. Right main and right acute marginal branch

15. Which major coronary artery and vessel supply the septal wall of the left ventricle? (LO 14.1)
 a. Left main and circumflex artery
 b. Left main and left anterior descending
 c. Left main and septal
 d. Right main and right acute marginal branch

16. Which major coronary artery and vessel supply the lateral wall of the left ventricle? (LO 14.1)
 a. Left main and circumflex artery
 b. Left main and left anterior descending
 c. Right main and septal
 d. Right main and right acute marginal branch

17. Which major coronary artery and vessel supply the anterior wall of the left ventricle? (LO 14.1)
 a. Left main and circumflex artery
 b. Left main and left anterior descending
 c. Right main and septal
 d. Right main and right acute marginal branch

18. Signs of myocardial ischemia may include (LO 14.2)
 a. ST segment elevation.
 b. ST segment depression only.
 c. ST segment depression and T wave inversion.
 d. pathologic Q wave.

19. Signs of myocardial injury may include (LO 14.2)
 a. ST segment elevation.
 b. ST segment depression only.
 c. ST segment depression and T wave inversion.
 d. pathologic Q wave.

20. Which of the following is the most common sign on a 12-lead ECG that an infarction has occurred? (LO 14.2)
 a. ST segment elevation.
 b. ST segment depression only.
 c. ST segment depression and T wave inversion.
 d. pathologic Q wave.

21. What two views are referred to when determining electrical axis? (LO 14.3)
   a. V1 and V2
   b. V3 and V4
   c. I and aVF
   d. III and aVR

22. When determining axis deviation, if lead I and lead aVF both have predominantly positive QRS complexes, the patient has (LO 14.3)
   a. normal axis.
   b. left axis deviation.
   c. right axis deviation.
   d. extreme right axis deviation.

23. When determining axis deviation, if the QRS complex in lead I is predominantly negative and the QRS in lead aVF is predominantly positive, the patient has (LO 14.3)
   a. normal axis.
   b. left axis deviation.
   c. right axis deviation.
   d. extreme right axis deviation.

24. When determining axis deviation, if lead I and lead aVF both have predominantly negative QRS complexes, the patient has (LO 14.3)
   a. normal axis.
   b. left axis deviation.
   c. right axis deviation.
   d. extreme right axis deviation.

25. When determining axis deviation, if the QRS complex in lead I is predominantly positive and the QRS in lead aVF is predominantly negative, the patient has (LO 14.3)
   a. normal axis.
   b. left axis deviation.
   c. right axis deviation.
   d. extreme right axis deviation.

26. Which leads are referred to when analyzing a 12-lead ECG for the presence of left ventricular hypertrophy? (LO 14.5)
   a. V2, V3, V5, and V6
   b. I, aVL, II, and III
   c. V1, V2, V5, and V6
   d. I, aVL, aVR, and V4

27. When totaled, how many millimeters is the minimum necessary to clinically suspect hypertrophy? (LO 14.5)
   a. 3
   b. 5
   c. 35
   d. 350

28. Which of the following most accurately describes the difference between LBBB and RBBB when viewing lead V1? (LO 14.4)
   a. The QRS complex is less than 0.12 second for RBBB and greater than 0.12 second for LBBB.
   b. The QRS complex is positive for LBBB and negative for RBBB.
   c. The QRS complex is negative for LBBB and positive for RBBB.
   d. The QRS complex is greater than 0.12 second for RBBB and less than 0.12 second for LBBB.

39. Identify the location of the AMI on this 12-lead ECG, and explain your answer. (LO 14.2)

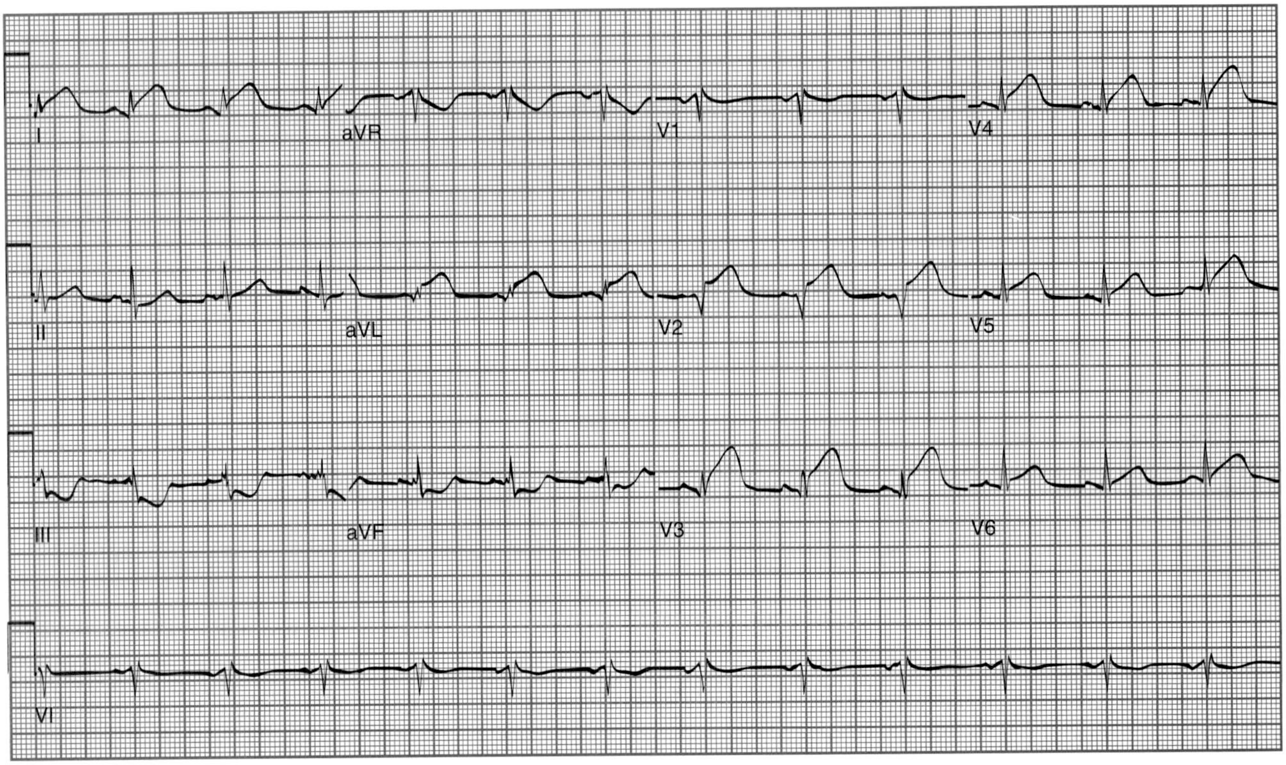

25mm/s 10mm/mV 150Hz

40. Identify the electrical axis, and explain your answer. (LO 14.3)

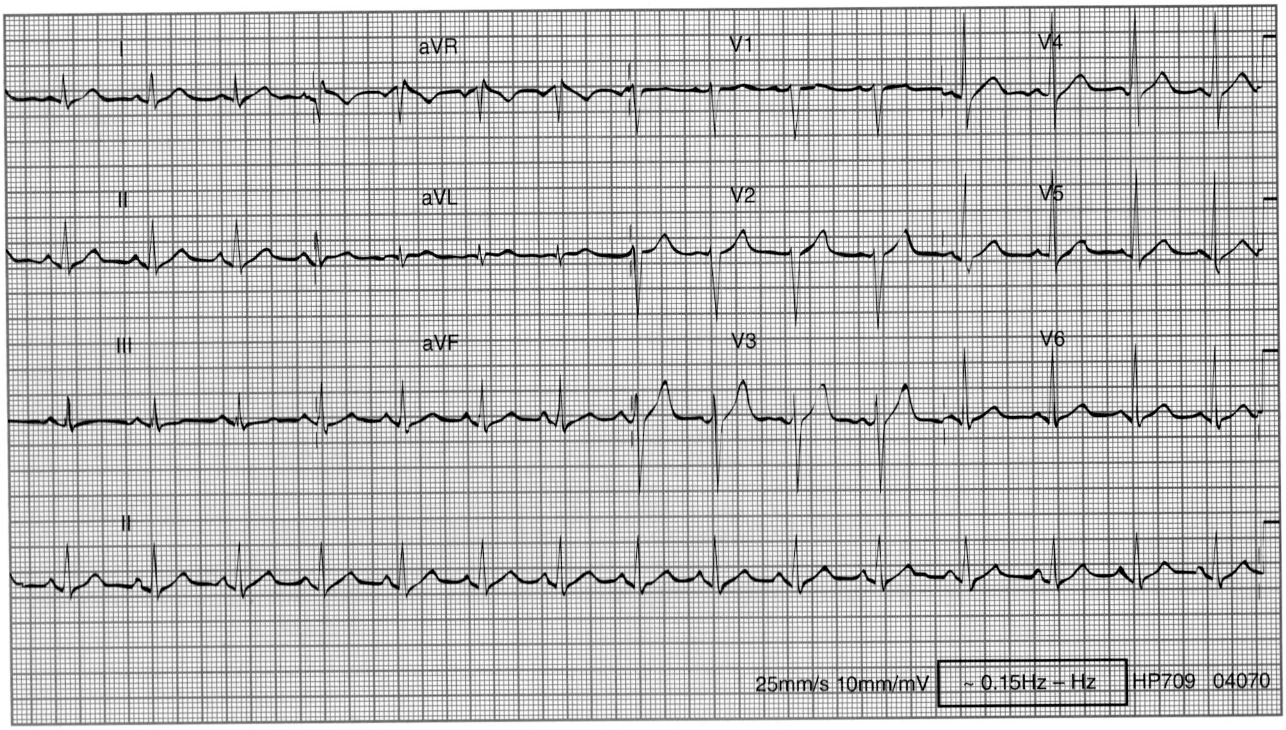

41. Identify the electrical axis, and explain your answer. (LO 14.3)

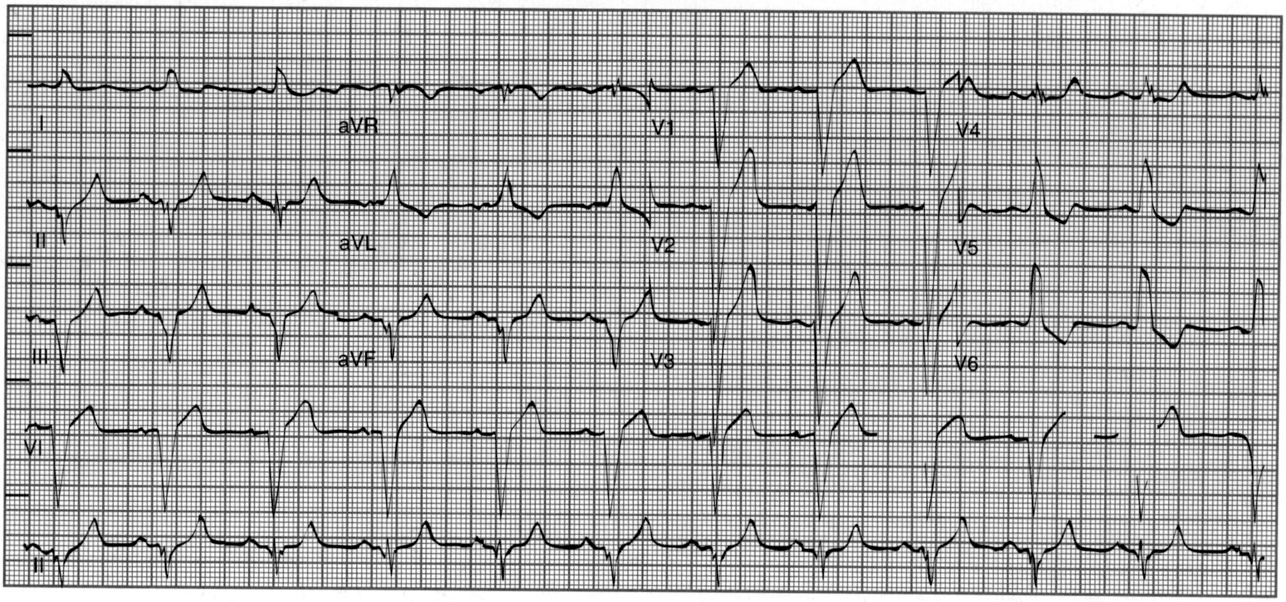

42. Identify the electrical axis, and explain your answer. (LO 14.3)

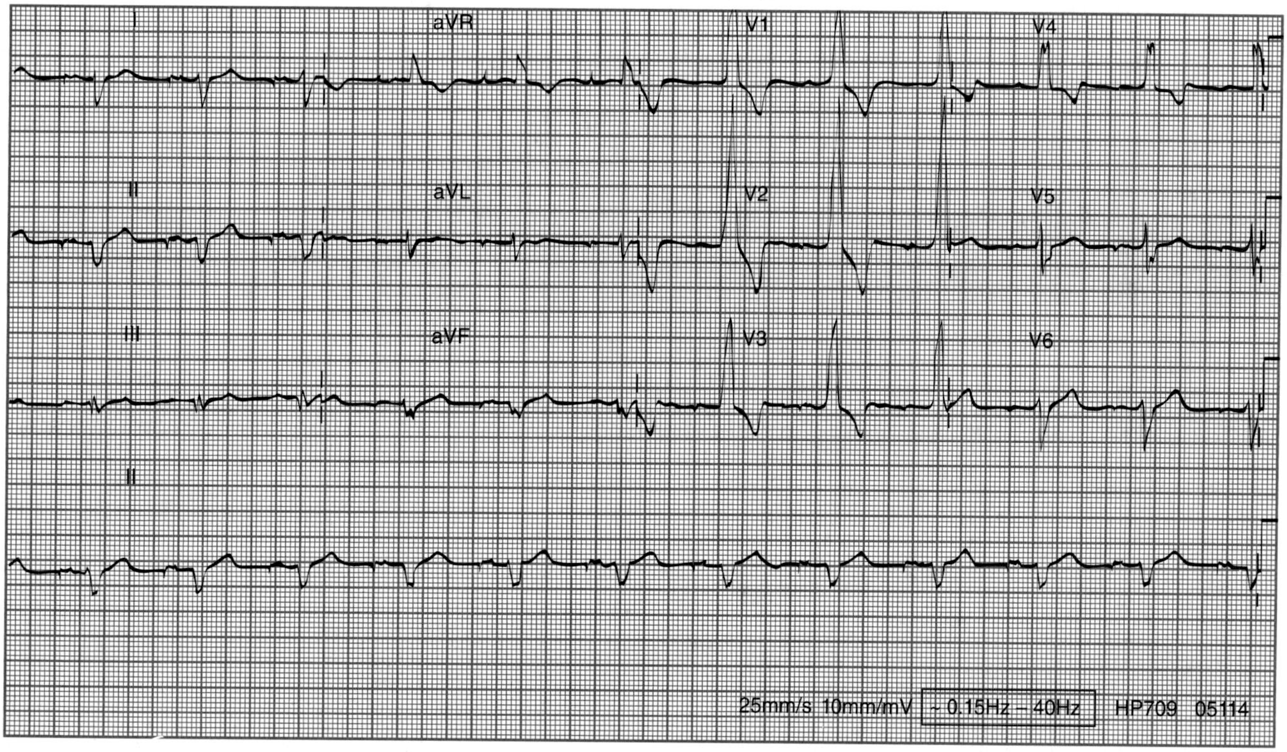

43. Identify the bundle branch block, and explain your answer. (LO 14.4)

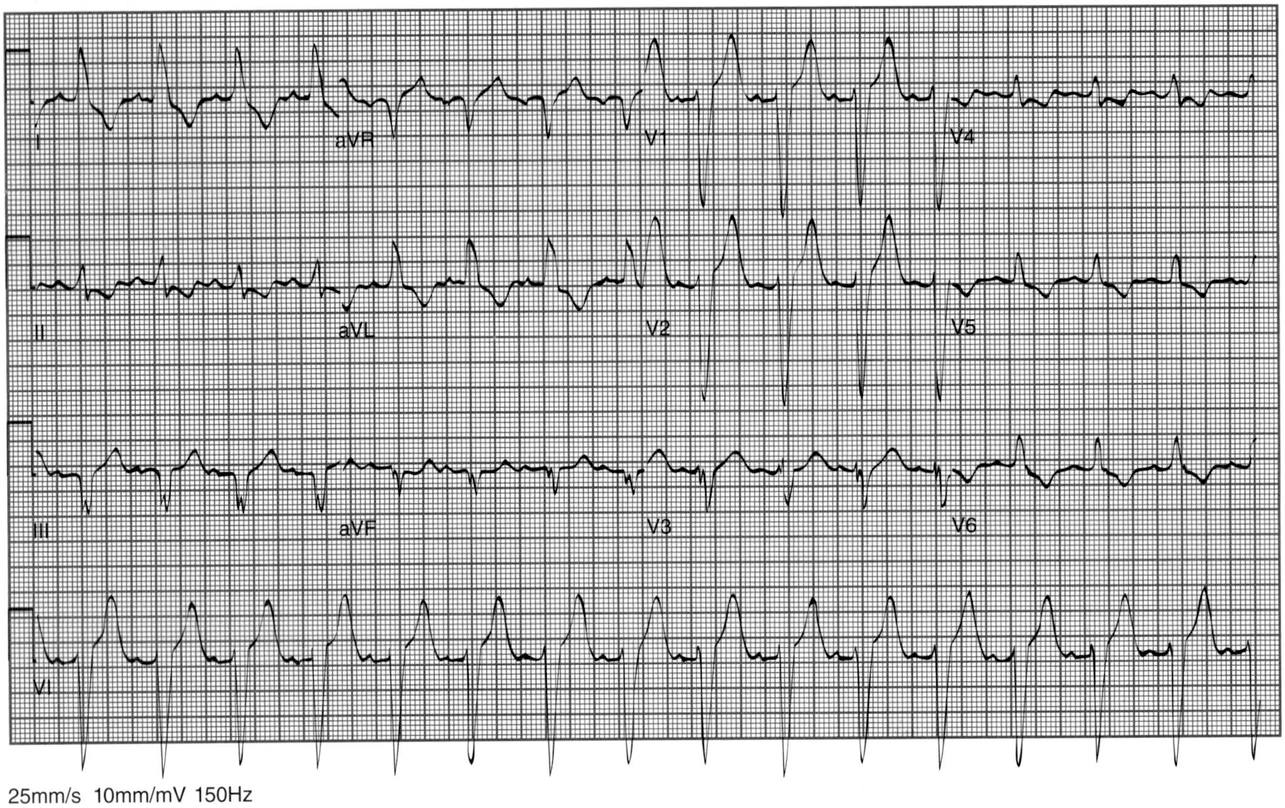

44. Identify the bundle branch block, and explain your answer. (LO 14.4)

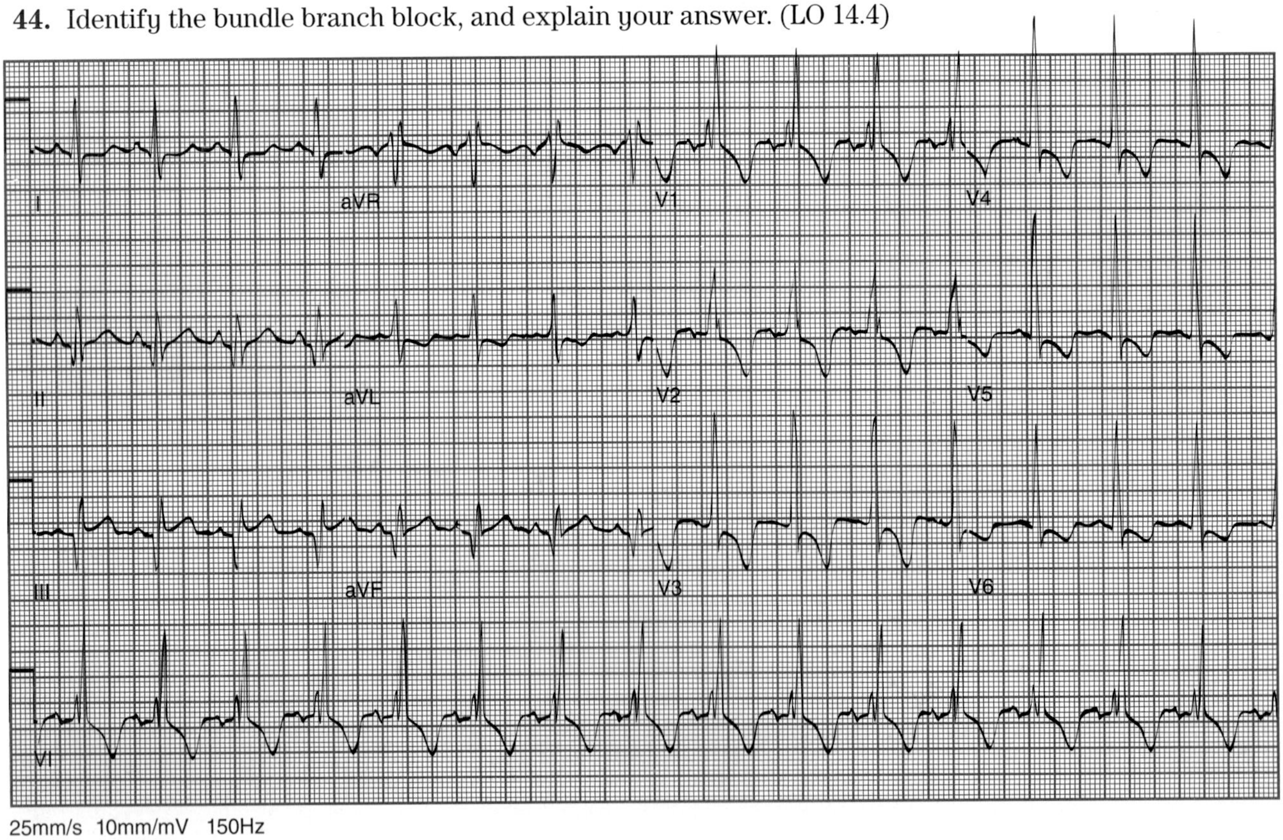

45. Review the figure and determine if left ventricular hypertrophy is present. Explain your answer. (LO 14.5)

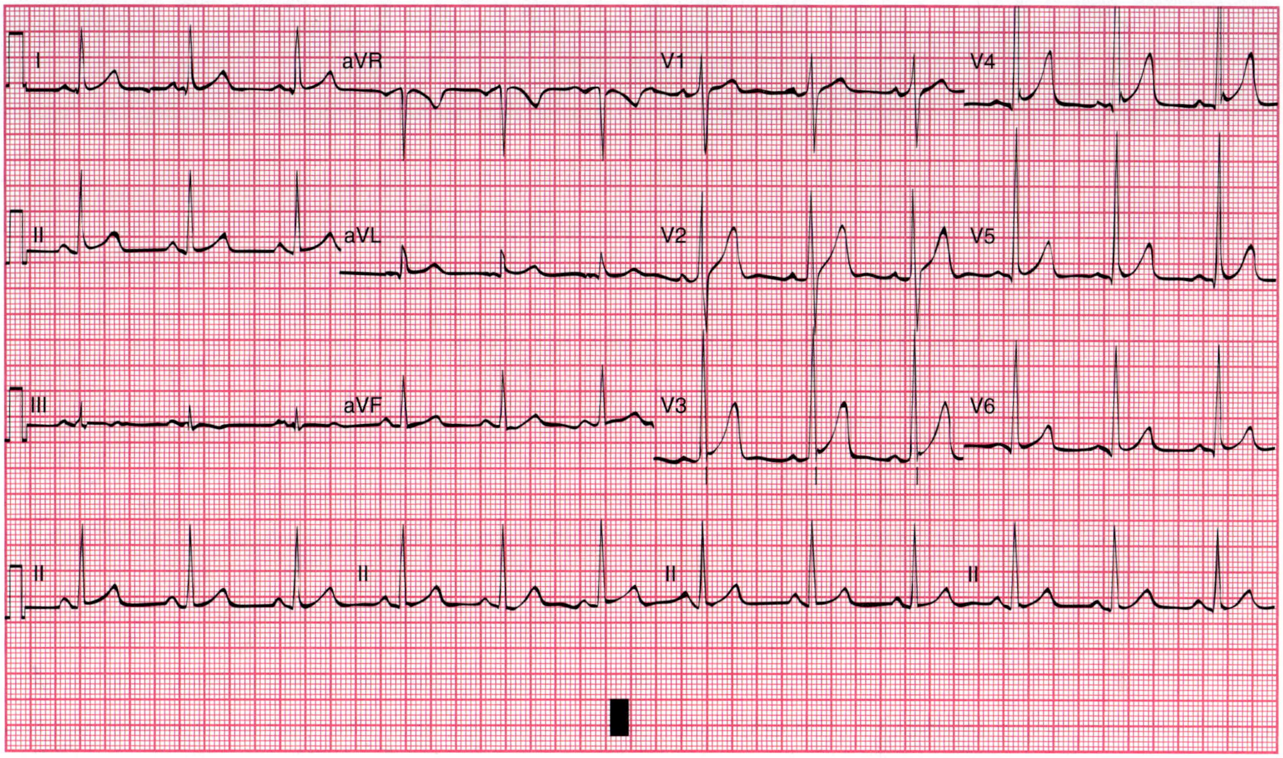

Putting It All Together

46. Circle the correct words and fill in the blanks to identify the following:

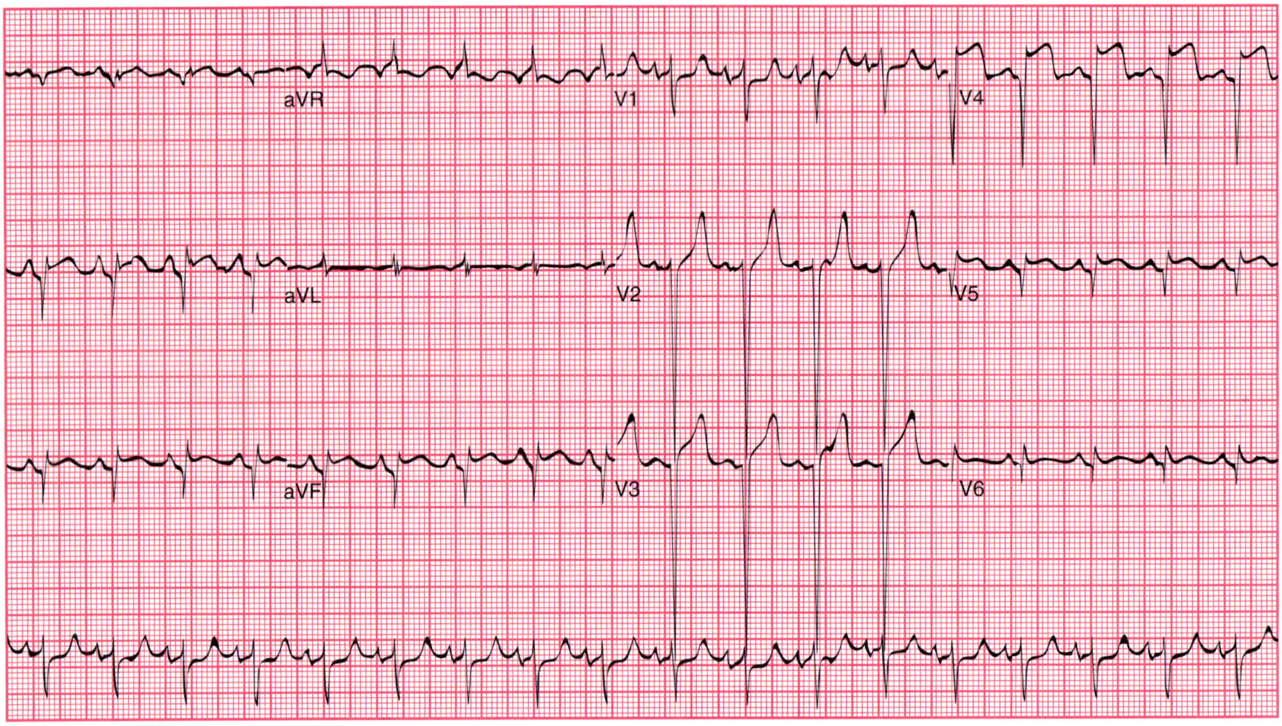

10mm/mV 150Hz

Electrical axis: Normal Left Right Extreme

BBB: Normal Right BBB Left BBB

LVH: Normal or LVH (with mm measurement) ______________

Leads with ST depression, T wave inversion, or none: ______________

Leads with ST elevation or none: ______________

Interpretation: ______________

47. Circle the correct words and fill in the blanks to identify the following:

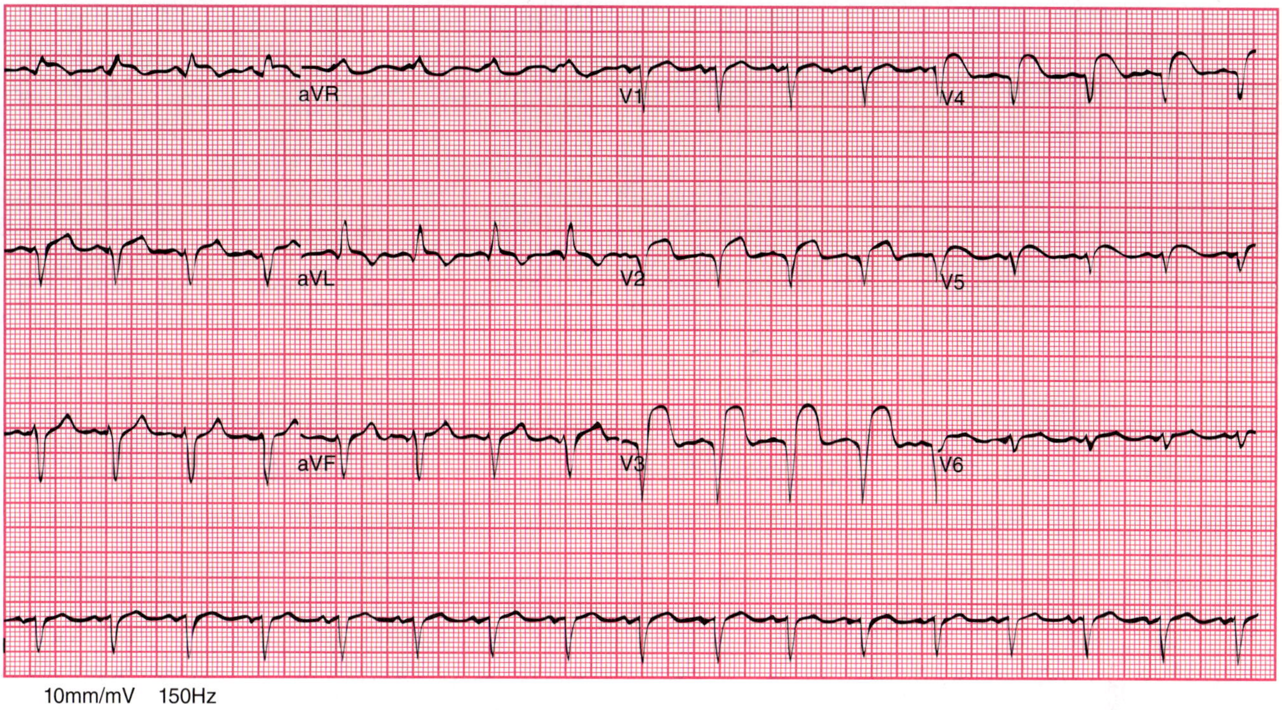

Electrical axis: Normal Left Right Extreme

BBB: Normal Right BBB Left BBB

Leads with ST elevation or none: ______________

LVH: Normal or LVH (with mm measurement) ______________

Leads with ST depression, T wave inversion, or none: ______________

Leads with ST elevation or none: ______________

Interpretation: ______________________________

48. Circle the correct words and fill in the blanks to identify the following:

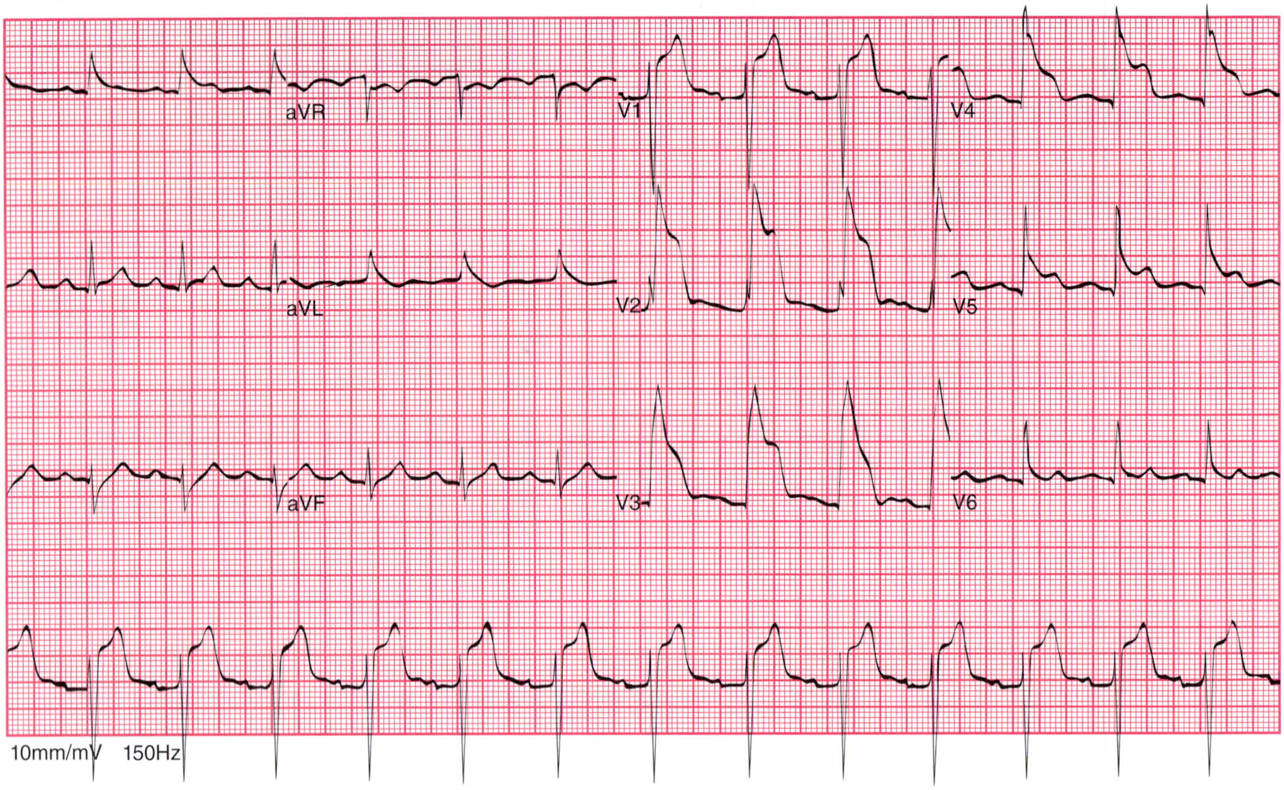

Electrical axis: Normal Left Right Extreme

BBB: Normal Right BBB Left BBB

Leads with ST elevation or none: ______________

LVH: Normal or LVH (with mm measurement) ______________

Leads with ST depression, T wave inversion, or none: ______________

Leads with ST elevation or none: ______________

Interpretation: ________________________________

49. Circle the correct words and fill in the blanks to identify the following:

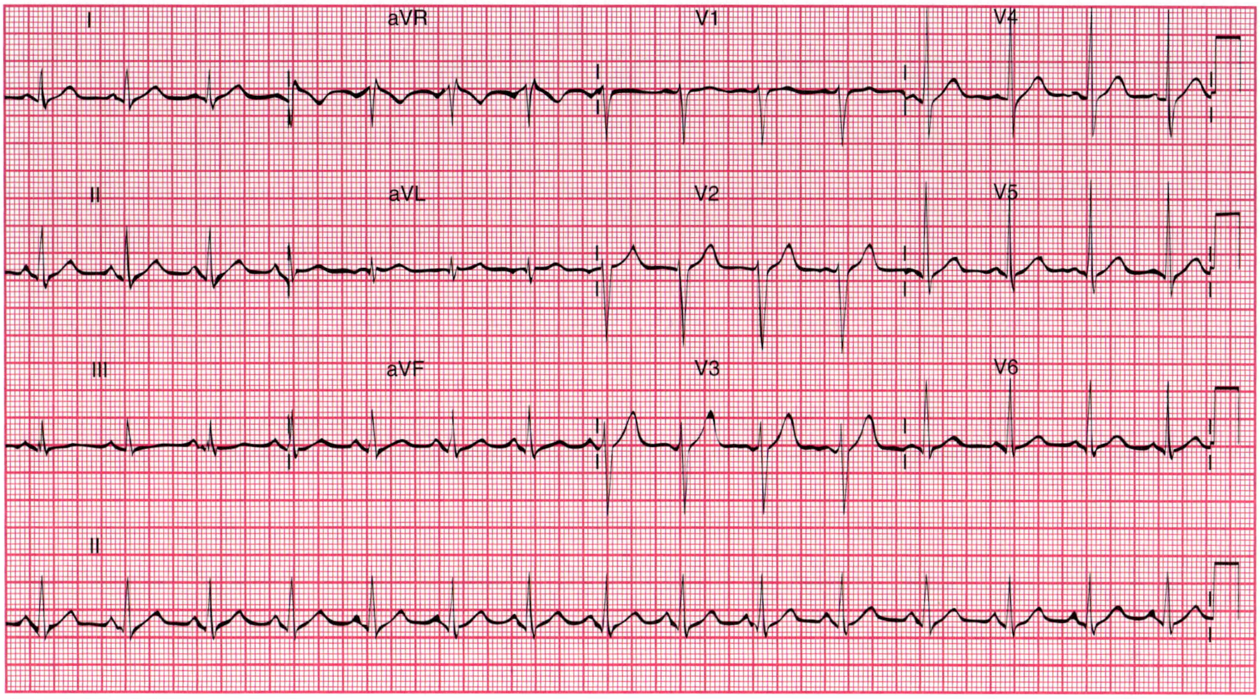

10mm/mV 150Hz

Electrical axis: Normal Left Right Extreme

BBB: Normal Right BBB Left BBB

LVH: Normal or LVH (with mm measurement) ______________

Leads with ST depression, T wave inversion, or none: ______________

Leads with ST elevation or none: ______________

Interpretation: ______________

50. Circle the correct words and fill in the blanks to identify the following:

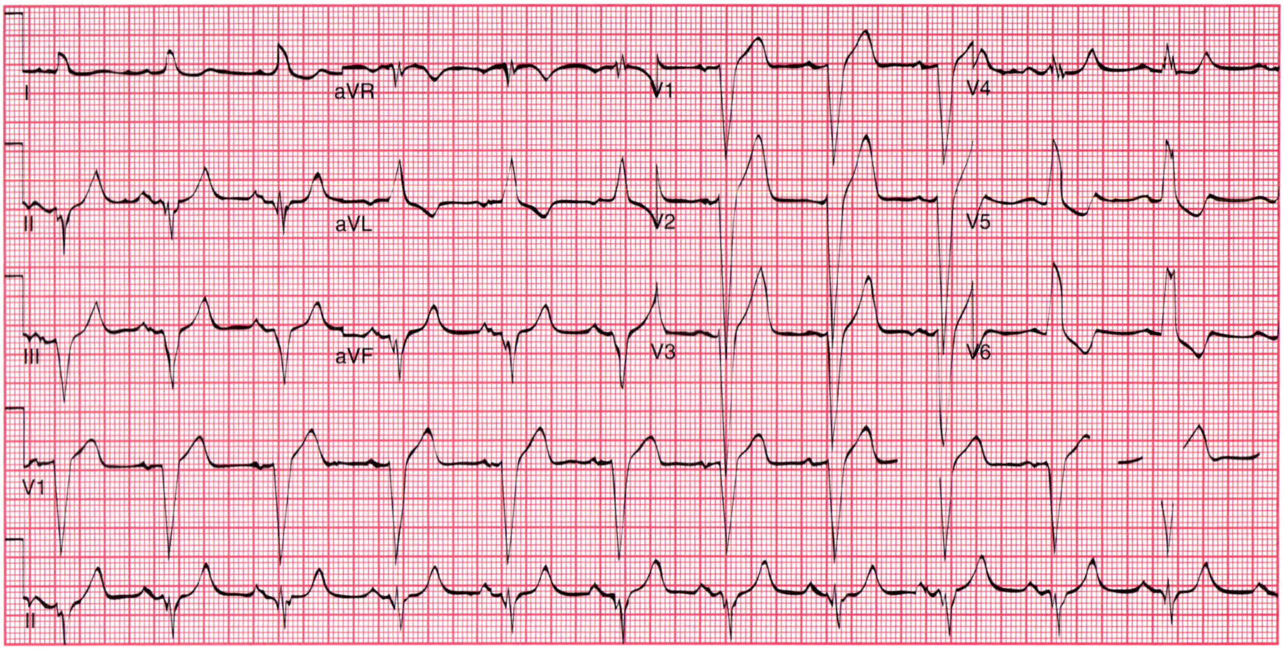

10mm/mV 150Hz

Electrical axis: Normal Left Right Extreme

BBB: Normal Right BBB Left BBB

LVH: Normal or LVH (with mm measurement) ____________

Leads with ST depression, T wave inversion, or none: ____________

Leads with ST elevation or none: ____________

Interpretation: ____________________________

51. Circle the correct words and fill in the blanks to identify the following:

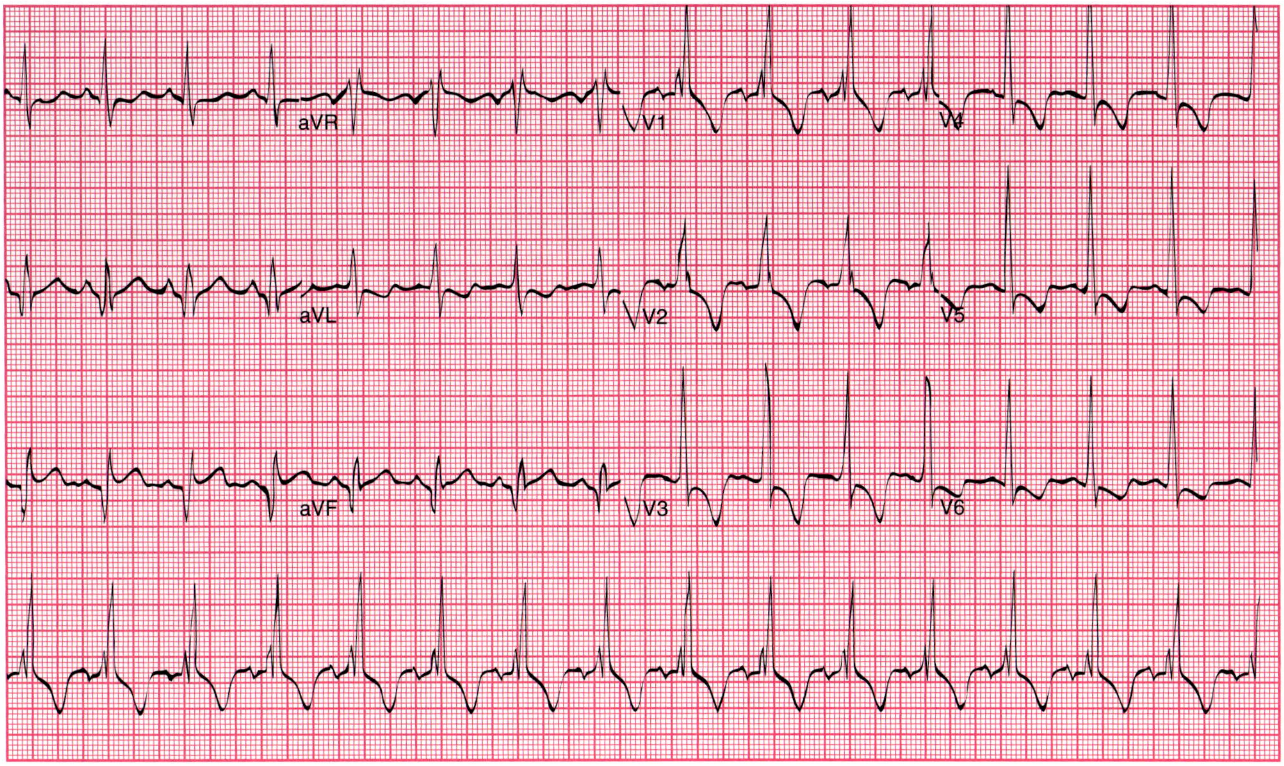

Electrical axis: Normal Left Right Extreme

BBB: Normal Right BBB Left BBB

LVH: Normal or LVH (with mm measurement) ____________

Leads with ST depression, T wave inversion, or none: ____________

Leads with ST elevation or none: ____________

Interpretation: ____________

Now that you have completed the material in the chapter text, go to Connect and complete any chapter activities you have not yet done.

Appendix A

Cardiovascular Medications

Beta Blockers

Drugs in this class include:

- Atenol**ol** (Tenormin)
- Metoprol**ol** (Toprol XL, Lopressor)
- Propranol**ol** (Inderal)
- Sotal**ol** (Betapace, Sotalex)
- Labetol**ol** (Normodyne, Trandate)
- Carvedil**ol** (Coreg)

Note: The names of the majority of drugs in this class end in *ol.*

Beta blockers are used to treat angina pectoris (chest pain caused by lack of blood/oxygen to the heart muscle), hypertension (high blood pressure), and various heart rhythm disturbances such as atrial fibrillation and PVCs.

Cardiac Glycosides

Drugs in this class include:

- Digoxin (Lanoxin, Digitek)
- Digitoxin (Crystodigin)

Digitalis, the most common and well known of the cardiac glycosides, is extracted from the foxglove plant. It has been used for over 100 years to treat atrial fibrillation and congestive heart failure. Digitalis increases the force of the heart's contractions and slows the heart rate. This medication is especially helpful in treating patients with congestive heart failure (CHF). Digoxin is a medication with a host of side effects (i.e., visual disturbances, various cardiac dysrhythmias, and even depression of the ST segment, also known as the *"digitalis effect,"* or *"dig dip"*).

Calcium Channel Blockers

Drugs in this class include:

- Amlodipine (Norvasc)
- Diltiazem (Cardizem)

- Verapamil (Calan, Isoptin)
- Nifedipine (Adalat, Procardia)

Calcium channel blockers are used to treat a variety of cardiac conditions including hypertension, angina pectoris, and certain types of rapid heart beat conditions such as atrial fibrillation and paroxysmal supraventricular tachycardia (SVT). They are also used to treat coronary artery spasms and after a heart attack for patients who cannot tolerate beta blockers.

ACE Inhibitors

Drugs in this class include:

- Enalapr**il** (Vasotec)
- Lisinopr**il** (Prinivil, Zestril)
- Captopr**il** (Capoten)
- Benazepr**il** (Lotensin)

Note: The names of the majority of drugs in this class end in *il*.

The angiotensin-converting enzyme (ACE) inhibitors work by inhibiting (blocking) the conversion of angiotensin I to angiotensin II in the lungs. Angiotensin II is a potent hormone that constricts arterioles and raises blood pressure. As a result, ACE inhibitors lower the blood pressure. ACE inhibitors are also used in the treatment of patients with congestive heart failure. They work by lowering the overall resistance in the vascular beds, making it easier for the heart to pump the blood.

Antiarrhythmic Medications

There are many different classes of antiarrhythmic medications because the electrical conduction system of the heart is so complex. Each class of medication affects the speed or way that electricity flows through the heart. Beta blockers, calcium channel blockers, and cardiac glycosides are antiarrhythmics. Two other classes of antiarrhythmic medications include sodium channel blockers and postassium channel blockers. Examples of medications that are used to treat arrhythmias, especially during cardiac care, include atropine, epinephrine, isuprel, and lidocaine.

Anticoagulants (Blood Thinners)

Drugs in this class include:

- Warfarin (Coumadin)
- Heparin
- Enoxaparin (Lovenox)

This group of drugs is extremely useful in the treatment of blood clot conditions. These medications are administered by a number of different methods, including orally or by injection. These medications prevent new blood clots from forming and existing blood clots from becoming larger. They *do not* lyse (break up or destroy) existing clots.

Oral Medications

Coumadin (warfarin) is the most commonly prescribed oral "blood thinner." It is prescribed in the treatment of heart valve conditions (including patients with artificial valves and for valve prolapse when blood is not flowing in the proper direction). It is also prescribed for other medical conditions in which blood clotting is a problem and embolization is a risk, including cardiac dysrhythmias such as atrial fibrillation.

Intravenous or Subcutaneous Medications

Heparin and Lovenox are very potent intravenous blood thinners. This type of thinner is generally used in an inpatient setting to quickly stop the development of an ongoing blood clot as seen in serious unstable angina, certain strokes, and acute pulmonary embolism. They have no effect on blood platelets.

Warfarin (as previously noted) is primarily used in the treatment of atrial fibrillation and in patients who have artificial metallic heart valves. Warfarin use significantly reduces the risk of embolism development in patients with atrial fibrillation.

Antiplatelet Agents

Drugs in this class include:

- Aspirin (Bayer)
- Clopidogrel (Plavix)
- Ticlopidine (Ticlid)

Antiplatelet medications decrease platelet aggregation (clumping) and inhibit thrombus (clot) formation. They are effective in the arterial circulation where anticoagulants (blood thinners) have little effect.

These medications may be used by patients with any of the following:

- Coronary artery disease
- Heart attack
- Angina (chest pain)
- Stroke and transient ischemic attacks (TIAs)
- Peripheral artery disease
- Angioplasty and stent placement
- Heart bypass surgery
- Atrial fibrillation, to prevent the formation of blood clots

Aspirin is a very potent antiplatelet agent that has been found to lower the risk of heart attacks and to improve the prognosis with a heart attack. Data have also shown a reduced stroke risk in patients who take prophylactic aspirin. It is a first-line drug administered to "chest pain" patients presenting for emergency care of acute coronary syndromes. Aspirin is routinely prescribed to men over 40 years and postmenopausal women to reduce their risk of clot formation.

Plavix (clopidogrel) keeps platelets in the blood from sticking together and forming clots. These clots are the direct cause of cardiovascular incidents such as heart attacks and strokes. Plavix is useful in angioplasty/coronary stent implantation to prevent postprocedure closure of the treated artery.

Fibrinolytics

Also known as "clot busters," these medications are most commonly used in an inpatient setting, where they rapidly dissolve clots wherever they are located; for example, inside a coronary artery (causing a heart attack) or inside a brain artery (causing a stroke). The clot is lysed quickly once the clot buster is administered. These drugs can also be used to treat large pulmonary embolisms and clots that are causing obstruction of a prosthetic (artificial) valve.

Because of the way clot busters work, they can increase the risk of bleeding elsewhere in the body (IV site, intracranial, etc.) when administered. Unfortunately, the people with the greatest need for these medications are also at the greatest risk for complications as a result of them.

Diuretics

Diuretics act by removing salt and water from the body through the kidneys (elimination). Diuretics are used primarily in the treatment of congestive heart failure (CHF) and are often used in the treatment of hypertension (high blood pressure). *Caution must be observed when treating patients with diuretics* as salt and water are not the only elements removed by the action of medications in this class. Other essential electrolytes, such as potassium, calcium, and magnesium, may be eliminated as well, which may contribute to the development of cardiac dysrhythmias.

Cholesterol-Lowering Agents (Statins)

Drugs in this class include:

- Atorvastatin (Lipitor)
- Pravastatin (Pravachol)
- Rosuvastatin (Crestor)
- Simvastatin (Zocor)

Cholesterol-lowering medications lower the LDL (low-density lipoprotein or “bad”) cholesterol in the blood. Some of these drugs also raise the HDL (high-density lipoprotein or “good”) cholesterol. This class of drugs has been shown to reduce the incidence of heart attack and death in patients with high cholesterol and coronary artery disease. Some statins may reverse atherosclerotic plaque within blood vessels, thereby reducing the potential for sudden cardiac death and potentially reducing the need for surgical intervention. There are always drawbacks: This category of medications is also potentially hepatotoxic, and high doses of statins may in some cases destroy the liver.

Nitrates

Drugs in this class include:

- Nitroglycerin (Nitor-Dur, Nitrolingual, Nitrostat)
- Isosorbide dinitrate (Dilatrate-SR, Isordil)
- Isosorbide mononitrate (ISMO)

Nitrates are the most commonly prescribed vasodilators, or medications that widen the blood vessels. They are frequently used for relief of ischemic chest pain in patients with coronary vascular disease and angina (chest pain). They work by relaxing smooth muscles, most notably the muscles of the heart and blood vessels. As a result, pressure on blood vessel walls is reduced, which allows more blood to circulate with less effort by the heart. Nitrates affect arteries as well as veins, but their vasodilatory effect is more pronounced on veins. Nitrates prevent and relieve angina by relieving vasoconstriction and increasing blood flow and oxygen to ischemic heart muscle.

Nitrates can be administered intravenously, sublingually (via metered spray or tablet), transdermally (ointments or skin patches), and orally.

Safety note: Never handle nitrates with your bare hands! Nitrates are absorbed easily through the skin.

Extra Precautions for Patients Taking Nitrates

- If a patient is already taking any medication to treat hypertension and/or **erectile dysfunction** (e.g., Viagra, Cialis, Levitra), the addition of nitrates can be dangerous. When taken in combination, these medications can increase the effects of nitrates on blood pressure, causing profound, irreversible hypotension, cardiac arrest, and even death.

Inotropic Agents (Cardiotonics)

Drugs in this class include:

- Adenosine (Adenocard)
- Dobutamine (Dobutrex)

Inotropes, or inotropic agents, affect the heart's contractile force. These medications strengthen the pumping action of the heart and, as a result, reduce cardiac workload (myocardial oxygen demand). They are commonly used to treat patients with heart failure or tachydysrhythmias. Cardiac glycosides such as digitalis are also considered inotropic agents.

Chemical Stress Testing Agents

There are two categories of chemical stress testing agents. The cardioactive agents have an effect on the heart, and the imaging agents allow the heart to be visualized during the test.

Cardioactive drugs include:

- Dobutamine (Dobutrex)—increase cardiac output and heart rate, coronary artery vasodilation
- Adenosine (Adenocard)—coronary artery vasodilation
- Persantine (Dipyridamole)—coronary artery vasodilation
- Regadenoson (Lexiscan)—coronary artery vasodilation

Imaging agents include:

- Cardiolite
- Thallium
- Myoview

Appendix B

Standard and Isolation Precautions

Key Components of Standard Precautions

Handwashing (or using an antiseptic hand rub)

- After touching blood, body fluids, secretions, excretions, and contaminated items.
- Immediately after removing gloves.
- Between patient contacts.

Gloves

- For contact with blood, body fluids, secretions, and contaminated items.
- For contact with mucous membranes and nonintact skin.

Masks, Goggles, Face Masks

- Protect mucous membranes of eyes, nose, and mouth when contact with blood and body fluids is likely.

Gowns

- Protect skin from blood or body fluid contact.
- Prevent soiling of clothing during procedures that may involve contact with blood or body fluids.

Soiled Linen

- Handle soiled linen to prevent soiled surfaces from touching skin or mucous membranes.
- Do not prerinse soiled linens.

Patient Care Equipment

- Handle soiled equipment in a manner to prevent contact with skin or mucous membranes and to prevent contamination of clothing or the environment.
- Clean reusable equipment prior to reuse.

Environmental Cleaning

- Routinely care for, clean, and disinfect equipment and furnishings in patient care areas.

Sharps

- Avoid recapping used needles.
- Avoid removing used needles from disposable syringes.
- Avoid bending, breaking, or manipulating used needles by hand.
- Place used sharps in approved puncture-resistant sharps containers.

Patient Resuscitation

- Use mouthpieces, resuscitation bags, or other ventilation devices to avoid mouth-to-mouth resuscitation.

Patient Placement

- Place patients who contaminate the environment or cannot maintain appropriate hygiene in private rooms.

Hand Hygiene Practices and Procedures

Recommended Practices

- Wash hands at the beginning of the workday. Wash your hands with soap and water whenever they are visibly contaminated with blood or other body fluids.
- If hands are not visibly contaminated, an alcohol-based hand rub can be used.
- Wash hands at the end of the workday before leaving the facility.

Indications for Hand Hygiene

- Before putting on and after removing gloves.
- Between patient contacts; between different procedures on the same patient.
- After touching blood, body fluids, secretions, excretions, and contaminated objects.
- After handling specimen containers or tubes.
- After restroom visits, eating, combing hair, handling money, and any other time your hands get contaminated.
- Before inserting any invasive device.
- After having contact with a patient's skin.
- After having contact with wound dressings (bandages).
- After having contact with inanimate objects near a patient.
- Before eating, applying cosmetics, or handling contact lenses.

Basic Steps for Handwashing

- Remove all rings and jewelry.
- Turn on water, and adjust temperature to warm.
- Wet your hands liberally without leaning your body against the sink area.
- Apply soap, and work up a good lather.
- Use circular motions while applying friction, being sure to interlace your fingers to clean between them for 2 minutes at the start of your workday, 15–30 seconds in between patients, and 1–2 minutes when hands are visibly soiled.

- Rinse each hand, allowing water to run from your wrists toward the fingertips, keeping fingers pointing downward. Contamination under fingernails should be removed with a tool designed for that purpose, such as an orange stick.
- Repeat the above steps if your hands are very soiled.
- Dry hands thoroughly by patting with paper towels; discard paper towels into waste receptacle.
- Turn off water with a clean, dry paper towel, if indicated.
- Clean the area using dry paper towels, if indicated.

Advantages of Alcohol-Based Hand Rubs (foam or gel)

- Kill bacteria and viruses more effectively and more quickly than handwashing with soap and water.
- Less damaging to the skin than soap and water, resulting in less skin irritation.
- Require less time than handwashing.
- Dispensers can be placed in more accessible areas.

Basic Steps for Alcohol-Based Hand Rubs

- Make sure there is no visible dirt or contamination.
- Apply ½ to 1 teaspoon of alcohol cleanser, either foam or gel, to one hand. Check the manufacturer's directions for the proper amount.
- Rub your hands together vigorously, making sure all surfaces are covered.
- Continue rubbing until your hands are dry.

Note: Many facilities have sensors that turn on water automatically when the hands are lowered to the faucet. Other facilities have a knee or foot device that is used to turn on the water.

TABLE B-1 **Personal Protective Equipment (PPE) Practices**

Type	When Used	Rules for Use
Gloves	For hand contact with blood, mucous membranes, and other potentially infectious materials or when nonintact skin is anticipated, when performing vascular access procedures, or when handling contaminated items or surfaces	• Does not replace handwashing. • Perform hand hygiene before applying and after removing gloves. • When removing gloves, do not touch the outside (contaminated) area of the gloves. • Keep gloved hands away from the face. • Avoid touching or adjusting other PPE. • Remove if torn, and perform hand hygiene before putting on new gloves. • Limit surfaces and items touched. • Extend gloves over isolation gown cuffs.

Gown	During procedures and patient care activities when contact of clothing/exposed skin with blood/body fluids, secretions, or excretions is anticipated	• To put on gown: – Put opening in the back. – Secure at neck and waist. • To remove gown: – Unfasten ties. – Peel gown away from neck and shoulder—do not touch outside. – Turn contaminated outside toward the inside. – Fold or roll into a bundle. – Discard in biohazard container.
Mask	During patient care activities likely to generate splashes or sprays of blood, body fluids, secretions, or excretions	• Fully cover nose and mouth. • Use respirator masks such as N95, N99, or N100 for airborne precautions. • To put on mask: – Place over nose, mouth, and chin. – Fit flexible nosepiece over nose bridge. – Secure on head with ties or elastic. – Adjust to fit. • To remove mask: – Untie the bottom tie, then untie the top tie. – Remove from face—do not touch the outside. – Discard in biohazard container.
Eye protection	During patient care activities likely to generate splashes or sprays of blood, body fluids, secretions, or excretions	• Goggles should fit snugly over and around the eyes. • Personal glasses are not an acceptable substitute. • Use a face shield that protects face, nose, mouth, and eyes if desired. • Use face shield to cover forehead, extend below chin, and wrap around side of face. • Position goggles over eyes and secure to the head using the earpieces or headband. • Position face shield over face and secure on brow with headband. • Remove goggles or face shield: – Grasp ear or head pieces with ungloved hands. – Lift away from face—do not touch outside. – Place in designated receptacle for reprocessing or disposal.

Isolation (Transmission-Based) Precautions

There are three categories of transmission-based precautions:

1. Contact precautions
2. Droplet precautions
3. Airborne precautions

Transmission-based precautions are used when the route(s) of transmission is (are) not completely interrupted using standard precautions alone. For some diseases that have multiple routes of transmission (e.g., severe acute respiratory syndrome, SARS), more than one transmission-based precautions category may be used. When used either singly or in combination, they are always used in addition to standard precautions.

Contact Precautions

Contact precautions are intended to prevent transmission of infectious agents, including important microorganisms, which are spread by direct or indirect contact with the patient or the patient's environment. Certain infections require the use of contact precautions, including patients infected or colonized with multi-drug-resistant organisms. Contact precautions also apply where the presence of excessive wound drainage, fecal incontinence, or other discharges from the body suggests an increased potential for extensive environmental contamination and risk of transmission.

A single-patient room is preferred for patients who require contact precautions. When a single-patient room is not available, consultation with infection control personnel is recommended to assess the various risks associated with other patient placement options (e.g., cohorting, keeping the patient with an existing roommate). In multipatient rooms, at least 3 feet of spatial separation between beds is advised to reduce the opportunities for inadvertent sharing of items between the infected/colonized patient and other patients.

Healthcare personnel caring for patients on contact precautions wear a gown and gloves for all interactions that may involve contact with the patient or potentially contaminated areas in the patient's environment. To contain pathogens, PPE should be donned upon room entry and discarded before exiting the patient room. This is especially necessary for pathogens that have been implicated in transmission through environmental contamination, such as vancomycin-resistant enterococci, *Clostridium difficile,* noroviruses, and other intestinal tract pathogens.

Droplet Precautions

Droplet precautions are intended to prevent transmission of pathogens that are spread through close respiratory or mucous membrane contact with respiratory secretions. Because these pathogens do not remain infectious over long distances in a healthcare facility, special air handling and ventilation are not required to prevent droplet transmission. Infectious agents for which droplet precautions are indicated include pertussis, influenza virus, adenovirus, rhinovirus, *Neisseria meningitides,* and group A streptococcus (for the first 24 hours of antimicrobial therapy).

A single-patient room is preferred for patients who require droplet precautions. When a single-patient room is not available, consultation with infection control personnel is recommended to assess the various risks associated with other patient placement options (e.g., cohorting, keeping the patient with an existing roommate).

Spatial separation of at least 3 feet and drawing the curtain between patient beds is especially important for patients in multibed rooms with infections transmitted by the droplet route.

Healthcare personnel wear a mask (a respirator is not necessary) for close contact with infectious patients; the mask is generally donned upon room entry. Patients on droplet precautions who must be transported outside of the room should wear a mask if tolerated and follow respiratory hygiene/cough etiquette.

Airborne Precautions

Airborne precautions prevent transmission of infectious agents that remain infectious over long distances when suspended in the air (e.g., rubeola virus [measles], varicella virus [chickenpox], *M. tuberculosis,* and possibly SARS-CoV). The preferred placement for patients who require airborne precautions is in an airborne infection isolation room (AIIR). An AIIR is a single-patient room that is equipped with special air handling and ventilation capacity that meet the American Institute of Architects/Facility Guidelines Institute (AIA/FGI) standards for AIIRs. Some states require the availability of such rooms in hospitals, emergency departments, and nursing homes that care for patients with *Mycobacterium tuberculosis.* A respiratory protection program that includes education about use of respirators, fit-testing, and user seal checks is required in any facility with AIIRs.

In settings where airborne precautions cannot be implemented due to limited engineering resources (e.g., physician offices), masking the patient, placing the patient in a private room (e.g., office examination room) with the door closed, and providing N95 or higher-level respirators or masks if respirators are not available for healthcare personnel will reduce the likelihood of airborne transmission until the patient is either transferred to a facility with an AIIR or returned to the home environment, as deemed medically appropriate.

Healthcare personnel caring for patients on airborne precautions wear a mask or respirator mask that is donned prior to room entry. Whenever possible, nonimmune healthcare workers should not care for patients with vaccine-preventable airborne diseases (e.g., measles, chickenpox, and smallpox).

Applications of Transmission-Based Precautions

Diagnosis of many infections requires laboratory confirmation. Because laboratory tests, especially those that depend on culture techniques, often require two or more days for completion, transmission-based precautions must be implemented while test results are pending based on the clinical presentation and likely pathogens. Use of appropriate transmission-based precautions at the time a patient develops symptoms or signs of transmissible infection, or arrives at a healthcare facility for care, reduces transmission opportunities.

Discontinuation of Transmission-Based Precautions

Transmission-based precautions remain in effect for limited periods of time, while the risk for transmission of the infectious agent persists or for the duration of the illness. For some diseases, such as pharyngeal or cutaneous diphtheria, or respiratory syncytial virus (RSV), transmission-based precautions remain in effect until culture or antigen-detection test results document eradication of the pathogen and, for RSV, symptomatic disease is resolved. For other diseases (e.g., *M. tuberculosis*), state laws/regulations and healthcare facility policies may dictate the duration of precautions. In immunocompromised patients, viral shedding can persist for prolonged periods of time (many weeks to months) and transmission to others may occur during that time; therefore, the duration of contact and/or droplet precautions may be prolonged for many weeks.

Application of Transmission-Based Precautions in Ambulatory and Home Care Settings

Although transmission-based precautions generally apply in all healthcare settings, exceptions exist. For example, in home care, AIIRs are not available. Furthermore, family members already exposed to diseases such as varicella and tuberculosis would not use masks or respiratory protection, but visiting phlebotomists or other healthcare workers would need to use such protection. Similarly, management of patients colonized or infected with multi-drug-resistant organisms may necessitate contact precautions in acute care hospitals and in some long-term care facilities when there is continued transmission, but the risk of transmission in ambulatory care and home care has not been defined. Consistent use of standard precautions may suffice in these settings, but more information is needed.

**The material in this section was adapted from Centers for Disease Control Guidelines for Isolation Precautions 2007 (www.cdc.gov).*

Appendix C

Medical Abbreviations, Acronyms, and Symbols

The following are common medical abbreviations, acronyms, and symbols. Always check the facility where you are employed for the acceptable medical abbreviations, acronyms, and symbols used. Avoid using abbreviations and symbols designated as Do Not Use by The Joint Commission (TJC) (www.jointcommission.org) or as Error-Prone by the Institute for Safe Medication Practices (www.ismp.org).

Medical Abbreviation	Term
Numbers	
1°	First degree
2°	Second degree
2DE	Two-dimensional echocardiography
3°	Third degree
A	
A&O X3	Alert and oriented to person, place, and date
a&w	Alive and well
AAA	Abdominal aortic aneurysm
ABG	Arterial blood gas
AC	Before eating or meal
ACLS	Advanced cardiac life support
ad lib	Ad libitum (as desired)

ADAT	Advance diet as tolerated
AEA	Above elbow amputation
AF	Atrial fibrillation
Afl or a flutter	Atrial flutter
Agit	Agitation
AHHD	Arteriosclerotic hypertensive heart disease
AICD	Automatic implanted cardiac defibrillator
AIDS	Acquired immunodeficiency syndrome
AIMI	Anteroinferior myocardial infarction
AIVR	Accelerated idioventricular rhythm
AKA, a k amputation	Above the knee amputation
a-line	Arterial line
Amb	Ambulate
a/n or abnl	Abnormal
a/o	Alert and oriented
AODM	Adult-onset diabetes mellitus
a-p	Anterior and posterior
a-p&lat	Anteroposterior and lateral
Appt	Appointment
Apw	Aortopulmonary window
ARDS	Acute respiratory distress syndrome
ARF	Acute renal failure
AS	Aortic stenosis
ASAP	As soon as possible
ASCVD or ASCVHD	Atherosclerotic cardiovascular disease
ASD	Atrial septal defect
ASHD	Atherosclerotic heart disease
ASHVD	Atherosclerotic hypertensive vascular disease
ASMI	Anteroseptal myocardial infaction

Medical Abbreviation	Term
ASVD	Arteriorsclerotic vascular disease
ASVHD	Arteriosclerotic vascular heart disease
AV, a-v	Atrioventricular
AVS	Arteriovenous shunt
AWMI	Anterior wall myocardial infarction
B	
BBB	Bundle branch block
BID	Twice a day
bil	Bilateral
BKA	Below the knee amputation
BP	Blood pressure
BPM or bpm	Beats per minute
BRP	Bathroom privileges
BS	Bowel or breath sounds
BW	Body weight
Bx	Biopsy
C	
c̄	With
C&S	Culture and sensitivity
CA	Cancer
CABG	Coronary artery bypass graft
CAD	Coronary artery disease
CAT	Computerized axial tomography
CBC	Complete blood count
CBG	Capillary blood gas
CC	Chief complaint
CCU	Cardiac care unit
CF	Cystic fibrosis

(Continued)

CHB	Complete heart block
CHF	Congestive heart failure
CI	Cardiac index
CNS	Central nervous system
CO	Cardiac output
c/o	Complaining of
COLD	Chronic obstructive lung disease
COPD	Chronic obstructive pulmonary disease
CP	Chest pain
CPAP	Continuous positive airway pressure
CPK	Creatine phosphokinase
CPK-mb	Creatine phosphokinase myocardial band
CPR	Cardiopulmonary resuscitation
CRF	Chronic renal failure
CT	Computerized tomography
CVA	Cerebrovascular accident
CVC	Central venous catheter
CVHD	Cardiovascular heart disease
CVP	Central venous pressure
CXR	Chest x-ray
D	
DAT	Diet as tolerated
DDx	Differential diagnosis
D5W	5% dextrose in water
DI	Diabetes insipidus
DIC	Disseminated intravascular coagulopathy
DIG	Digoxin
DJD	Degenerative joint disease

Medical Abbreviation	Term
DKA	Diabetic ketoacidosis
DM	Diabetes mellitus
DNR	Do not resuscitate
DOA	Dead on arrival
DOB	Date of birth
DOD	Date of discharge
DOE	Dyspnea on exertion
DTR	Deep tendon reflexes
DVT	Deep venous thrombosis
DX or Dx	Diagnosis
E	
EBL	Estimated blood loss
ECG or EKG	Electrocardiogram
ET	Endotracheal
ETOH	Ethanol (alcohol)
ETT	Endotracheal tube
Eval	Evaluation
F	
FBS	Fasting blood sugar
fekg	Fetal electrocardiogram
fem pop, fem-pop	Femoral popliteal
FEV	Forced expiratory volume
FTT	Failure to thrive
FU	Follow up
FUO	Fever of unknown origin
Fx	Fracture

(*Continued*)

G	
GI	Gastrointestinal
gm or g	Gram
Gr	Grain; 1 grain = 60 to 65 mg
GSW	Gunshot wound
gt or gtt	Drops
GTT	Glucose tolerance test
GU	Genitourinary
GXT	Graded exercise tolerance (stress test)
H	
HA	Headache
HAV	Hepatitis A virus
HBP	High blood pressure
HCT	Hematocrit
HDL	High density lipoprotein
HEENT	Head, eyes, ears, nose, throat
Hep A	Hepatitis A
Hep B	Hepatitis B
Hep lock or hep-lock	Heparin lock
Hgb	Hemoglobin
H/H, H&H	Hemoglobin/hematocrit
HIV	Human immunodeficiency virus
HO	History of
HOB	Head of bed
HOH	Hard of hearing
HPI	History of present illness
HR	Heart rate
HSV	Herpes simplex virus

Medical Abbreviation	Term
HTN	Hypertension
Hx	History
I	
I&D	Incision and drainage
I&O	Intake and output
IASD	Interatrial septal defect
ICS	Intercostal space
ICU	Intensive care unit
ID	Infectious disease, identification, or intradermal
IDDM	Insulin-dependent diabetes mellitus
IHSS	Idiopathic hypertropic subaortic stenosis
IM	Intramuscular
IMCU	Intermediate medical care unit
IMV	Intermittent mandatory ventilation
INF	Intravenous nutritional fluid
IPPB	Intermittent positive pressure breathing
IRBBB	Incomplete right bundle branch block
IRDM	Insulin-resistant diabetes mellitus
ITP	Idiopathic thrombocytopenic purpura
IV	Intravenous
IVC	Inferior vena cava
IVP	Intravenous pyelogram
IWMI	Inferior wall myocardial infarction
J	
JVD	Jugular venous distention
JODM	Juvenile-onset diabetes mellitus

(*Continued*)

K	
KOR	Keep open rate
KVO	Keep vein open
L	
L	Left
LAD	Left axis deviation or left anterior descending
LAE	Left atrial enlargement
LAHB	Left anterior hemiblock
LAP	Left atrial pressure
LBBB	Left bundle branch block
LLL	Left lower lobe
LMP	Last menstrual period
LOC	Loss of consciousness or level of consciousness
LP	Lumbar puncture
LPN	Licensed practical nurse
LUL	Left upper lobe
LUQ	Left upper quadrant
LV	Left ventricle
LVAD	Left ventricular assist device
LVEDP	Left ventricular end diastolic pressure
LVF	Left ventricular failure
LVH	Left ventricular hypertrophy
LWMI	Lateral wall myocardial infarction
M	
MAP	Mean arterial pressure
MAST	Medical antishock trousers
MI	Myocardial infarction or mitral insufficiency
mL	Milliliter

Medical Abbreviation	Term
MLE	Midline episiotomy
mm	Millimeter
MRI	Magnetic resonance imaging
MRSA	Methicillin-resistant *Staphylococcus aureus*
msec	Millisecond
MSSA	Methicillin-sensitive *Staphylococcus aureus*
MVA	Motor vehicle accident
N	
n&v, n/v	Nausea and vomiting
n/a	Not applicable
NAD	No active disease
NAS	No added salt
NCV	Nerve conduction velocity
NED	No evidence of recurrent disease
NG	Nasogastric
NGT	Nasogastric tube
NIDDM	Non-insulin-dependent diabetes mellitus
NKA	No known allergies
NKDA	No known drug allergies
NMR	Nuclear magnetic resonance
NPO	Nothing by mouth
NRM	No regular medication
NSAID	Non-steroidal anti-inflammatory drugs
NSR	Normal sinus rhythm
NT	Nasotracheal
NTG	Nitroglycerine
NV&D	Nausea, vomiting, and diarrhea

(*Continued*)

O	
OD	Overdose
OOB	Out of bed
OR	Operating room
P	
P	Para
PA	Posteroanterior
PAC	Premature atrial contraction or complex
PaO_2	Peripheral arterial oxygen content
PAP	Pulmonary artery pressure
PAT	Paroxysmal atrial tachycardia
PC	After eating
PCWP	Pulmonary capillary wedge pressure
PDA	Patent ductus arteriosus
PDR	*Physicians' Desk Reference*
PE	Pulmonary embolus, physical exam, or pleural effusion
PEEP	Positive end expiratory pressure
PEMI	Posterior wall myocardial infarction
PFT	Pulmonary function tests
PI	Pulmonic insufficiency disease
PJC	Premature junctional contraction or complex
PMH	Previous medical history
PMI	Point of maximal impulse
PND	Paroxysmal nocturnal dyspnea
Pneumo	Pneumothorax
PO	By mouth
POD	Postop day
PP	Postprandial
PR	By rectum

Medical Abbreviation	Term
PRBC	Packed red blood cells
Pre-op or preop	Preoperative
PRN	As needed
PS	Pulmonic stenosis
PSVT	Paroxysmal supraventricular tachycardia
PT	Prothrombin time or physical therapy
Pt	Patient
PTCA	Percutaneous transluminal coronary angioplasty
PTT	Partial thromboplastin time
PUD	Peptic ulcer disease
PVC	Premature ventricular contraction or complex
PVD	Peripheral vascular disease
PVI	Peripheral vascular insufficiency
PVT	Paroxysmal ventricular tachycardia
PWP	Pulmonary wedge pressure
Q	
q	Every
q4h, q6h, . . .	Every 4 hours, every 6 hours, etc.
qh	Every hour
qid	Four times a day
QNS	Quantity not sufficient
R	
R	Right
RA	Rheumatoid arthritis or right atrium
RAD	Right axis deviation
RAE	Right atrial enlargement
RAP	Right atrial pressure

(*Continued*)

RBBB	Right bundle branch block
RBC	Red blood cell
RDA	Recommended daily allowance
RLL	Right lower lobe
RML	Right middle lobe
R/O	Rule out
ROM	Range of motion
ROS	Review of systems
RRR	Regular rate and rhythm
RT	Respiratory or radiation therapy
RTC	Return to clinic
RUL	Right upper lobe
RV	Residual volume
RVH	Right ventricular hypertrophy
Rx	Treatment
Rxn	Reaction
S	
s̄	Without
SA	Sinoatrial
SBE	Subacute bacterial endocarditis
SEM	Systolic ejection murmur
SG	Swan-Ganz
SGA	Small for gestational age
SICU	Surgical intensive care unit
sig	Write on label
SIMV	Synchronous intermittent mandatory ventilation
sl	Sublingual
SOAP	Subjective, objective, assessment, plan
SOB	Shortness of breath

Medical Abbreviation	Term
SR	Sinus rhythm
ST	Sinus tachycardia
stat	Immediate
Subcut	Subcutaneous
SVT	Supraventricular tachycardia
Synch	Synchronized
Syst	Systolic
Sx	Symptoms
T	
TB	Tuberculosis
TIA	Transient ischemic attack
tid	Three times a day
TKO	To keep open
TLC	Total lung capacity
TNTC	Too numerous to count
TO	Telephone order
TPN	Total parenteral nutrition
TV	Tidal volume
tw	Twice a week
TX	Treatment, transplant
U	
UGI	Upper gastrointestinal
URI	Upper respiratory infection
US	Ultrasound
V	
V1	Chest lead I
V2	Chest lead II
V3	Chest lead III

(*Continued*)

V4	Chest lead IV
V5	Chest lead V
V6	Chest lead VI
VC	Vital capacity
VF or vfib	Ventricular fibrillation
VO	Verbal or voice order
V/Q	Ventilation-perfusion
VS	Vital signs
VSS	Vital signs stable
VT	Ventricular tachycardia
W	
WD	Well developed
WN	Well nourished
WNL	Within normal limits
WPW	Wolff-Parkinson-White
X	
X	times (e.g., X3 episodes of vomiting)
XRT	X-ray therapy
Y	
yo	Years old

Error-Prone Abbreviations

Many medication errors have occurred as a result of misinterpretation of abbreviations and symbols. As a result, the Joint Commission (TJC) and the Institute for Safe Medical Practice (ISMP) have created lists of abbreviations that should not be used. Although many of the commonly used abbreviations are listed, some prescribers still use them, so you need to know what they mean. In your own work, however, use only the accepted and standard abbreviations to help reduce the chance of misinterpretation and errors. This section lists common error-prone abbreviations that should not be used. The official ISMP error-prone list can be viewed at www.ismp.org/Tools/errorproneabbreviations.pdf.

Abbreviations	Meaning	Common Error	Recommended Correction
ad	right ear	Interpreted as right eye	Write out *right ear*
as	left ear	Interpreted as left eye	Write out *left ear*
au	both ears	Interpreted as both eyes	Write out *both ears*
DC, d/c	discontinue, discharge	Interpreted as discontinue medication when intended as discharge order	Write out *discontinue* or *discharge*
hs	at bedtime	Interpreted as half strength	Write out *bedtime* or *half strength*
od	right eye	Interpreted as right ear	Write out *right eye*
os	left eye	Interpreted as left ear	Write out *left eye*
ou	both eyes	Interpreted as both ears	Write out *both eyes*
qd	every day	Interpreted as qid (four times a day)	Write out *every day*
qhs	every night at bedtime	Interpreted as qid (four times a day)	Write out *nightly*
qn	every night	Interpreted as every hour	Write out *bedtime* or *nightly*
sc, sq, sub-q	subcutaneous	Interpreted as sublingual and every	Write out *subcutaneous* or *subcut*
ss	sliding scale or ½	Interpreted as 55	Write out *sliding scale* or ½ or *one-half*
U, u	unit	Interpreted as 0 or 4	Write out *unit*
ud, udt	as directed	Interpreted as unit dose	Write out *as directed*
Doses and Additional Information			
Trailing zeros (2.0 mg)	2 mg	Interpreted as 20 mg	Eliminate the use of trailing zeros when expressing whole numbers for doses
Missing zero before decimal point (.4 mg)	0.4 mg	Interpreted as 4 mg	Express doses less than a whole number with a zero before the decimal point
Period after abbreviations (mg.)	mg	The period may be interpreted as the number 1	Do not use a period after abbreviations

(*Continued*)

No space between dose and abbreviations (500 mg)	500 mg	Interpreted as 50,000	Use a space between dose and abbreviations
Missing commas in large doses (10,000 units)	10,000 units	Interpreted as 1,000 or 100,000	Use commas or write out the words (10,000 units or ten thousand units)
Symbols			
ʒ	dram	Interpreted as the number 3	Use the metric system of measurement
♏	minim	Interpreted as mL	Use the metric system of measurement
> and <	greater than and less than	Interpreted as the opposite	Write out *greater than* or *less than*
/	slash mark	Interpreted as the number 1	Write *per* instead of slash mark
@	"at" symbol	Interpreted as the number 2	Write out *at*
&	"and" symbol	Interpreted as the number 2	Write out *and*
+ or and (+)	"plus" sign or handwritten "and" sign	Interpreted as the number 4	Write out *and*

Appendix D

Anatomical Terms

Anatomical terms are used to describe the location of body parts and various body regions. In order to correctly use these terms, it is assumed that the body is in the anatomical position. See Figures D-1 and D-2 and Table D-1.

Figure D-1 Directional terms provide mapping instructions for locating organs and body parts.

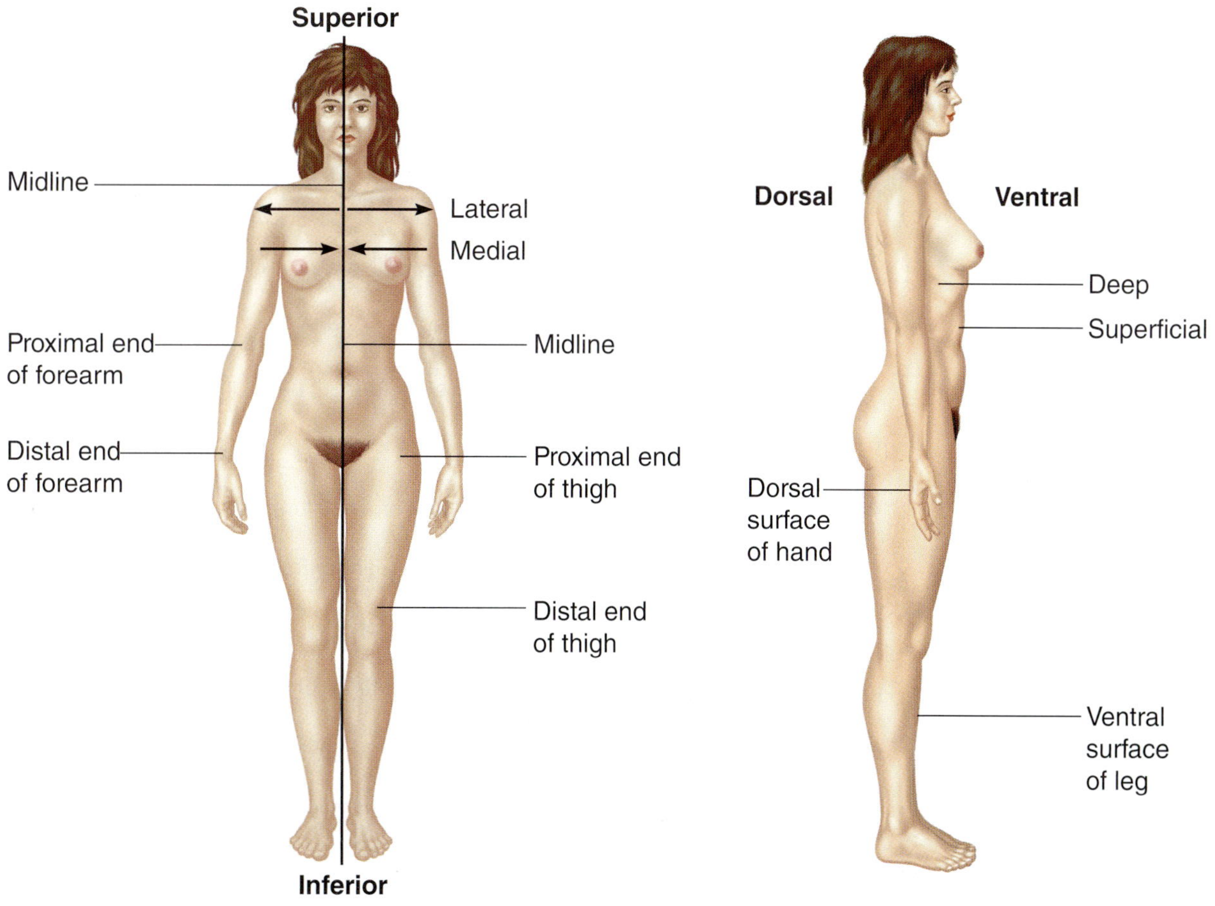

Figure D-2 Spatial terms are based on imaginary cuts or planes through the body.

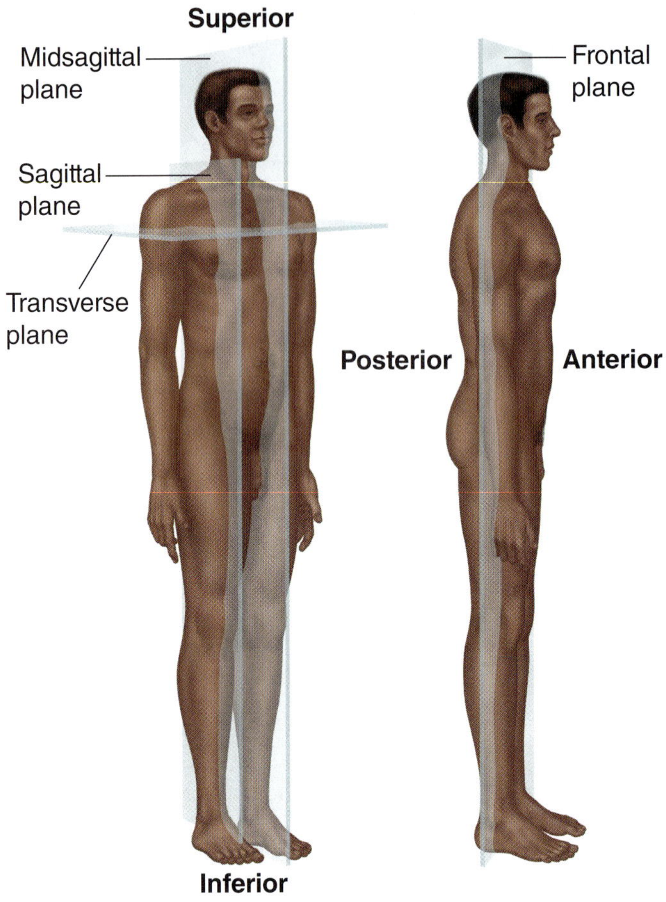

TABLE D-1 Anatomical Terms

Term	Definition
Anterior	Toward the front of the body; ventral
Caudal	Below, behind, or closer to the feet; posterior
Coronal plane	Divides into front (ventral) and back (dorsal) parts; frontal plane
Cranial	Toward the head; superior
Deep	Inward from a point of attachment or away from the surface of the body
Distal	Farther away from a point of attachment or from the center of the body
Dorsal	Toward the back of the body; posterior
External	Outward or movement toward the exterior of a hollow form
Frontal plane	Divides the body into front (ventral) and back (dorsal) parts; coronal plane
Horizontal plane	Divides the body into superior (top) and inferior (bottom); transverse plane

Term	Definition
Inferior	Below or closer to the feet
Internal	Inward or movement toward the middle of a hollow form
Lateral	To the side
Medial	Closer to the midline of the body
Midline	Vertical line that divides the body into exact left and right halves
Midsagittal plane	Divides the body into equal left and right sides
Parietal	Near the side or top
Peripheral	Near the surface or outside
Posterior	Toward the back of the body; dorsal
Proximal	Closer to a point of attachment or to the center of the body
Sagittal plane	Divides the body into left and right sides
Superficial	Close to the surface
Superior	Above or closer to the head
Transverse plane	Divides the body into superior (top) and inferior (bottom); horizontal plane
Ventral	Toward the front of the body; anterior
Visceral	Inside or internal

Glossary

A

action potential The change in the electrical potential of the heart muscle when it is stimulated.

acute coronary syndrome (ACS) This is a broad term that refers to unstable angina, ST segment elevation MI (STEMI), and non-ST segment elevation MI (NSTEMI). ACS is usually associated with intracoronary plaque changes or thrombosis, where blood flow is suddenly stopped.

advanced cardiac life support (ACLS) A set of clinical interventions for the urgent treatment of cardiac arrest and other life-threatening medical emergencies, as well as the knowledge and skills to deploy those interventions.

alternating current (AC) interference Unwanted markings on the ECG caused by other electrical current sources.

ambulate To walk; ambulating is walking.

anatomically contiguous lead Two or more leads looking at the same part of the heart, or numerically consecutive chest leads.

angina An oppressive pain or pressure in the chest when the heart muscle does not receive enough oxygen due to partial or complete blockage of a coronary artery.

angiogram An invasive procedure during which x-rays are taken of a blood vessel after injection of a radiopaque substance.

angioplasty Surgical repair of blood vessels.

angle of Louis A ridge about an inch or so below the suprasternal notch where the main part of the sternum and the top of the sternum, known as the manubrium, are attached.

anorexia Decreased or loss of appetite.

anterior axillary line An imaginary vertical line starting at the front axilla that extends down the left side of the chest.

antidysrhythmic Type of medication given to prevent cardiac rhythm abnormalities.

aorta The largest artery of the body; transports blood from the left ventricle of the heart to the entire body.

aortic semilunar valve Valve located in the aorta that prevents the backflow of blood into the left ventricle.

apnea The absence of breathing.

arrhythmia Irregular rhythm or abnormal heart rate.

arteriosclerosis An abnormal thickening and hardening of the arterial walls with resulting loss of elasticity.

artifact Unwanted marks on the ECG tracing caused by activity other than the heart's electrical activity.

ascites Abnormal collection of serous fluid within the abdomen (peritoneal cavity). This may occur secondary to congestive heart failure.

asystole A condition in which no rhythm or electrical current is traveling through the cardiac conduction system.

atherosclerotic plaque Fatty deposits accumulated due to elevated glucose levels.

atrial kick The extra blood that can be ejected into the ventricles by the atria as a result of the electrical impulse slowing as it enters the AV node.

atriobiventricular pacing A sequential pacemaker stimulation of the atria and then both ventricles, rather than just the lower right ventricle. Also known as *biventricular pacing.*

atrioventricular (AV) Related to the atria and ventricles of the heart.

atrioventricular (AV) node Delays the electrical impulse to allow the atria to complete their contraction.

atrioventricular delay The measurement from the atrial spike to the ventricular spike, or from the beginning of the P wave to the ventricular spike on a pacemaker tracing.

atrioventricular sequential pacing A pacemaker stimulation of the atria and then the lower part of the right ventricle in a sequence that mimics the normal cardiac conduction system and allows for atrial kick.

atrium (pl. atria) Top two chambers of the heart.

augmented lead Normally small ECG lead tracings that are increased in size by the ECG machine in order to be interpreted.

auscultated blood pressure Blood pressure determined while listening with a stethoscope.

auscultation Listening to the body sounds, such as heart, lung, and stomach, using a stethoscope.

automatic external defibrillator (AED) A lightweight, portable device that recognizes abnormal rhythm and determines if the rhythm is considered a "shockable rhythm."

automaticity The ability of the heart to initiate an electrical impulse without being stimulated by an independent source.

autonomic nervous system (ANS) A system that is in charge of the body's automatic functions, such as the heart rate.

AV Atrioventricular; related to the atria and ventricles.

AV junction The AV node and surrounding tissue, including the bundle of His.

axis deviation Changes that occur on a 12-lead ECG due to orientation or position of the heart within the chest.

B

Bachmann's bundle The structure that relays the electrical impulse from the SA node to the left atrium in a normal heart.

beta blockers Drugs used to treat hypertension.

bigeminy Pattern in which every other complex is a premature beat (PVC).

biphasic A waveform that has positive (upward) and negative (downward) deflections (phases) on the ECG tracing.

bipolar lead A type of ECG lead that measures the flow of electrical current in both directions at the same time.

blocked or nonconducted impulse Impulse occurs too soon after the preceding impulse, causing a period when no other impulses can occur in the ventricles.

body mechanics Using movements that maintain proper posture and avoid muscle and bone injuries.

bolus A concentrated amount of medication or fluid to be administered over a prescribed short period of time.

bradycardia A slow heart rate, usually less than 60 beats per minute.

bundle branch block Impulse is delayed or blocked within the bundle branches of the normal conduction pathway.

bundle branches Left and right branches of the bundle of His that conduct impulses down either side of the interventricular septum to the left and right ventricles.

bundle of His (atrioventricular or AV bundle) Located next to the AV node; provides the transfer of the electrical impulse from the atria to the ventricles.

C

Cardiac Care Unit (CCU) A specialized patient care location for patients with cardiovascular disorders that require cardiac monitoring.

cardiac cycle The contraction and relaxation of the heart.

cardiac enzymes (cardiac markers or cardiac biomarkers) Chemicals found in the bloodstream that are indicators of myocardial cell death (infarction). Common examples include troponin, CK-MB, and myoglobin.

Examples of Cardiac Enzyme Tests and Peak Serum Level

Blood Test	Benefit	Peak Level in Blood
Troponin	Most specific	12 hours
CK-MB	Good test if there is not any skeletal muscle damage	10–24 hours
Myoglobin	Not specific to the heart but useful in nontrauma-related cardiac patients due to early presence in bloodstream	2 hours

cardiac output The volume of blood the heart pumps each minute.

cardiac output parameters Observation guidelines used to assess the blood supply to the vital organs of the body to maintain normal function.

cardiogenic shock Inadequate flow of arterial blood, typically as a result of left heart failure.

cardiologist A physician who specializes in the study of the heart.

cardiopulmonary resuscitation (CPR) The provision of ventilations (breaths) and chest compressions (blood circulation) for a person who shows no signs of breathing or having a heartbeat.

cardiovascular Related to the heart and blood vessels (veins and arteries).

cardiovascular disease (CVD) Disease related to the heart and blood vessels (veins and arteries).

cardiovascular technologist An individual who has advanced skills and can assist physicians with invasive cardiovascular diagnostic tests, such as angioplasty or heart surgery.

cardioversion The use of electricity to change an abnormally fast or cardiac dysrhythmia to a normal rhythm.

cerebrovascular accident (CVA) A stroke. Caused by a hemorrhage in the brain or more often by a clot lodged in a cerebral artery.

chemical stress echocardiogram A stress echocardiogram in which the heart is stressed by chemicals, rather than physical exercise.

chemical stress test Stress test performed after administering medications that cause the heart rate to increase or the coronary blood vessels to dilate; performed on patients who cannot perform the exercise required in a regular stress test.

chordae tendineae Structures that connect the atrioventricular (tricuspid and mitral) valves to the papillary muscles and prevent them from opening in the wrong direction.

circumflex artery One of the primary branches of the left coronary artery, which winds around, supplying blood to the lateral wall of the left ventricle.

Code Blue An alert that notifies healthcare providers that a patient is unresponsive and needs assistance immediately.

collateral blood vessels Side-by-side, as in small vessels providing additional blood flow to a region of tissue.

complexes Atrial or ventricular contractions as they appear on the ECG; complete ECG waveforms.

conductivity The ability of the heart cells to receive and transmit an electrical impulse.

congestive heart failure (CHF) Failure of the heart to pump an adequate amount of blood to the body tissues.

contiguous leads Referring to similar views of the heart (e.g., II, III, and aVF inferior leads, or numerically consecutive chest leads).

contractility The ability of the heart muscle cells to shorten in response to an electrical stimulus.

coronary angiography An x-ray visualization of the coronary vessels after a radiopaque dye is injected into the patient.

coronary artery bypass graft (CABG) surgery Surgical intervention performed by taking a grafted or transplanted blood vessel and attaching it to the heart at a point beyond an occluded coronary artery to reestablish blood flow.

coronary artery disease (CAD) Narrowing of the arteries of the heart, causing a reduction of blood flow.

coronary circulation The circulation of blood to and from the heart muscle.

coronary vascular disease (CVD) Narrowing of the coronary blood vessels, causing a reduction in the blood flow to the heart.

coupling Two PVCs that occur back to back.

crash cart A cart or tray containing emergency medication and equipment that can be easily transported to the location of an emergency for life support.

D

defibrillator A machine that produces and sends an electrical shock to the heart in an attempt to correct the electrical pattern of the heart.

delta wave A widening at the beginning of the QRS complex due to ventricular pre-excitation.

deoxygenated blood Blood that has little or minimal oxygen (oxygen-poor blood).

depolarization The electrical activation of the cells of the heart that initiates contraction of the heart muscle.

dextrocardia When the heart is on the opposite or right side of the chest.

diabetes mellitus (DM) A condition characterized by a lack of production of insulin, resulting in elevated glucose (sugar) in the blood stream.

diastole The phase of the cardiac cycle when the heart is expanding and refilling; also known as the relaxation phase.

diastolic blood pressure The blood pressure measured when the heart relaxes, representing the minimum amount of pressure exerted against the vessel walls at all times; the number corresponding to the last Korotkoff sound heard when performing an auscultated blood pressure.

direct contact A mode of transmission of infection that occurs from one person to another.

dissociative Not related at all; the atria and the ventricles beat entirely independently of each other.

dysrhythmia Abnormal heartbeat.

E

ECG monitor technician An individual who has the technical knowledge and skills to view and evaluate the electrical tracings of patients' hearts on an oscilloscope and, when necessary, alert the appropriate healthcare professional to treat abnormalities.

echocardiogram Noninvasive diagnostic test that uses sound to study the heart, heart valves, and blood vessels.

echocardiography Noninvasive diagnostic testing that uses ultrasound to study the heart and blood vessels.

ectopicim pulse An electrical impulse that comes from outside of the normal pacemaker site or electrical conduction pathway.

eICU Electronic Intensive Care Unit; an off-site unit of the hospital that monitors patients remotely through wired or wireless connections.

Einthoven triangle A triangle formed by three of the limb electrodes—the left arm, the right arm, and the left leg; it is used as a reference for the first six leads of the 12-lead ECG.

electrical capture Evidence on an ECG tracing, including the spacing of spikes and waveforms.

electrocardiogram (ECG) A tracing of the heart's electrical activity recorded by an electrocardiograph.

electrocardiograph An instrument used to record the electrical activity of the heart.

electrocardiograph (ECG) technician An individual who has the technical skills and knowledge to record an ECG and prepare it for the physician.

electrocardiology The study of the heart's electrical activity.

electrodes Small sensors placed on the skin to detect the electrical activity from the heart.

electronic pacemaker A man-made source of electrical current causing depolarization of the myocardium; artificial pacemakers are electronic.

emphysema Decreased respiratory function usually caused by smoking, chronic bronchitis, or old age.

enhanced external counter pulsation (EECP) Treatment for chronic angina patients who do not have other options due to health status. This procedure is performed five days a week for several weeks, with the intent of developing collateral blood vessels—essentially creating a "natural" bypass around narrowed or blocked arteries.

ER Emergency room; patient care location that provides urgent care.

ethics Standards of behavior and concepts of right and wrong.

excitability The ability of the heart muscle cells to respond to an impulse or stimulus; also called *irritability*.

F

failure to depolarize The pacing activity of a pacemaker continues to occur without evidence that the electrical activity has depolarized or captured the myocardium. Also called *loss of capture*.

failure to pace Pacemaker does not send electrical impulses to the myocardium; also known as *malfunction*.

failure to sense The pacemaker does not recognize or sense the patient's own inherent cardiac electrical activity. Also known as *malsensing*.

false positive When a diagnostic test indicates that disease is present but, in reality, no disease is present. A false positive is never considered a negative result. It is a positive result, albeit a falsely positive one.

fibrinolytic agent Medications administered to break down the fibrin in a blood clot, essentially dissolving it.

focus (pl. foci) A cardiac cell or group of cells that produces an ectopic beat.

frequent PVC Six or more PVCs per minute.

G

gain A control on the ECG machine that increases or decreases the size of the deflections on the ECG tracing.

galvanometer An instrument is used to detect electrocardiograph waves.

gamma camera A camera that records the gamma radiation emitted by the radioactive tracers in a patient's blood.

gate A selective technique in which a gamma camera is triggered by specific events captured by a three-lead ECG monitor.

H

healthcare provider The scope of practice of each healthcare provider will determine the extent of the interpretation and treatment of each of the cardiac dysrhythmias or conditions. Each specific scope is determined by the licensure of each state. For example: Prescribing a medication is the responsibility of the physician. But some state practices allow nurse practitioners and physician assistants to prescribe medication under the guidance of the physician.

hepatitis Inflammation of the liver usually caused by a virus.

hertz (Hz) A unit of frequency measured in cycles (or events) per second.

HIV (human immunodeficiency virus) The virus that causes AIDS (acquired immune deficiency syndrome).

Holter Proper name given to one type of ambulatory monitor, named after Norman Holter, inventor of the procedure and machine.

Holter monitor An instrument that records the electrical activity of the heart during a patient's normal daily activities; also known as an *ambulatory monitor*.

homeostasis The state of balance the body attempts to maintain by the regulation of body processes.

hypercoagulopathy An increased ability of the blood to form clots.

hypertension High blood pressure.

hypertrophy Abnormal thickening of the ventricular wall due to chronic pressure overload; is often caused by hypertension.

hyperventilation To breathe at an increased rate and depth of inspiration and expiration.

hypotension A lower than normal blood pressure that can cause reduction of blood flow to vital organs.

I

ICU Intensive Care Unit; a specialized patient care location for patients who require monitoring and constant patient care.

indirect contact A mode of transmission of infection involving fomites (objects) or vectors (person, animal, or microorganism).

infarction A lack of oxygen to body tissue due to a blocked blood vessel.

inherent rhythm The patient's own heart rhythm.

inhibited Electrical current is stopped from being sent to the myocardium.

input Data entered into an ECG machine, usually through electrodes on the skin surface.

intercostal space (ICS) The space between two ribs.

interpolated PVC A PVC that occurs during the normal R-R interval without interrupting the underlying rhythm.

interval The period of time between two activities within the heart.

interventricular septum A partition or wall (septum) that divides the right and left ventricles.

invasive Procedure that requires entrance into a body cavity, tissue, or blood vessel.

ischemia Lack of blood supply to an area of tissue due to a blockage in the circulation to that area.

isoelectric The period when the electrical tracing of the ECG is at zero or a straight line, and no positive or negative deflections are seen.

isolation precautions The second level of steps taken to prevent the spread of infection; some examples include separating the infected patient from others and using personal protective equipment.

IV fluid challenge Administration of IV fluid (i.e., 0.9% NaCl) to offset the effect of administered medication or to treat for hypovolemia. Often referred to as a fluid resuscitation.

J

J point A point on the QRS complex where the depolarization is completed and repolarization starts.

junctional escape rhythm A rhythm that occurs when the SA node fails to initiate the electrical activity and one of the backup pacemaker sites takes over.

L

law Rules of conduct enforced by a controlling authority such as the government.

leads Covered wires that conduct the electrical impulse from the electrodes to the ECG machine.

left anterior descending artery One of the primary branches of the left main coronary artery supplying blood to the anterior wall of the left ventricle.

left atrium The left upper chamber of the heart, which receives blood from the lungs.

left ventricle The left lower chamber of the heart, which pumps oxygenated blood through the body. It is the biggest and strongest chamber, known as the workhorse of the heart.

libel Writing defamatory words about someone; this is both illegal and unethical.

limb lead An ECG lead placed on an arm or a leg.

loss of capture The pacing activity continues to occur without evidence that the electrical activity has depolarized or captured the myocardium. Also called *failure to depolarize*.

M

malfunctioning Failure of a pacemaker to send electrical impulses to the myocardium; also called *failure to pace*.

marginal artery One of the primary branches of the right coronary artery, providing blood to the inferior wall of the left ventricle.

malsensing The pacemaker does not recognize or sense the patient's own inherent cardiac electrical activity; also called *failure to sense*.

maximal exercise Target heart rate of 220 minus the age of the patient.

mechanical capture The heart's ability to respond to electrical impulses delivered by a natural or electronic pacemaker.

medical professional liability Legal responsibility of healthcare professionals for their performance.

midaxillary line An imaginary vertical line that starts at the middle of the axilla (armpit) and extends down the side of the chest.

midclavicular line An imaginary line on the chest that runs vertically through the center of the clavicle.

midscapular line Imaginary line on the back that runs vertically through the center of the scapula.

millimeter (mm) A unit of measurement to indicate time on the ECG tracing. Time is measured on the horizontal axis.

millivolt (mV) A unit of measurement to indicate voltage on the ECG tracing. Voltage is measured on the vertical axis.

mitral (bicuspid) valve Valve with two cusps or leaflets located between the left atrium and left ventricle; it prevents backflow of blood into the left atrium.

morphology Overall form and structure.

multichannel recorder An ECG machine that monitors all 12 leads but records three leads at a time and switches leads automatically, recording each of the four sets of three leads.

multifocal PVC Varied shapes and forms of the PVCs, suggesting more than one irritable focus.

myocardial Pertaining to the heart (*cardia*) muscle (*myo*).

myocardial infarction (MI) (heart attack) A blockage of one or more of the coronary arteries causing lack of oxygen to the heart and death of the muscle tissue.

myocardial injury Injury to the cardiac muscle caused by prolonged reduction or interruption of blood flow.

myocardial ischemia A reduction in blood flow and oxygen to the myocardium for a short period of time.

N

neurological Pertaining to the nervous system, its diseases, and its functions.

neuropathy Nerve damage that causes vascular and autonomic nervous system problems, with loss of ability to maintain blood pressure and loss or impaired sensation. Common cause is chronic diabetes mellitus.

noninvasive Procedure that does not require entrance into a body cavity, tissue, or blood vessel.

non-ST segment elevation MI (NSTEMI) A type of heart attack in which the classic signs and symptoms are not present. Caused by incomplete occlusion of a coronary artery.

normotensive Normal blood pressure.

nuclear stress test A stress test in which radionuclides (radioactive tracers) are administered to trace the path of blood through the heart.

O

occasional PVC Less than six PVCs per minute.

oscilloscope A monitor or television-type device that shows the tracing of the electrical activity of the heart.

output display The part of the ECG machine that displays the tracing for the electrical activity of the heart, usually in an electronic or printed form on a 12-lead ECG machine.

oversensing The pacemaker senses electrical current from other muscle movements or electrical activity outside of the body as the electrical current in the patient's heart.

oxygenated blood Blood having oxygen (oxygen-rich blood).

P

pacemaker Refers to a natural or man-made source of electrical current causing depolarization of the myocardium.

pacemaker competition Competition between the pacemaker generator and the heart's inherent rate over control of the myocardium.

pacing spike A thin spike on the ECG tracing that results from the pacemaker stimulation impulse.

pallor Pale skin.

palpitations Fast heartbeat sensation felt by the patient, which may or may not be associated with complaints of chest pain.

papillary muscles Muscles in the ventricles that anchor the chordae tendineae and atrioventricular valves.

paraspinous line Imaginary line on the spine that runs vertically through the side of the spine.

parasympathetic The branch of the autonomic nervous system (ANS) that helps to slow the heart rate.

paroxysmal event Witnessed change in any cardiac rhythm, including starting, stopping, or both.

pathologic Q wave A Q wave that measures 0.04 second or wider in duration and/or is 1/3 or more the height of the R wave in that lead.

percutaneous coronary intervention (PCI) Another name for angioplasty. This minimally invasive procedure is performed with a sheath and catheter to inject dye for fluoroscopic examination to determine the specific location of a narrowed or occluded artery. Once this portion of the procedure is performed, a catheter with a balloon is inserted, and the balloon is placed at the location of the obstruction and inflated. The intent is to outwardly compress the plaque and reestablish blood flow to the region of tissue distal to the occlusion.

percutaneous transluminal coronary angioplasty (PTCI) Similar to PCI, but now it is specific to a coronary vessel. A catheter with a balloon is inserted, placed at the location of the obstructed coronary artery, and inflated. The intent is to outwardly compress the plaque and reestablish blood flow to the region of tissue distal to the occlusion.

perfusion Supplying nutrients and oxygen to the organs and tissues by way of blood flow through the vessels.

pericardium A two-layered sac of tissue enclosing the heart.

personal protective equipment (PPE) Devices such as gloves, gowns, face masks or shields, and eye protection designed to protect a healthcare worker from sources of infection.

physiologic Q wave A normal Q wave, measuring less than 0.04 second in duration and less than 1/3 the height of the R wave in that lead.

polarization The state of cellular rest in which the inside is negatively charged and the outside is positively charged.

posterior axillary line Imaginary line on the back that runs vertically from the shoulder down on the outer edge of the rib cage.

posterior descending artery One of the primary branches of the right coronary artery providing blood to the posterior wall of the heart.

precordial lead A type of lead placed on the chest in front of the heart; known as a V lead.

premature ventricular complex (PVC) An ectopic impulse originating in either ventricle that occurs too early in the cycle.

pulmonary artery Large artery that transports deoxygenated blood from the right ventricle to the lungs. This is the only artery in the body that carries deoxygenated blood.

pulmonary circulation The transportation of blood to and from the lungs; blood is oxygenated in the lungs during pulmonary circulation.

pulmonary edema Abnormal collection of fluid within the pleural space (lungs) due to congestive heart failure (left ventricle).

pulmonary embolism A blocked artery in the lungs, usually caused by a blood clot.

pulmonary semilunar valve A valve found in the pulmonary artery that prevents backflow of blood into the right ventricle during pulmonary circulation.

pulmonary veins Transport oxygenated blood back into the left atrium of the heart. These are the only veins in the body that carry oxygenated blood.

Purkinje fibers The fibers within the heart that distribute electrical impulses from cell to cell throughout the ventricles.

Purkinje network Spreads the electrical impulse throughout the ventricles by means of the Purkinje fibers.

Q

QS complex A deep Q/S wave with no preceding R wave. Can indicate a left bundle branch block.

quadgeminy Pattern in which every fourth complex is a premature complex (for example, PVC).

R

R-on-T PVC PVC occurs on the downslope of the T wave or the vulnerable period of the ventricular refractory period.

radiologist A physician who specializes in the use of radioactive substances to diagnose and treat disease.

rales (crackles) Noisy breath sounds during inhalation caused by retained airway secretions. When caused by pulmonary edema, rales are heard as very short, soft, bubbling lung sounds.

rate pressure product (RPP) Systolic blood pressure multiplied by the heart rate; also known as *double product.*

renal Pertaining to the kidneys.

renal infarction A lack of oxygen to kidney tissue due to a blocked blood vessel.

repolarization The return of heart muscle cells to their resting electrical state, causing the heart muscle to relax.

restenosis When a blood vessel that has been treated with angioplasty returns to a blocked state or becomes reoccluded.

retrograde Moving backward.

rhythm The regularity of an occurrence such as the heartbeat.

right atrium The right upper chamber of the heart, which receives blood from the body.

right ventricle The right lower chamber of the heart, which pumps blood to the lungs.

run of ventricular tachycardia Three or more PVCs in a row at a rate of greater than 100 bpm. Also known as *triplet PVCs* or *salvo.*

S

salvo Three or more PVCs in a row at a rate exceeding 100 bpm; also called *triplet PVCs* or *run of ventricular tachycardia.*

segment A portion or part of the electrical tracing produced by the heart.

seizure An interruption of the electrical activity in the brain that causes involuntary muscle movement and sometimes unconsciousness.

semilunar valve A valve with half-moon-shaped cusps that open and close, allowing blood to travel only one way; located in the pulmonary artery and the aorta.

septal artery Branch from the left anterior descending artery providing blood to the interventricular septum.

serial ECG comparison Multiple and frequent ECG tracings recorded at intervals based upon the patient's condition and compared to monitor changes.

SICU Surgical Intensive Care Unit; a specialized patient care location for care of patients after surgery.

signal processing The process within the ECG machine that amplifies the electrical impulse and converts it to a mechanical action on the output display.

single-channel recorder An ECG machine that records one lead tracing at a time.

sinoatrial (SA) node An area of specialized cells in the upper right atrium that initiates the heartbeat.

skin rasp A rough piece of material used to abrade (scrape) the skin prior to electrode placement.

slander Making derogatory remarks about someone that jeopardizes his or her reputation or means of livelihood; slander is both illegal and unethical.

somatic tremor Voluntary or involuntary muscle movement; also known as *body tremor.*

speed control A control on the ECG machine that regulates how fast or slow the paper runs during the tracing.

ST segment elevation MI (STEMI) Classic MI with expected ST segment deviation and development of pathologic Q wave.

standard precautions Procedures, such as performing hand hygiene and wearing gloves, used with all patients that are designed to prevent the spread of infection.

stat Immediately.

stent A small, metal mesh tube that opens up inside a coronary artery to keep it patent.

stress ECG Another name for exercise electrocardiography.

stress echocardiogram A test that combines an exercise stress test with an echocardiogram to assess left ventricular wall motion both before and immediately after exercise.

stroke volume The volume of blood ejected by one or both ventricles with each contraction.

submaximal exercise Target heart of 220 minus the age multiplied by a percentage between 60 and 85.

sudden cardiac arrest A condition in which the heart stops beating suddenly, often without warning, due to a failure of its electrical system.

suprasternal notch The dip you feel at the anterior base of the neck just above the manubrium, where the clavicle attaches to the sternum.

supraventricular An ectopic focus originating above the ventricles in the atria or junctional region of the heart.

sympathetic The branch of the autonomic nervous system (ANS) that causes an increase in the heart rate.

syncope Loss of consciousness (fainting).

systemic circulation The pathways for pumping blood throughout the body and back to the heart.

systole The contraction phase of the cardiac cycle, during which the heart is pumping blood out to the pulmonary (lungs) and systemic (body) circulation.

systolic blood pressure The blood pressure measured when the left ventricle of the heart contracts; the number corresponding with the first Korotkoff sound heard when performing an auscultated blood pressure.

T

tachycardia A fast heart rate, usually greater than 100 beats per minute.

target heart rate (THR) Heart rate measurement needed to truly exercise the heart.

technician An individual who has the knowledge and skills to carry out technical procedures.

technologist An individual who specializes in a field of science.

telemedicine A monitoring system in which ECG tracings are communicated from a patient outside a medical facility to the physician via a telephone or digital system.

telemetry The transmission of data electronically to an unattached or distant location.

thrombolytic agent Medications administered intravenously that possess the ability to lyse or dissolve a clot.

thrombus A blood clot that forms on the wall in a diseased area of the endocardium or on the wall of an injured blood vessel.

TJC The Joint Commission (formerly the Joint Commission on Accreditation of Healthcare Organizations, or JCAHO); organization that establishes patient safety goals for healthcare facilities.

Torsades de Pointes Type of ventricular tachycardia in which depolarization impulses move from one ventricle to the other, resulting in a "twisted ribbon" appearance on the ECG tracing.

tricuspid valve Valve located between the right atrium and right ventricle; it prevents backflow of blood into the right atrium.

trigeminy Pattern in which every third complex is a premature beat (PVC).

triggered Caused to occur; for example, electrical impulses are caused to occur if a pacemaker fails to detect the heart's normal contractions.

triplet PVCs Three or more PVCs in a row at a rate exceeding 100 bpm; also called *salvo* or *run of ventricular tachycardia.*

tunica adventitia Tough, fibrous, outermost layer of the artery, responsible for keeping the vessel open.

tunica intima Innermost layer of the artery; single-cell layer of endothelial cells that comes in direct contact with the blood.

tunica media Middle layer of the artery; comprised of smooth muscle. This layer is responsible for dilation and constriction of the vessel walls so it plays a major role in maintaining blood pressure.

U

underlying rhythm The heart rhythm that would be present if the abnormal impulses were ignored or removed from the tracing.

undersensing The pacemaker is unable to detect any electric activity and never turns off.

unifocal PVC Early complex that has shape suggesting only one irritable focus present.

unipolar lead A type of ECG lead that measures the flow of electrical current in one direction only.

unstable angina (pre-infarction angina) A warning sign that the disease that has been causing angina has worsened. Signs and symptoms are less predictable, last longer, and are more painful than previously experienced.

V

vagal tone A constant tension on the vagus nerve that causes the heart to beat more slowly.

vena cava (pl. venae cavae) Largest vein in the body, which provides a pathway for deoxygenated blood to return to the heart; its upper portion, the superior vena cava, transports blood from the head, arms, and upper body; and its lower portion, the inferior vena cava, transports blood from the lower body and legs.

vital signs Temperature, pulse, respirations, blood pressure, and pain assessment.

volume expander IV solution administerred to fill fluid volume or replace the space that blood normally takes up. The context referred to in this book is referring to inert fluids, specifically 0.9% NaCl. It is given to increase blood volume in the hypotensive or potentially hypotensive patient in an effort to maintain homeostasis.

W

wandering baseline Artifact in which the tracing drifts away from the center of the graph paper. Also known as *baseline shift.*

Wolfe-Parkinson-White syndrome A type of supraventricular tachycardia in which an extra electrical pathway between an atrium and a ventricle short-circuits the normal pathway, resulting in paroxysmal tachycardia events. This syndrome also affects the morphology of the QRS complex. As a result of the abnormal conduction pathway, the QRS complex begins early and measures abnormally wide (0.12 second or greater) with a classic "delta" wave.

Photo Credits

Design Elements

Clinical Thinking: © Cn Boon/Alamy RF; Patient Education & Communication: © Helder Almeida/Dreamstime.com; Safety & Infection Control: © mauhorng/iStockphoto.com; Troubleshooting: © Comstock/Alamy RF; Law & Ethics: © ericsphotography/Getty Images RF; Interpret-TIP: © Total Care Programming, Inc.

Chapter 1

Figure 1.1: © James Davies/Alamy; 1.3: © BSIP/Newscom; 1.4: © Sheila Terry/SPL/Science Source; 1.5: © Chris Bjornberg/Science Source; 1.6: © Ron Thompson/Rapport Press/Newscom; 1.7: Aerotel Medical Systems (1998) LTD; 1.8: © Paul Burns/Corbis RF; 1.9a: © McGraw-Hill Education/Jill Braaten, photographer; 1.9b: © Lillian Mundt; 1.10: © Total Care Programming, Inc.; 1.13a: © Jeffrey Coolidge/Getty Images RF.

Chapter 3

Figure 3.7: © Art Directors & TRIP/Alamy; 3.8, 3.9: Courtesy of GE Healthcare Systems; 3.11a: © Dr. P. Marazzi/SPL/Science Source; 3.11b: © Lillian Mundt; 3.12a: © Total Care Programming, Inc.; 3.12b: Courtesy of Tempo Medical Products; 3.13: © Total Care Programming, Inc.

Chapter 4

Figures 4.1, 4.5, 4.10: © Total Care Programming, Inc.

Chapter 5

Figures 5.1, 5.2: © Total Care Programming, Inc.

Chapter 11

Figure 11.1: © 2014 Welch Allyn® All rights reserved; 11.2: © BSIP/Newscom; 11.4: © Collection CNRI/Phototake.

Chapter 12

Figure 12.1: Aerotel Medical Systems (1998) LTD; 12.2: © 2014 SCHILLER AG; 12.3, 12.4: © Total Care Programming, Inc.; 12.5: © BSIP SA/Alamy; 12.6: © Total Care Programming, Inc.; 12.7a-b: © Card Guard AG/Life Watch Holding Corp.; 12.8, 12.9: Aerotel Medical Systems (1998) LTD; 12.11: © Total Care Programming, Inc.

Chapter 13

Figure 13.9: © Dynamic Graphics/Jupiterimages RF; 13.10: © Horizon International Images Limited/Alamy; 13.13: © EECP is a registered® trademark of Vasomedical, Inc. Westbury, NY.

Index

A

B

C

D

E

F

G

H

I

J

L

M

N

O

P

Q

R

S

T

U